Updates in Pediatric Sleep and Child Psychiatry

Updates in Pediatric Sleep and Child Psychiatry

Special Issue Editors

Ujjwal Ramtekkar
Anna Ivanenko

MDPI • Basel • Beijing • Wuhan • Barcelona • Belgrade

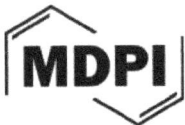

MDPI

Special Issue Editors

Ujjwal Ramtekkar
Department of Psychiatry Ohio State University
USA

Anna Ivanenko
Northwestern University
USA

Editorial Office
MDPI
St. Alban-Anlage 66
4052 Basel, Switzerland

This is a reprint of articles from the Special Issue published online in the open access journal *Medical Sciences* (ISSN 2076-3271) from 2017 to 2018 (available at: https://www.mdpi.com/journal/medsci/special_issues/updates_in_pediatric_sleep).

For citation purposes, cite each article independently as indicated on the article page online and as indicated below:

LastName, A.A.; LastName, B.B.; LastName, C.C. Article Title. *Journal Name* **Year**, *Article Number*, Page Range.

ISBN 978-3-03897-938-8 (Pbk)
ISBN 978-3-03897-939-5 (PDF)

Contents

About the Special Issue Editors

Ujjwal Ramtekkar, MD, MPE, MBA is a child and adolescent psychiatrist at Nationwide Children's Hospital and Assistant Professor at the Ohio State University, USA. He also serves as the associate medical director for Partners for Kids, one of the largest pediatric accountable care organization in the country. His clinical and research interests include sleep in psychiatric disorders, neurodevelopmental disorders, telehealth and population health outcomes research.

Anna Ivanenko, MD, PhD, is child and adolescent psychiatrist and a sleep medicine specialist. Dr. Ivanenko is a Professor of Clinical Psychiatry and Behavioral Sciences at the Feinberg School of Medicine, Northwestern University, Division of Child and Adolescent Psychiatry, Ann and Robert H Lurie Children's Hospital of Chicago. Her clinical and research interests focus on the interface between sleep, emotional and behavioral development and psychopathology in children. She has been publishing and presenting on the topics of childhood sleep disorders and psychiatric disturbances.

Preface to "Updates in Pediatric Sleep and Child Psychiatry"

The bidirectional relationship between sleep disorders and psychiatric symptoms is becoming increasingly important for the scientific and clinical community. Thus, there is a growing need to address the overlap between sleep and psychopathology in pediatric patients, especially in the context of the revised DSM-5 Diagnostic and Statistical Manual of Mental Disorders. Also, there is a growing trend for a multidisciplinary management approach of co-morbid medical and psychiatric conditions.

In this special issue, we aim to address these aforementioned under-represented topics. The articles written on a wide range of topics by leading authorities in the field of pediatric neurology, child psychiatry, and pediatric sleep medicine will be a great resource for clinicians to enhance their knowledge on pediatric sleep and psychiatry.

We would like to acknowledge the authors for their outstanding contributions and to thank all reviewers who took time to provide constructive feedback to enhance the quality and clarity of the articles published. Finally, we would like to extend sincere gratitude towards the managing editor and publication team at MDPI for their assistance and direction in successfully publishing this special issue.

Ujjwal Ramtekkar, Anna Ivanenko
Special Issue Editors

medical sciences

MDPI

Article

Assessment and Treatment of Pediatric Sleep Problems: Knowledge, Skills, Attitudes and Practices in a Group of Community Child Psychiatrists

Ali Anwar [1], Michael D. Yingling [1], Alicia Zhang [1], Ujjwal Ramtekkar [2] and Ginger E. Nicol [1,*]

[1] Department of Psychiatry, Washington University School of Medicine, 660 S. Euclid Ave., Campus Box 8134, St. Louis, MO 63110, USA; s.anwar@wustl.edu (A.A.); yinglinm@wustl.edu (M.D.Y.); aliciazhang@wustl.edu (A.Z.)
[2] Compass Health Network, University of Missouri Columbia School of Medicine, 3 Hospital Plaza Dr., Columbia, MO 65212, USA; uramtekkar@compasshn.org
* Correspondence: nicolg@wustl.edu

Received: 4 January 2018; Accepted: 20 February 2018; Published: 23 February 2018

Abstract: As part of a university-based quality improvement project, we aimed to evaluate child psychiatrists' knowledge, skills, attitudes, and practices regarding assessment and treatment of pediatric sleep problems. We developed a nine-question survey of knowledge, skills, attitudes, and practices regarding assessing for and treating sleep complaints in pediatric patients, and administered this survey to child psychiatrists in training and in practice in the state of Missouri. Respondents reported sleep hygiene as the first-line treatment strategy, followed by the use of supplements or over-the-counter remedies. The most common barriers to evidence-based assessment and treatment of sleep problems were the lack of ability to obtain reliable history, and parental preference for medications over behavioral approaches for sleep concerns. These results suggest potential opportunities for enhancing knowledge regarding validated assessment tools and non-pharmacological treatment options for sleep problems. Additional research is needed to further assess the quality and type of sleep education provided in child psychiatry training programs.

Keywords: child psychiatry; sleep problems; medical education

1. Background

Sleep problems are a common complaint amongst individuals suffering from psychiatric illness [1–3]. There has been emerging evidence in recent years about the complex relationship between sleep and psychiatric disorders that has suggested the existence of a bidirectional relationship [4]. Sleep is part of the symptom criteria in the Diagnostic and Statistical Manual of Mental Disorders, Fifth Edition (DSM-V) for numerous major psychiatric conditions, including those first observed in childhood. Sleep disorders are more common in youth who may attempt suicide or engage in high-risk self-harming behavior [5,6]. Even in psychiatric disorders where sleep disruption is not a major symptom marker, sleep is still thought to play a role in the development and maintenance of dysfunctional symptoms. For example, attention deficit hyperactivity disorder ADHD symptoms are commonly presented complaints in outpatient child psychiatric practices. Children with ADHD can have more bedtime resistance, more issues with initiation of sleep, more nighttime awakenings, difficulties with morning awakenings, sleep-disordered breathing, and daytime sleepiness [7]. Sleep apnea itself is associated with symptoms of hyperactivity, impulsivity, inattention, and poor academic performance [8,9]. Studies have suggested that there may be a higher prevalence of restless legs syndrome and periodic limb movement syndrome in children with ADHD [10]. Autism spectrum disorder is another condition where sleep is not part of the symptom criteria, but sleep problems are common. An estimated 40–80% of children with autism spectrum disorder have sleep problems [11]. Sleep disturbances are common in major mood disorder diagnoses, from decreased need for sleep in bipolar mood disorders to hypersomnia or varying degrees of insomnia in major depression. Finally, insomnia is a frequent complaint in schizophrenia, and can have negative effects on quality of life and cognition. It has even been suggested that sleep deficits may be a precursor of psychosis [12]. Many psychiatric medications that are often prescribed can have an impact on sleep as well. Selective serotonin reuptake inhibitors (SSRIs) are among the most commonly used medications to treat depression and anxiety, and have been known to cause restless legs syndrome or periodic limb movements [13].

Despite the importance of sleep in day-to-day functioning and development, and the role that sleep plays in the development and maintenance of psychiatric conditions, many physicians across various specialties have limited education on adequately screening, diagnosing, and treating sleep problems. In 2001, Owens et al. surveyed 828 physicians on their knowledge about sleep disorders in the pediatric population. Most of the surveyed physicians were primary care physicians, about 75% of them being pediatricians. Less than half of the participants responded that they felt confident in screening for sleep problems in children. Only 25% of participants felt confident in treating sleep in children. The authors of this study felt that this may be due to gaps in basic knowledge about pediatric sleep disorders. They referenced prior studies that documented the limited amount of didactics and other teaching on pediatric sleep disorders in medical school and in residency. The lack of emphasis on sleep issues in pediatric textbooks was also mentioned as a contributor to the gaps in knowledge [14].

Adding to challenges in treating pediatric sleep complaints is the limited data supporting the use of prescription medications for this indication in children. In 2010, Stojanovski et al. looked at trends in medications prescribed for sleep problems in US pediatric outpatients. The survey included 35% pediatricians, 24% psychiatrists, 13% general/family practice physicians, 4% neurologists, and 23% other specialists. They found that more than 80% of visits where sleep problems were reported led to the use of a prescription medication. Furthermore, medications that physicians used to treat sleep problems were those primarily used in psychiatric conditions and had limited evidence for safety and efficacy in children [15]. Despite the prevalence of sleep complaints in children with psychiatric disorders, and the common use of psychotropic medications to treat pediatric sleep problems, there remains a paucity of research assessing the practices and preferences of pediatric psychiatrists.

Given the prominence of sleep disturbances in children who come to clinical attention for psychiatric complaints, we aimed to assess clinician practices in this population in our region. We aimed to evaluate current knowledge, skills, attitudes, and practices across a range of clinician experience related to assessment and treatment of sleep problems in the pediatric psychiatric population. Our goal was to identify potential areas for intervention and/or further education of physicians to improve current practice.

2. Materials and Methods

2.1. Knowledge, Skills, Attitudes and Practices Survey

We developed a simple nine-question survey (see Supplementary materials) as part of a quality improvement project conducted at Washington University School of Medicine between January and June 2017, to evaluate psychiatric clinician knowledge, skills, attitudes, and practices regarding assessing for and treating sleep complaints in pediatric patients. Questions were generated based on a review of existing literature regarding current guidelines [16,17], community provider knowledge and practices, and the research team's previous experience working with pediatric sleep disorders [18]. All survey responses were anonymous.

2.2. Participants

The questionnaire was distributed in person at a regional child psychiatry organization meeting (Greater St. Louis Area Regional Organization for Child & Adolescent Psychiatry, GSL ROCAP), as well as to general psychiatry and child psychiatry trainees at Washington University School of Medicine. GSL ROCAP members unable to attend meetings in person were emailed the survey.

2.3. Statistical Analysis

Data were analyzed using SPSS software (v.22; IBM Corp., Armonk, NY, USA). All available data from all participants were used. Descriptive statistics (mean, frequencies, and proportions) were generated for survey responses. Likert scale items were converted from text value to numerical rating (e.g., 1 = not at all; 3 = very much). Responses to each survey question are reported as number (n) and percentage of clinicians with a response in each category for a given question.

3. Results

A total of 55 clinicians (31.6%) out of 174 contacted responded to the survey. Respondents were 1–5 years in practice ($n = 4$, 7.3%), 6–10 years in practice ($n = 7$, 12.7%), and 10–15 years in practice ($n = 11$, 20.0%). Most participants practiced in an outpatient setting: 61.8% ($n = 34$) reported working in an academic outpatient clinic; 49.1% ($n = 27$) reported working in a community mental health clinic; and 23.6% ($n = 13$) reported working in a private outpatient clinic. Note that participants were able to select multiple clinical settings if they worked in more than one.

The majority of participants ($n = 50$, 90.9%) reported that they assess for sleep problems in all of their patients, with 78.6% ($n = 44$) reporting that they assess for sleep problems at every clinical visit. When participants were asked to rate their confidence in their ability to assess sleep problems on a scale of 1–5, with 1 being poor confidence and 5 being excellent confidence, 41.8% ($n = 23$) chose 3 (moderate confidence), 41.8% ($n = 23$) chose 4 (good confidence), and 16.4% ($n = 9$) chose 5 (excellent confidence). In total, 72.2% ($n = 13$) of participants who have been in practice for at least 15 years said they had good or excellent confidence (4 or 5) in their ability to assess sleep problems. Only 33.3% ($n = 5$) of participants still in training said they had good or excellent confidence (4 or 5) in their assessment of sleep problems (Figure 1).

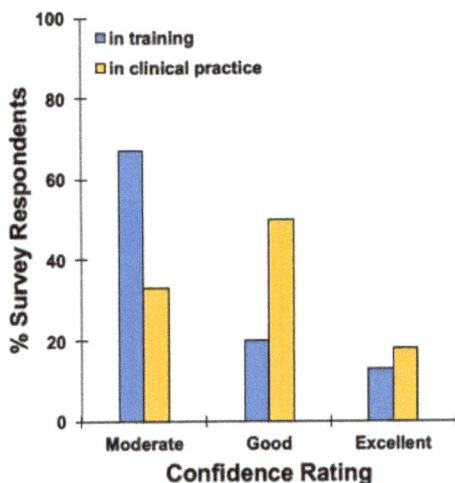

Figure 1. Respondent self-report of confidence in assessing pediatric sleep concerns by level of clinical experience.

One survey participant reported using a specific sleep questionnaire, while the overwhelming majority (n = 54, 98.2%) reported assessing for sleep problems as part of their clinical interview. Difficulty in obtaining accurate information from the patient or adult caregiver was reported as a barrier to assessing sleep problems by 45.5% (n = 25) of respondents; 41.8% (n = 23) reported limited time during the clinical visit as a major barrier to obtaining accurate information regarding sleep problems.

When asked which treatment strategy (sleep hygiene, alpha-2 agonists, over-the-counter supplements, atypical antipsychotics, sedatives/hypnotics, sedating antidepressants, or other) was viewed as most important, almost all participants (n = 54, 98.2%) ranked sleep hygiene as most important. Participants still in training (n = 15) all ranked sleep hygiene as most important. Over-the-counter supplements (e.g., melatonin, valerian) were most-ranked second (n = 39, 70.9%) and alpha-2 agonists (clonidine and guanfacine) were most-ranked third (n = 25, 45.5%). Participants still in training ranked over-the-counter supplements as second most important (n = 12, 80%) compared with 67.5% (n = 27) of participants who had completed training (Figure 2).

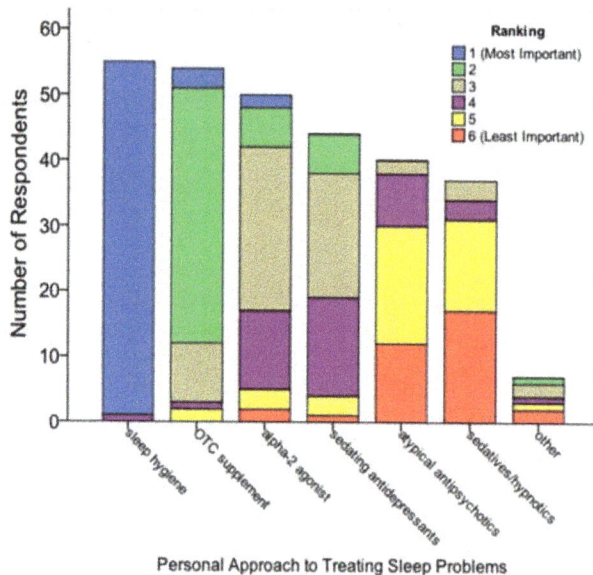

Figure 2. Ranked importance of clinical approaches to sleep problems.

Anticipated non-compliance with recommendations (52.7%, n = 29) and patient/guardian preference for medications (32.7%, n = 18) were the most selected reasons for barriers to using sleep hygiene as a first-line treatment for sleep problems.

4. Discussion

To our knowledge, this is the first study to report on the skills, attitudes, and practices of child psychiatric providers regarding pediatric sleep concerns. A better understanding of clinician perspectives on this matter is important in identifying knowledge gaps and developing educational strategies for improving adherence to best practices. While the majority of our respondents reported routinely assessing for sleep concerns in their patients, they also noted that major barriers to assessment were limited time and difficulty in obtaining accurate information. Despite this rather universal report of challenges in assessment, only one respondent reported routinely using a validated sleep assessment tool to screen for sleep problems. The majority of our respondents also reported first-line use of low-risk treatment approaches with modest evidence, including education on sleep hygiene and recommending use of over-the-counter supplements such as melatonin. However, the importance of other treatment approaches was variably ranked, with no respondents reporting use of non-pharmacological strategies other than sleep hygiene. In addition, while nearly all respondents ranked sleep hygiene as being "very important" in their treatment approach, patient/guardian preference for medications and anticipated non-compliance were reported as significant barriers to using it as a first-line intervention. Finally, we observed a difference in confidence and knowledge based on number of years in practice, with more seasoned clinicians having greater confidence in assessment abilities. These results suggest potential opportunities for educating psychiatric providers on assessment tools and behavioral approaches for sleep problems in children.

Limited time for assessment and difficulty obtaining accurate information were identified as the biggest barriers by those surveyed in this study. Although clinical screening for sleep difficulties cannot take the place of gold standard sleep assessments, particularly for the evaluation of disorders such as obstructive sleep apnea, validated sleep questionnaires completed by the patient/guardian in the waiting room prior to the visit may address barriers to screening reported by our respondents. Validated self-report questionnaires commonly used in the pediatric sleep assessment include the Pediatric Sleep Questionnaire (PSQ), the Pediatric Daytime Sleepiness Scale (PDSS), the BEARS (B = Bedtime Issues, E = Excessive Daytime Sleepiness, A = Night Awakenings, R = Regularity and Duration of Sleep, S = Snoring), and the Ten Item Sleep Screener. The PSQ is a 49-item questionnaire for parents that is divided into behavioral, sleepiness, and snoring domains. This can be used for patients aged 2–18 years. It has sensitivity and specificity of 0.81 and 0.87, respectively [19]. The PDSS is an eight-item questionnaire where items are scored on a Likert scale rating system. It is used to measure excessive sleepiness in children and has been shown to have good internal consistency [20]. The BEARS pediatric sleep screening tool assesses sleep disorders in children aged 2–18 years. It has parent-directed and child-directed questions that evaluate five domains including bedtime problems, excessive daytime, awakenings during the night, regularity and duration of sleep, and snoring. Questions are distinct for toddlers/preschoolers (2–5 years), school-aged children (6–12 years), and adolescents (13–18 years) [21]. Another pediatric sleep screening tool is the Ten Item Sleep Screener which asks such questions as "Does the child snore lightly or loudly at night?"; "Does the child wake up frequently in the night?"; "Does the child have a difficult temperament (irritable or easily frustrated)?" [22]. Additional studies evaluating the validity of these screening tools compared with gold standard assessments would be helpful in this population.

The fact that respondents ranked pharmacological interventions as having limited and varying importance in their clinical practices is likely a reflection of the lack of evidence supporting the use of medications for the treatment of insomnia and other sleep-related problems in children [1]. Participants in our survey overwhelmingly ranked sleep hygiene as the most important intervention in addressing sleep problems, but noted important barriers to using it consistently as a first-line treatment approach. Cognitive behavioral therapy for insomnia (CBT-I) is a structured behavioral intervention that has been shown to be effective and have fewer risks than medication [23], but was not listed by any respondents as a primary treatment strategy. This suggests a limited knowledge of or ability to provide evidence-based behavioral treatments such as CBT-I, which could be usefully included in psychotherapy education during training.

Although not directly addressed by our survey, others have posited that low confidence in and knowledge of treatment for pediatric sleep problems—particularly in child psychiatry trainees—is related to the lack of a universally-adapted pediatric sleep curriculum in residency training [18]. In 2002, Krahn et al. surveyed 98 program directors of general psychiatry residencies in the USA, and observed a lack of standardized approaches to sleep education in training programs. They reported that 82% of participating programs had sleep lectures as part of didactics. However, only 44% offered a sleep medicine elective, and the majority did not have a faculty member that was a sleep medicine specialist [24]. Similarly, Khawaja et al. surveyed 39 chief psychiatry residents, and found that about 90% reported that their training programs offered didactic sleep education. However, only 38% of programs had faculty that were trained in sleep medicine, and only 34% offered a sleep medicine elective [25]. No programs reported a structured curriculum devoted specifically to pediatric sleep concerns. These findings highlight the need to further study the effectiveness of current sleep education approaches for psychiatric trainees, with a focus on those going into pediatric psychiatry.

This study was subject to important limitations. In particular, this was a small quality improvement project aiming to assess clinical practices within the Eastern Missouri region, and may not be generalizable to practitioners in other regions. Most of the participants were either in training or had been in practice for 15 years or more, with low representation of early career psychiatrists (1–5 years in practice). Additionally, we did not assess current training practices nor query respondents on their educational experiences during training with respect to assessment and treatment of pediatric sleep concerns. Finally, we did not specifically assess for knowledge of psychotherapeutic approaches to pediatric sleep problems. A larger sample size with a better representation of clinicians at different stages of their careers, assessing for training experiences, and knowledge of behavioral approaches other than sleep hygiene is necessary to further assess for knowledge gaps and develop targeted educational approaches for pediatric sleep training in child psychiatry training. However, our study did provide some insight into potential areas for quality improvement in assessment of sleep problems and future directions for research and clinician education.

Supplementary Materials: The following are available online at http://www.mdpi.com/2076-3271/6/1/18/s1, Sleep Problems Survey.

Acknowledgments: The authors would like to thank Amanda Ricchio, for administrative assistance in collecting data and in manuscript preparation, and the clinicians who responded to the survey.

Author Contributions: A.A. was the project leader and was responsible for developing the survey with support from G.E.N. and U.R., and in collecting survey response data. M.D.Y. provided expertise in the management and analysis of data. A.A, G.E.N. and M.D.Y. had access to all the data and analyzed the data. A.A., M.D.Y. and G.E.N. were responsible for the decision to submit the report, and drafted it. A.Z. provided assistance in developing the manuscript and interpreting the results of analyses. All authors read, critically revised, and approved the report. The corresponding author, G.E.N., confirms that she had full access to all the data in the study and takes responsibility for the integrity of the data and the accuracy of the data analysis.

Conflicts of Interest: G.E.N. has received research funding from the National Institute of Mental Health (NIMH), Otsuka America, Inc., Alkermes, The Sidney R. Baer, Jr. Foundation, the Center for Brain Research in Mood Disorders (CBRiMD) at Washington University. A.A., M.D.Y., A.Z. and U.R. have nothing to disclose.

References

1. Ramtekkar, U.; Ivanenko, A. Sleep in children with psychiatric disorders. *Semin. Pediatr. Neurol.* **2015**, *22*, 148–155. [CrossRef] [PubMed]

2. Ivanenko, A.; Crabtree, V.M.; Obrien, L.M.; Gozal, D. Sleep complaints and psychiatric symptoms in children evaluated at a pediatric mental health clinic. *J. Clin. Sleep Med.* **2006**, *2*, 42–48. [PubMed]

3. Ivanenko, A.; Johnson, K. Sleep disturbances in children with psychiatric disorders. *Semin. Pediatr. Neurol.* **2008**, *15*, 70–78. [CrossRef] [PubMed]

4. Krystal, A.D. Psychiatric disorders and sleep. *Neurol. Clin.* **2012**, *30*, 1389–1413. [CrossRef] [PubMed]

5. Franic, T.; Kralj, Z.; Marcinko, D.; Knez, R.; Kardum, G. Suicidal ideations and sleep-related problems in early adolescence. *Early Interv. Psychiatry* **2014**, *8*, 155–162. [CrossRef] [PubMed]

6. Goldstein, T.R.; Bridge, J.A.; Brent, D.A. Sleep disturbance preceding completed suicide in adolescents. *J. Consult. Clin. Psychol.* **2008**, *76*, 84–91. [CrossRef] [PubMed]

7. Cortese, S.; Faraone, S.V.; Konofal, E.; Lecendreux, M. Sleep in children with attention-deficit/hyperactivity disorder: Meta-analysis of subjective and objective studies. *J. Am. Acad. Child Adolesc. Psychiatry* **2009**, *48*, 894–908. [CrossRef] [PubMed]

8. Hunter, S.J.; Gozal, D.; Smith, D.L.; Philby, M.F.; Kaylegian, J.; Kheirandish-Gozal, L. Effect of sleep-disordered breathing severity on cognitive performance measures in a large community cohort of young school-aged children. *Am. J. Respir. Crit. Care Med.* **2016**, *194*, 739–747. [CrossRef] [PubMed]

9. Galland, B.; Spruyt, K.; Dawes, P.; McDowall, P.S.; Elder, D.; Schaughency, E. Sleep disordered breathing and academic performance: A meta-analysis. *Pediatrics* **2015**, *136*, e934–e946. [CrossRef] [PubMed]

10. Tsai, M.H.; Hsu, J.F.; Huang, Y.S. Sleep problems in children with attention deficit/hyperactivity disorder: Current status of knowledge and appropriate management. *Curr. Psychiatry Rep.* **2016**, *18*, 76. [CrossRef] [PubMed]

11. Cortesi, F.; Giannotti, F.; Ivanenko, A.; Johnson, K. Sleep in children with autistic spectrum disorder. *Sleep Med.* **2010**, *11*, 659–664. [CrossRef] [PubMed]

12. Lunsford-Avery, J.R.; Orr, J.M.; Gupta, T.; Pelletier-Baldelli, A.; Dean, D.J.; Smith Watts, A.K.; Bernard, J.; Millman, Z.B.; Mittal, V.A. Sleep dysfunction and thalamic abnormalities in adolescents at ultra high-risk for psychosis. *Schizophr. Res.* **2013**, *151*, 148–153. [CrossRef] [PubMed]

13. Hoque, R.; Chesson, A.L., Jr. Pharmacologically induced/exacerbated restless legs syndrome, periodic limb movements of sleep, and REM behavior disorder/REM sleep without atonia: Literature review, qualitative scoring, and comparative analysis. *J. Clin. Sleep Med.* **2010**, *6*, 79–83. [PubMed]

14. Owens, J.A. The practice of pediatric sleep medicine: Results of a community survey. *Pediatrics* **2001**, *108*, E51. [CrossRef] [PubMed]

15. Stojanovski, S.D.; Rasu, R.S.; Balkrishnan, R.; Nahata, M.C. Trends in medication prescribing for pediatric sleep difficulties in US outpatient settings. *Sleep* **2007**, *30*, 1013–1017. [CrossRef] [PubMed]

16. Morgenthaler, T.I.; Owens, J.; Alessi, C.; Boehlecke, B.; Brown, T.M.; Coleman, J., Jr.; Friedman, L.; Kapur, V.K.; Lee-Chiong, T.; Pancer, J.; et al. Practice parameters for behavioral treatment of bedtime problems and night wakings in infants and young children. *Sleep* **2006**, *29*, 1277–1281. [PubMed]

17. Moturi, S.; Avis, K. Assessment and treatment of common pediatric sleep disorders. *Psychiatry* **2010**, *7*, 24–37. [PubMed]

18. Ramtekkar, U.P. Sleep problems in children: Training, practices, and attitudes of child psychiatry residents. In *Proceeding of the Prescribing Wellness across the Lifespan, Proceedings of the American Psychiatric Association 166th Annual Meeting, San Francisco, CA, USA, 18–22 May 2013*; American Psychiatric Association: San Francisco, CA, USA, 2013.

19. Chervin, R.D.; Hedger, K.; Dillon, J.E.; Pituch, K.J. Pediatric sleep questionnaire (PSQ): Validity and reliability of scales for sleep-disordered breathing, snoring, sleepiness, and behavioral problems. *Sleep Med.* **2000**, *1*, 21–32. [CrossRef]

20. Drake, C.; Nickel, C.; Burduvali, E.; Roth, T.; Jefferson, C.; Pietro, B. The pediatric daytime sleepiness scale (PDSS): Sleep habits and school outcomes in middle-school children. *Sleep* **2003**, *26*, 455–458. [PubMed]

21. Owens, J.A.; Dalzell, V. Use of the 'BEARS' sleep screening tool in a pediatric residents' continuity clinic: A pilot study. *Sleep Med.* **2005**, *6*, 63–69. [CrossRef] [PubMed]

22. Spruyt, K.; Gozal, D. Pediatric sleep questionnaires as diagnostic or epidemiological tools: A review of currently available instruments. *Sleep Med. Rev.* **2011**, *15*, 19–32. [CrossRef] [PubMed]

23. Wu, J.Q.; Appleman, E.R.; Salazar, R.D.; Ong, J.C. Cognitive behavioral therapy for insomnia comorbid with psychiatric and medical conditions: A meta-analysis. *JAMA Intern. Med.* **2015**, *175*, 1461–1472. [CrossRef] [PubMed]

24. Krahn, L.E.; Hansen, M.R.; Tinsley, J.A. Psychiatric residents' exposure to the field of sleep medicine: A survey of program directors. *Acad. Psychiatry* **2002**, *26*, 253–256. [CrossRef] [PubMed]

25. Khawaja, I.S.; Dieperink, M.E.; Thuras, P.; Kunisaki, K.M.; Schumacher, M.M.; Germain, A.; Amborn, B.; Hurwitz, T.D. Effect of sleep skills education on sleep quality in patients attending a psychiatry partial hospitalization program. *Prim. Care Companion CNS Disord.* **2013**, *15*. [CrossRef] [PubMed]

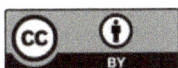

medical sciences

MDPI

Review

Pharmacological Approach to Sleep Disturbances in Autism Spectrum Disorders with Psychiatric Comorbidities: A Literature Review

Sachin Relia [1,*] and Vijayabharathi Ekambaram [2,*]

1 Department of Psychiatry, University of Tennessee Health Sciences Center, 920, Madison Avenue, Suite 200, Memphis, TN 38105, USA
2 Department of Psychiatry, University of Oklahoma Health Sciences Center, 920, Stanton L Young Blvd, Oklahoma City, OK 73104, USA
* Correspondence: srelia@uthsc.edu (S.R.); vijayabharathi-ekambaram@ouhsc.edu (V.E.);
Tel.: +1-901-448-4266 (S.R.); +1-405-271-5251 (V.E.); Fax: +1-901-297-6337 (S.R.); +1-405-271-3808 (V.E.)

Received: 15 August 2018; Accepted: 17 October 2018; Published: 25 October 2018

Abstract: Autism is a developmental disability that can cause significant emotional, social and behavioral dysfunction. Sleep disorders co-occur in approximately half of the patients with autism spectrum disorder (ASD). Sleep problems in individuals with ASD have also been associated with poor social interaction, increased stereotypy, problems in communication, and overall autistic behavior. Behavioral interventions are considered a primary modality of treatment. There is limited evidence for psychopharmacological treatments in autism; however, these are frequently prescribed. Melatonin, antipsychotics, antidepressants, and α agonists have generally been used with melatonin, having a relatively large body of evidence. Further research and information are needed to guide and individualize treatment for this population group.

Keywords: autism spectrum disorder; sleep disorders in ASD; medications for sleep disorders in ASD; comorbidities in ASD

1. Introduction

Autism is a developmental disability that can cause significant emotional, social, and behavioral dysfunction. According to the Diagnostic and Statistical Manual (DSM-V) classification [1], autism spectrum disorder (ASD) is characterized by persistent deficits in domains of social communication, social interaction, restricted and repetitive patterns of behavior, interests, or activities. The term autism spectrum disorder has replaced the earlier terminology of pervasive developmental disorder in the classification systems of DSM-IV TR [2]. There is greater variability in clinical presentation of ASD, depending upon each individual's intelligence quotient (IQ) level. Intelligence quotient is a major determinant in determining the degree of impairment among individuals with ASD. In DSM-V, ASD is categorized as low-functioning autism with below average intelligence quotient (<70) and high-functioning autism with above average intelligence quotient ($\geq$70) [1].

Studies have documented individuals with low-functioning autism experience significant impairments in their ability to function and exhibit serious behavioral disturbances, self-injurious behaviors, and socially inappropriate behaviors, and these individuals have higher predisposition to sleep–wake disturbances compared to their counterparts with high-functioning autism [3–5]. Overall, it is estimated that about 1 in 59 children suffer from ASD [6]. Sleep disorders occur frequently in autism spectrum disorder, with some studies reporting a prevalence between 50%–80% [7].

Studies have suggested low-functioning autism with increased severity, such as language deficits, increases the likelihood of sleep problems and can worsen the severity of sleep problems in these individuals [8,9]. There is also a lack of available data in low-functioning autism because of challenges in obtaining actigraphy and polysomnography studies in these members of the population [10].

Various potential mechanisms, including delayed melatonin peak, reduced rhythm amplitude, reduced ferritin, and increased periodic limb movements in sleep, have been hypothesized as a cause of sleep problems in ASD [11–13]. Sleep problems in individuals with ASD have also been associated with poor social interaction, increased stereotypy, problems in communication, and overall autistic behavior [14].

It is well established that psychiatric morbidities frequently co-occur in autism spectrum disorders and play a major role in sleep dysregulation. Conditions like anxiety and attention-deficit hyperactivity disorder (ADHD) in the ASD population can increase arousals, delay sleep onset latencies, and contribute to insomnia. Seizures and gastrointestinal disorders (like diarrhea) can cause frequent awakenings, sleep deprivation, and disruption in the sleep cycle [15].

Though sleep problems account for the most common reason for medications being prescribed, even in younger children, it is interesting to note that no medication is U.S. Food and Drug Administration (FDA)-approved for treatment of sleep disorders in children. In a community survey, approximately 75% of practitioners had recommended nonprescription medications and about 50% had prescribed a sleep medication during a six-month practice period [16].

Generally, behavioral interventions should be considered primary modalities of treatment and should be initiated before considering pharmacotherapy. The functioning level of autism (high- vs. low-functioning) should be taken into consideration before determining treatment approaches. The basic tenets of behavioral interventions do not differ greatly for children and adolescents with autism. Even, booklet-delivered behavioral interventions specifically designed for autism have been developed and shown to be effective [17,18]. A behavioral sleep medicine toolkit outlining evaluation and treatment of insomnia in children with ASD has also been developed by the Autism Treatment Network (ATN) [19]. Furthermore, applied behavior analysis (ABA) and parent-based education have also shown improvement in sleep disorders in ASD [15].

Medications should be considered if behavioral interventions are ineffective or difficult to be implemented, especially in individuals with low-functioning autism, and should be used in combination with nonpharmacological strategies, which result in more sustained improvement [20]. Furthermore, medications should be initiated at the lowest effective dose and increased only if necessary. To decrease the risk of rebound insomnia, medication should be closely monitored and tapered gradually. Of particular concern, adolescents should be screened for alcohol and drug use, due to the additive effects of sedative hypnotic medications and recreational substances. Timing is crucial in the treatment of sleep disorders, as most hypnotic medications have their onset of action within 30 min and peak within 1–2 h. Therefore, dosing too early or too late would result in limited efficacy. Since over-the-counter (OTC) preparations are commonly used, an inquiry should be made to check concurrent use of OTC agents.

2. Melatonin

Melatonin is one of most common agents recommended for treatment of sleep difficulties and children with ASD. In a community survey of pediatricians, the majority had recommended a nonprescription medication for treatment of pediatric insomnia, with about 15% having recommended melatonin [16]. Melatonin is a hormone primarily synthesized in the pineal gland, with a major function to regulate circadian and core body temperature rhythms. Dim light melatonin onset (DLMO) is the single most accurate marker for assessing circadian pacemaker rhythms [21]. It is rapidly distributed to body tissues including the cerebrospinal fluid, bile, and saliva, where concentrations greatly exceed those found in the blood. Melatonin levels generally decline with advancing age. Its production is inhibited (by light) and is regulated by a circuitous pathway through the suprachiasmatic nuclei. Endogenous melatonin has both chrono biotic and sedative–hypnotic effects [22]. It has also been described that pharmacokinetic profiles of endogenous and supplemental melatonin in children with ASD are normal and comparable to typically developing children [23].

Several studies, including open-label data, uncontrolled trials to control trials, and meta-analysis, have been conducted in patients with ASD, establishing the efficacy of melatonin. Since it is considered a dietary supplement, its safety has not been thoroughly evaluated by the FDA. It is generally regarded as safe, despite lack of rigorous data pertaining to its use. Recommendations regarding use in children and adolescents are also mixed. National Institutes of Health (NIH) states that "Important questions remain about its usefulness, how much to take, when to take it, and its long-term safety" [24]. Because of its effects on other hormones, melatonin might interfere with development during adolescence. American Academy of Pediatrics states, "Melatonin appears to be effective in reducing time to sleep onset in adults (and, based on considerably less data, in children) for initial insomnia. This effect appears to last for days to weeks but not long-term. Thus, melatonin is not recommended for long-term use" [25]. By contrast, the Australian Sleep Health Foundation states that melatonin "may benefit children who are developing normally as well as children with Attention Deficit Hyperactivity Disorder, autism, other developmental disabilities or visual impairment" [26]. Here, we examine the efficacy studies regarding use of melatonin in children with autism spectrum disorders.

A key retrospective study, describing the use of melatonin in 107 subjects (2–18 years) utilizing a 3–6 mg dose, demonstrated that sleep concerns were no longer present for approximately 25% of the parents at follow-up after 1.8 years [27].

In another open-label trial, Malow and colleagues evaluated the efficacy of melatonin in 24 children aged 3–10 years, utilizing doses up to 9 mg. This study demonstrated that sleep onset latency was reduced by an average of 21.3 min (from 42.9 to 21.6 min, $p < 0.0001$), but there was no significant difference in total sleep duration, sleep efficiency, or night waking after 14 weeks of therapy. The study also demonstrated improvements in behavior and reduction in stereotypical and compulsive phenomena [28].

On the other hand, in another smaller placebo-controlled trial of 18 subjects, aged 2–15 years with ASD or fragile X syndrome, the melatonin group demonstrated significant improvements in total sleep duration and sleep onset time compared to the placebo group. Particularly, total sleep duration was increased by 21 min ($p = 0.057$) and sleep onset latency was decreased by 42 min ($p = 0.017$) [29].

There are limited data evaluating the efficacy of a controlled release formulation. In a double-blind crossover trial involving 51 subjects aged 2–18 years, where more than half of the subjects had ASD, melatonin 5 mg (1 and 4 mg immediate and controlled release, respectively) was found to reflect an increased mean total sleep duration (from 503.60 to 534.80 min, $p < 0.01$) and decreased sleep onset latency (65.18 to 32.48 min, $p < 0.01$) [30].

In a meta-analysis which included five randomized double-blind placebo-controlled crossover trials with 57 subjects with ASD and quantitative data sleep parameters, pooled data indicated that melatonin increased total sleep duration by an average of 73 min ($p < 0.01$) and decreased sleep onset latency by an average of 66 min ($p < 0.001$) [31]. However, there was no appreciable benefit for night wakings.

In another study, involving 146 children, using placebo-controlled intervention, 0.5–12, immediate release melatonin in a stepwise fashion, demonstrated only a small increase of 23 min in total sleep time but a much larger 38 min reduction in sleep latency. Additionally, melatonin had no demonstrable effect on night wakings [17].

Melatonin is available in different over-the-counter formulations ranging 1–10 milligrams in the United States and Canada, but in some countries, a prescription may be needed. Most commonly, a dose of 1–3 mg is recommended to be administered 30–60 min before intended bedtime [31]. However, if a circadian rhythm issue is identified, a lower dose (0.5–1 mg) administered earlier (3–4 h before bedtime) is recommended. An effective dose is not related to age or weight. Given the availability of different brands and the fact that strict regulations are not applicable to over-the-counter medications by the FDA, a concern is often raised regarding actual content of melatonin in the different formulations. In a recent study conducted in Ontario, which examined the melatonin content of different OTC formulations, actual melatonin content ranged from −83% to +478% of the labelled content. Furthermore, serotonin (5-hydroxytryptamine), a related indoleamine and controlled substance used in the treatment of several neurological disorders, was also identified in several supplements [32].

Melatonin is generally tolerated fairly well. Most studies published to date have not reported any serious safety concerns [28,29,33,34] (Table 1). Generally reported adverse effects include morning drowsiness, increased enuresis, headache, dizziness, and hypothermia. Some studies have reported suppression of the hypothalamic pituitary axis HPA axis with long term use and potential for precocious puberty on discontinuation [35]. Patients with a poor response have been shown to be poor CYP1A2 metabolizers.

Melatonin receptor agonists act selectively at MT1 and MT2 melatonin receptors and have demonstrated usefulness in children with autism spectrum disorder [36]. Ramelteon, the only drug in this class, has FDA approval for treatment of insomnia in adults. Side effects mainly include dizziness and fatigue and caution is advised for concomitant administration with Fluvoxamine.

Table 1. Selected medications for sleep referenced in the publications on autism spectrum disorder (ASD) and psychiatric comorbidities.

Medication	Dosing Range	Common Side Effects	Clinical Use
Melatonin	1–3 mg	Nausea, headache, dizziness, hypothermia	Effective in children with developmental disorders, Autism spectrum disorders, Jet Lag
Antipsychotics Olanzapine Risperidone	2.5–10 mg 0.25–2 mg	Daytime drowsiness, weight gain, hypercholesterolemia, diabetes Mellitus, prolactin elevation	Effective in comorbid maladaptive behaviors including irritability, aggression and self-injury
Antidepressants Trazodone *	20–50 mg (adult dose)	Dizziness, morning drowsiness, priapism, hypotension	Useful with comorbid depression
Alpha-adrenergic agonist Clonidine (immediate release) Guanfacine (immediate release)	0.05–0.225 mg 0.5–2 mg	Hypotension, bradycardia, irritability, dry mouth, REM suppression. Abrupt discontinuation causing rebound hypertension and rebound REM	Sleep initiation and maintenance insomnia
Antihistamine Diphenhydramine Trimeprazine Niaprazine (not approved for use in USA)	0.5 mg/kg up to 25 mg 45–90 mg 1 mg/kg/day three times daily	Sedation and anticholinergic effects, including fever, blurred vision, dry mouth, constipation, urinary retention, tachycardia and confusion	Transient insomnia
Sedative and Hypnotics Clonazepam	0.25–0.5 mg	Sedation, headaches, dizziness, cognitive impairment, rebound insomnia, physical and behavioral dependence	Parasomnias, periodic limb movement disorder, nocturnal biting
Iron supplements Oral Iron	6 mg elemental iron/kg/day	Metallic taste, vomiting, nausea, constipation, diarrhea, black/green stools	Sleep disturbances, Periodic limb movements of sleep, restless legs syndrome
Alzheimer's medications Donepezil	1.25–5 mg	Gastrointestinal symptoms, vivid dreams, insomnia, bradycardia, hypotension	Increased REM sleep percentage and decreased REM latency

* Adult data. REM: Rapid eye movement.

3. Antipsychotics

Antipsychotics as a class have the largest body of evidence for treatment of behavioral difficulties, including aggression and irritability for treatment in autism spectrum disorder. These are usually prescribed for mood and behavioral comorbidities and secondarily have a beneficial effect for sleep. Antipsychotics have traditionally been categorized as typical and atypical antipsychotics.

Typical antipsychotics, including haloperidol, fluphenazine, and thioridazine, are associated with higher incidence of extrapyramidal side effects and daytime somnolence. Newer, second-generation antipsychotics, including olanzapine, risperidone, and quetiapine, have a lower propensity for extrapyramidal side effects and are generally less sedating. There are limited efficacy and tolerability data for treatment of insomnia in children for this medication class. Few studies examining the effect on sleep architecture have shown that slow wave sleep is increased by olanzapine, ziprasidone, and Risperidone, whereas rapid eye movement (REM) suppression is greatest for ziprasidone and Risperidone [37]. Of the atypicals, risperidone and olanzapine have been prescribed for sleep disturbances in children [38] (Table 1). These agents are prescribed off label for treatment of insomnia and are not recommended to be prescribed routinely for this indication, especially as a first line pharmacotherapeutic agent. In particular, a guideline has been issued by the Canadian Academy of Child and Adolescent Psychiatry against its use for insomnia treatment in children, adults, or the elderly as a first line agent [39]. Other countries have also aimed to limit the number of prescriptions which may be allowed by government-subsidized programs.

4. Antidepressants

Limited data exist regarding use and efficacy of sedating antidepressants, selective serotonin reuptake inhibitors (SSRI) and tricyclic antideprssants (TCA), for treatment of sleep disturbances in children with autism spectrum disorder. These may be beneficial if insomnia is associated with comorbid psychiatric disorders. For example, sedating antidepressant such as mirtazapine and trazodone may be beneficial in a child with comorbid depression. These antidepressants promote sleep by antagonizing the effect of wake-promoting neurotransmitters, such as histamine, acetylcholine, noradrenaline, and serotonin. Most of these antidepressants suppress REM sleep and result in residual daytime sedation. Trazodone, in particular, is frequently preferred and used in psychiatric practice. Its efficacy has mainly been demonstrated in adults with psychiatric disorders (Table 1). Trazodone is a 5-HT2A/C antagonist and is one of the most sedating antidepressants with significant morning hangover effect. Fluoxetine, on the other hand, is generally associated with insomnia. The doses used for treatment of insomnia are generally lower compared to doses used for treatment of mood disorders. Selective serotonin reuptake inhibitors and tricyclic antidepressants can also be used if obsessional thoughts and anxiety significantly interfere with sleep onset. Amongst the TCAs, amitriptyline, imipramine, and doxepin are most sedating and used for treatment of insomnia in adults [40].

5. Anticonvulsants

Again, the data are limited regarding the use of anticonvulsants in the treatment of insomnia in this population group. Most of the trials have examined irritability and aggression and have reported improvement in these domains. The adverse events noted in these studies have ranged from insomnia to sedation [41]. Sedation is generally dose-related and tolerance is known to occur. The agents that have commonly been used in this category include valproate, lamotrigine, gabapentin, and carbamazepine. Gabapentin, in particular, has also demonstrated efficacy in adults with restless legs syndrome [42].

6. α-Adrenergic Agonists

The use of alpha agonist as off-label prescription has increased over the time. The prescription pattern in cohorts of children and adolescents (aged 4–18 years, $n = 282{,}875$) studied from 2009 to 2011 showed that about 68% of them received alpha agonists (shorter acting agents) as off-label medication for diagnosis of autism, primarily based on evidence from clinical trials without FDA approval. The study also revealed about 12% of them received alpha agonists for diagnosis of sleep and anxiety disorders without any evidence from randomized control trial in children [43].

Clonidine and guanfacine are the two primary alpha agonists used often as off-label medications for treating sleep disorder in autism.

Clonidine, an antihypertensive medication, is a central and peripheral a-adrenergic agonist which acts by stimulating presynaptic neurons, thereby decreasing noradrenergic release from the nerve terminals [44]. The two open-label retrospective studies in children and adolescents (aged 4–16 years) with autism and neurodevelopmental disorders documented that clonidine (dosing range: 0.05–0.225 mg/day) effectively improved sleep initiation and maintenance insomnia with good tolerability and few adverse events [45,46]. The potential side effects of clonidine include hypotension, bradycardia, irritability, dry mouth, and REM suppression, and its abrupt discontinuation can cause rebound hypertension and rebound REM [46,47].

Guanfacine, a selective α2A adrenergic receptor agonist, acts by stimulating postsynaptic alpha2A receptors in the prefrontal cortex (PFC) and in turn increases the noradrenergic transmission and connectivity of PFC networks [48]. Though immediate release guanfacine (dosing range: 0.5–2 mg/day) is frequently used off label for sleep disturbances in the pediatric population, there were no clinical trials conducted to determine its effectiveness [43,49,50]. Interestingly, a recent randomized, placebo-controlled trial of extended release guanfacine did not significantly improve sleep habits in Autism [51]. By contrast, a decrease in total sleep time was reported on polysomnography in placebo-controlled trial of extended release guanfacine [52].

7. Alzheimer's Medications

Several Alzheimer's medications have been studied for treating autism. Post mortem brain studies from individuals with autism have documented abnormalities in the cholinergic system and a connection between Alzheimer's disease and autism has been proposed by many researchers [53,54]. One of the Alzheimer medications, donepezil, was found to be effective in improving behavioral and attention issues in autism.

Donepezil acts by selective reversible inhibition of acetylcholinesterase enzyme and increases cholinergic transmission in the synaptic cleft. In addition, in previous studies, donepezil was found to increase REM sleep in healthy and demented adults [55,56].

REM sleep is important for the promotion of cortical plasticity in developing brain. In children with autism, REM sleep abnormalities, such as immature organization, decreased quantity, and abnormal twitches, have been described [57]. In animal models, therapeutic augmentation of REM sleep has shown positive behaviors and improvement in learning [58]. Association of REM sleep augmentation and donepezil (dosing range: 1.25–5 mg/day) was studied in a small case series of children with autism (n = 5). This study demonstrated an increase in REM sleep percentage and decrease in REM latency with use of donepezil [59]. However, the findings of the study are limited due its small sample size. The potential side effects of donepezil include gastrointestinal symptoms such as nausea, vomiting, diarrhea, vivid dreams, insomnia, bradycardia, and hypotension [60].

8. Antihistamines

In the survey mailed to pediatricians (n = 671) by the American Academy of Pediatrics (AAP), antihistamines were found to be the most commonly reported nonprescription medication for sleep disorders [16]. Randomized controlled studies in typically developing children have documented improvement in transient insomnia with antihistamines. Diphenhydramine, a first-generation antihistamine, is prescribed often (dosing range: 0.5 mg/kg up to a maximum of 25 mg/day) by practitioners for sleep problems. It acts as a competitive histamine (H1) receptor blocker in the central and peripheral nervous system, causing a sedative and hypnotic effect. Another H1 receptor antagonist, Trimeprazine (dosing range: 45–90 mg/day), has also been shown to improve nocturnal awakenings in children with chronic sleep disturbances. The potential side effects include sedation and anticholinergic effects, including fever, blurred vision, dry mouth, constipation, urinary retention, tachycardia, and confusion [48,49]. Despite widespread use of antihistamines, the clinical trials in patients with autism spectrum disorder have been limited. A European open-label study documented niaprazine, a piperazine derivative, which also acts as an antihistamine (dosing range: 1 mg/kg/day three times daily), to be effective in improving sleep problems in children with autism and with mild to moderate intellectual disability. Niaprazine has not been approved for use in the United States [61].

9. Sedative and Hypnotics

Benzodiazepines (BZDs) are frequently prescribed in adults with insomnia. However, they are prescribed less frequently in the pediatric population because of their side-effects profile includes sedation, headaches, dizziness, cognitive impairment, rebound insomnia, and physical and behavioral dependence. There have only been limited studies in pediatrics, which have shown improvement in sleep disorders with use of BZDs.

The mechanism of action of BZDs is primarily to bind to α and γ subunits of the gamma aminobutyric acid (GABA) chloride receptor, inducing a conformational change in the receptor complex, and facilitating GABA. The inhibitory action of GABA on the central nervous system causes sedative, anxiolytic, and muscle-relaxing effects [62]. Because of BZDs' muscle-relaxant property, they should be used cautiously in children with a sleep-related breathing disorder. Benzodiazepines are also well known to alter normal sleep state architecture and there has been polysomnographic evidence of atypical sleep spindles and slow wave sleep suppression with chronic BZD use.

The only benzodiazepine studied in sleep disorders in children with Autism was clonazepam. Clonazepam, an intermediate acting BZD, was found to be effective in treating parasomnias, partial arousals, periodic limb movement disorder, and nocturnal biting in children with developmental disabilities [49]. Its half-life ranges between 18–39 h, with time to peak level of 1–2 h, and it has a primary renal elimination [62]. A small case study of children ($n = 11$) with autism and REM behavior disorder (RBD) found clonazepam (dosing range: 0.25–0.5 mg/day) to be effective in improving sleep disturbances. It was well tolerated in most of the participants, except one paradoxical response in a child [57].

The nonbenzodiazepines, zaleplon, zolpidem, and eszopiclone, often called as 'Z-drugs', have similar pharmacology to BZDs, but are not chemically related to BZD. They act at benzodiazepine-1 subtype in the GABA receptor complex. All Z-drugs have a relatively short life. In contrast to BZD, they do not cause significant residual daytime sedation, cognitive, or memory impairment [63]. In addition, they do not typically cause rebound insomnia (an exacerbation of insomnia on abrupt cessation of a hypnotic) with abrupt discontinuation, which is one of the worsening adverse effects of BZD. Zaleplon and zolpidem have been used in children but data on the use of eszopiclone are limited [47]. Clearance of nonbenzodiazepine receptor agonist drugs in children is three times higher than in adults, which can cause medication ineffectiveness and may even lead to terrifying sleep states, like sleepwalking and sleep-related hallucinations [47]. There were no clinical trials available for this category of medications in autism.

10. Oral Iron Supplement

Serum ferritin, a storage form of iron (level below 50 ng/mL), was associated with restless legs syndrome (RLS) [64]. In a retrospective chart review study of children with autism spectrum disorder ($n = 9791$), significantly low serum ferritin levels were identified and associated with several sleep disorders, including periodic limb movements of sleep (27 ng/mL), sleep fragmentations (24 ng/mL), and poor sleep efficiency (7 ng/mL) [13].

Iron deficiency states were documented in the pathophysiology of RLS and the severity of iron deficiency states was correlated with the severity of RLS. Iron plays a major role in the dopamine production pathway; it acts as a cofactor for a rate limiting enzyme tyrosine hydroxylase in the dopamine production cycle. In patients with RLS, low cerebrospinal iron levels and low iron in the substantia nigra on magnetic resonance imaging were noted. Iron supplementation was found to be effective in the treatment of low ferritin with sleep disorders. The RLS foundation medical advisory board recommends iron therapy for low ferritin level below 50 ng/mL [64].

An open-label trial of oral iron supplement (6 mg elemental iron/kg/day) for 8 weeks in children with autism showed improvement in the sleep disturbance scale with an increase in serum ferritin level [65]. Potential side effects of oral iron include metallic taste, vomiting, nausea, constipation, diarrhea, and black/green stools [66].

11. Conclusions

In summary, sleep difficulties frequently co-occur in children with autism spectrum disorder and medications are often prescribed. However, limited evidence exists regarding the use and efficacy of medications for the treatment of sleep disorders in this population group. Melatonin has demonstrated good efficacy in open-label and placebo-controlled trials; however, long term effects still need to be thoroughly explored. Despite evidence and widespread use of medications to treat sleep disorders in this population group, no medications are FDA-approved for this indication. Identification and management of psychiatric comorbidities is important to achieve favorable outcomes. There is a need for more information and protocols needed to guide management for this population group.

Acknowledgments: S.R. and V.E. take responsibility for the integrity of the data and the accuracy of the data analysis.

Conflicts of Interest: The authors declare no conflict of interest.

References

1. *Diagnostic and Statistical Manual of Mental Disorders (DSM-V) 5*; American Psychiatric Association: Arlington, VA, USA, 2013.
2. American Psychiatric Association. *Diagnostic and Statistical Manual of Mental Disorders (DSM-IV-TR)*, 4th ed.; Text Revision; American Psychiatric Association Press: Washington, DC, USA, 2000.
3. Kanne, S.M.; Gerber, A.J.; Quirmbach, L.M.; Sparrow, S.S.; Cicchetti, D.V.; Saulnier, C.A. The role of adaptive behavior in autism spectrum disorders: Implications for functional outcome. *J. Autism Dev. Disord.* **2011**, *41*, 1007–1018. [CrossRef] [PubMed]
4. Ni Chuileann, S.; Quigley, J. Assessing recollection and familiarity in low functioning autism. *J. Autism Dev. Disord.* **2013**, *43*, 1406–1422. [CrossRef] [PubMed]
5. Sajith, S.G.; Clarke, D. Melatonin and sleep disorders associated with intellectual disability: A clinical review. *J. Intellect. Disabil. Res.* **2007**, *51*, 2–13. [CrossRef] [PubMed]
6. Baio, J.; Wiggins, L.; Christensen, D.L.; Maenner, M.J.; Daniels, J.; Warren, Z.; Kurzius-Spencer, M.; Zahorodny, W.; Robinson Rosenberg, C.; White, T.; et al. Prevalence of Autism Spectrum Disorder among Children Aged 8 Years—Autism and Developmental Disabilities Monitoring Network, 11 Sites, United States, 2014. *MMWR Surveill. Summ.* **2018**, *67*, 1–23. [CrossRef] [PubMed]
7. Richdale, A.L.; Schreck, K.A. Sleep problems in autism spectrum disorders: Prevalence, nature, & possible biopsychosocial aetiologies. *Sleep Med. Rev.* **2009**, *13*, 403–411. [CrossRef] [PubMed]
8. Adams, H.L.; Matson, J.L.; Cervantes, P.E.; Goldin, R.L. The relationship between autism symptom severity and sleep problems: Should bidirectionality be considered? *Res. Autism Spectr. Disord.* **2014**, *8*, 193–199. [CrossRef]
9. Tudor, M.E.; Hoffman, C.D.; Sweeney, D.P. Children with autism: Sleep problems and symptom severity. *Focus Autism Other Dev. Disabil.* **2012**, *27*, 254–262. [CrossRef]
10. Allik, H.; Larsson, J.O.; Smedje, H. Sleep patterns in school-age children with Asperger syndrome or high-functioning autism: A follow-up study. *J. Autism Dev. Disord.* **2008**, *38*, 1625–1633. [CrossRef] [PubMed]
11. Patzold, L.M.; Richdale, A.L.; Tonge, B.J. An investigation into sleep characteristics of children with autism and Asperger's Disorder. *J. Paediatr. Child Health* **1998**, *34*, 528–533. [CrossRef] [PubMed]
12. Richdale, A.L. Sleep problems in autism: Prevalence, cause, and intervention. *Dev. Med. Child Neurol.* **1999**, *41*, 60–66. [CrossRef] [PubMed]
13. Youssef, J.; Singh, K.; Huntington, N.; Becker, R.; Kothare, S.V. Relationship of serum ferritin levels to sleep fragmentation and periodic limb movements of sleep on polysomnography in autism spectrum disorders. *Pediatr. Neurol.* **2013**, *49*, 274–278. [CrossRef] [PubMed]

14. Limoges, E.; Mottron, L.; Bolduc, C.; Berthiaume, C.; Godbout, R. Atypical sleep architecture and the autism phenotype. *Brain* **2005**, *128*, 1049–1061. [CrossRef] [PubMed]

15. Cohen, S.; Conduit, R.; Lockley, S.W.; Rajaratnam, S.M.; Cornish, K.M. The relationship between sleep and behavior in autism spectrum disorder (ASD): A review. *J. Neurodev. Disord.* **2014**, *6*, 44. [CrossRef] [PubMed]

16. Owens, J.A.; Rosen, C.L.; Mindell, J.A. Medication use in the treatment of pediatric insomnia: Results of a survey of community-based pediatricians. *Pediatrics* **2003**, *111*, e628–e635. [CrossRef] [PubMed]

17. Gringras, P.; Gamble, C.; Jones, A.P.; Wiggs, L.; Williamson, P.R.; Sutcliffe, A.; Montgomery, P.; Whitehouse, W.P.; Choonara, I.; Allport, T.; et al. Melatonin for sleep problems in children with neurodevelopmental disorders: Randomised double masked placebo controlled trial. *BMJ* **2012**, *345*, e6664. [CrossRef] [PubMed]

18. Montgomery, P.; Stores, G.; Wiggs, L. The relative efficacy of two brief treatments for sleep problems in young learning disabled (mentally retarded) children: a randomised controlled trial. *Arch. Dis. Child.* **2004**, *89*, 125–130. [CrossRef] [PubMed]

19. Strategies to Improve Sleep in Children with Autism Spectrum Disorders. Available online: http://www.autismspeaks.org/science/resources-programs/autism-treatment-network/tools-you-can-use/sleep-tool-kit (accessed on 22 October 2018).

20. Mindell, J.A.; Kuhn, B.; Lewin, D.S.; Meltzer, L.J.; Sadeh, A. Behavioral treatment of bedtime problems and night wakings in infants and young children. *Sleep* **2006**, *29*, 1263–1276. [PubMed]

21. Pandi-Perumal, S.R.; Srinivasan, V.; Spence, D.W.; Cardinali, D.P. Role of the melatonin system in the control of sleep: Therapeutic implications. *CNS Drugs* **2007**, *21*, 995–1018. [CrossRef] [PubMed]

22. Owens, J.A.; Mindell, J.A. Pediatric insomnia. *Pediatr. Clin. North Am.* **2011**, *58*, 555–569. [CrossRef] [PubMed]

23. Goldman, S.E.; Adkins, K.W.; Calcutt, M.W.; Carter, M.D.; Goodpaster, R.L.; Wang, L.; Shi, Y.; Burgess, H.J.; Hachey, D.L.; Malow, B.A. Melatonin in children with autism spectrum disorders: Endogenous and pharmacokinetic profiles in relation to sleep. *J. Autism Dev. Disord.* **2014**, *44*, 2525–2535. [CrossRef] [PubMed]

24. Melatonin: In Depth. Available online: https://nccih.nih.gov/health/melatonin#hed1 (accessed on 22 October 2018).

25. Melatonin. Available online: https://www.aap.org/en-us/professional-resources/Psychopharmacology/Pages/Melatonin.aspx (accessed on 22 October 2018).

26. Melatonin and Children. Available online: https://www.sleephealthfoundation.org.au/public-information/fact-sheets-a-z/melatonin-and-children.html (accessed on 22 October 2018).

27. Andersen, I.M.; Kaczmarska, J.; McGrew, S.G.; Malow, B.A. Melatonin for insomnia in children with autism spectrum disorders. *J. Child Neurol.* **2008**, *23*, 482–485. [CrossRef] [PubMed]

28. Malow, B.; Adkins, K.W.; McGrew, S.G.; Wang, L.; Goldman, S.E.; Fawkes, D.; Burnette, C. Melatonin for sleep in children with autism: A controlled trial examining dose, tolerability, and outcomes. *J. Autism Dev. Disord.* **2012**, *42*, 1729–1737. [CrossRef] [PubMed]

29. Wirojanan, J.; Jacquemont, S.; Diaz, R.; Bacalman, S.; Anders, T.F.; Hagerman, R.J.; Goodlin-Jones, B.L. The efficacy of melatonin for sleep problems in children with autism, fragile X syndrome, or autism and fragile X syndrome. *J. Clin. Sleep Med.* **2009**, *5*, 145–150. [PubMed]

30. Wasdell, M.B.; Jan, J.E.; Bomben, M.M.; Freeman, R.D.; Rietveld, W.J.; Tai, J.; Hamilton, D.; Weiss, M.D. A randomized, placebo-controlled trial of controlled release melatonin treatment of delayed sleep phase syndrome and impaired sleep maintenance in children with neurodevelopmental disabilities. *J. Pineal Res.* **2008**, *44*, 57–64. [CrossRef] [PubMed]

31. Rossignol, D.A.; Frye, R.E. Melatonin in autism spectrum disorders: A systematic review and meta-analysis. *Dev. Med. Child Neurol.* **2011**, *53*, 783–792. [CrossRef] [PubMed]

32. Erland, L.A.; Saxena, P.K. Melatonin natural health products and supplements: Presence of serotonin and significant variability of melatonin content. *J. Clin. Sleep Med.* **2017**, *13*, 275–281. [CrossRef] [PubMed]

33. Garstang, J.; Wallis, M. Randomized controlled trial of melatonin for children with autistic spectrum disorders and sleep problems. *Child Care Health Dev.* **2006**, *32*, 585–589. [CrossRef] [PubMed]

34. Giannotti, F.; Cortesi, F.; Cerquiglini, A.; Bernabei, P. An open-label study of controlled-release melatonin in treatment of sleep disorders in children with autism. *J. Autism Dev. Disord.* **2006**, *36*, 741–752. [CrossRef] [PubMed]

35. Luboshitzky, R.; Lavi, S.; Thuma, I.; Lavie, P. Increased nocturnal melatonin secretion in male patients with hypogonadotropic hypogonadism and delayed puberty. *J. Clin. Endocrinol. Metab.* **1995**, *80*, 2144–2148. [CrossRef] [PubMed]

36. Stigler, K.A.; Posey, D.J.; McDougle, C.J. Ramelteon for insomnia in two youths with autistic disorder. *J. Child Adolesc. Psychopharmacol.* **2006**, *16*, 631–636. [CrossRef] [PubMed]

37. Krystal, A.D.; Goforth, H.W.; Roth, T. Effects of antipsychotic medications on sleep in schizophrenia. *Int. Clin. Psychopharmacol.* **2008**, *23*, 150–160. [CrossRef] [PubMed]

38. Meltzer, L.J.; Mindell, J.A.; Owens, J.A.; Byars, K.C. Use of sleep medications in hospitalized pediatric patients. *Pediatrics* **2007**, *119*, 1047–1055. [CrossRef] [PubMed]

39. Association, CP. First-Line Treatment for Insomnia 2015. Available online: https://www.cpa-apc. org/first-line-treatment-for-insomnia-should-not-include-routine-use-of-antipsychotics-say-canadian-psychiatrists/ (accessed on 22 October 2018).

40. Wichniak, A.; Wierzbicka, A.; Jernajczyk, W. Sleep and antidepressant treatment. *Curr. Pharm. Des.* **2012**, *18*, 5802–5817. [CrossRef] [PubMed]

41. Hellings, J.A.; Weckbaugh, M.; Nickel, E.J.; Cain, S.E.; Zarcone, J.R.; Reese, R.M.; Hall, S.; Ermer, D.J.; Tsai, L.Y.; Schroeder, S.R.; et al. A double-blind, placebo-controlled study of valproate for aggression in youth with pervasive developmental disorders. *J. Child Adolesc. Psychopharmacol.* **2005**, *15*, 682–692. [CrossRef] [PubMed]

42. Aurora, R.N.; Kristo, D.A.; Bista, S.R.; Rowley, J.A.; Zak, R.S.; Casey, K.R.; Lamm, C.I.; Tracy, S.L.; Rosenberg, R.S. The treatment of restless legs syndrome and periodic limb movement disorder in adults—An update for 2012: Practice parameters with an evidence-based systematic review and meta-analyses: An American Academy of Sleep Medicine Clinical Practice Guideline. *Sleep* **2012**, *35*, 1039–1062. [CrossRef] [PubMed]

43. Fiks, A.G.; Mayne, S.L.; Song, L.; Steffes, J.; Liu, W.; McCarn, B.; Margolis, B.; Grimes, A.; Gotlieb, E.; Localio, R.; et al. Changing patterns of alpha agonist medication use in children and adolescents 2009–2011. *J. Child Adolesc. Psychopharmacol.* **2015**, *25*, 362–367. [CrossRef] [PubMed]

44. Jamadarkhana, S.; Gopal, S. Clonidine in adults as a sedative agent in the intensive care unit. *J. Anaesthesiol. Clin. Pharmacol.* **2010**, *26*, 439–445. [PubMed]

45. Xue, M.; Brimacombe, M.; Chaaban, J.; Zimmerman-Bier, B.; Wagner, G.C. Autism spectrum disorders: Concurrent clinical disorders. *J. Child Neurol.* **2008**, *23*, 6–13. [CrossRef]

46. Ingrassia, A.; Turk, J. The use of clonidine for severe and intractable sleep problems in children with neurodevelopmental disorders—A case series. *Eur. Child Adolesc. Psychiatry* **2005**, *14*, 34–40. [CrossRef] [PubMed]

47. Pelayo, R.; Yuen, K. Pediatric sleep pharmacology. *Child Adolesc. Psychiatr. Clin. N. Am.* **2012**, *21*, 861–883. [CrossRef] [PubMed]

48. Wang, M.; Ramos, B.P.; Paspalas, C.D.; Shu, Y.; Simen, A.; Duque, A.; Vijayraghavan, S.; Brennan, A.; Dudley, A.; Nou, E.; et al. α2A-adrenoceptors strengthen working memory networks by inhibiting cAMP-HCN channel signaling in prefrontal cortex. *Cell* **2007**, *129*, 397–410. [CrossRef] [PubMed]

49. Hollway, J.A.; Aman, M.G. Pharmacological treatment of sleep disturbance in developmental disabilities: A review of the literature. *Res. Dev. Disabil.* **2011**, *32*, 939–962. [CrossRef] [PubMed]

50. Arnold, L.E. *Contemporary Diagnosis and Management of ADHD*, 3rd ed.; Handbooks in Health Care Co.: Newton, PA, USA, 2002; pp. 98–99.

51. Politte, L.C.; Scahill, L.; Figueroa, J.; McCracken, J.T.; King, B.; McDougle, C.J. A randomized, placebo-controlled trial of extended-release guanfacine in children with autism spectrum disorder and ADHD symptoms: An analysis of secondary outcome measures. *Neuropsychopharmacology* **2018**, *43*, 1772–1778. [CrossRef] [PubMed]

52. Rugino, T.A. Effect on Primary Sleep Disorders when children with ADHD are administered guanfacine extended release. *J. Atten. Disord.* **2018**, *22*, 14–24. [CrossRef] [PubMed]

53. Sokol, D.K.; Maloney, B.; Long, J.M.; Ray, B.; Lahiri, D.K. Autism, Alzheimer disease, and fragile X: APP, FMRP, and mGluR5 are molecular links. *Neurology* **2011**, *76*, 1344–1352. [CrossRef] [PubMed]

54. Perry, E.K.; Lee, M.L.; Martin-Ruiz, C.M.; Court, J.A.; Volsen, S.G.; Merrit, J.; Folly, E.; Iversen, P.E.; Bauman, M.L.; Perry, R.H.; et al. Cholinergic activity in autism: Abnormalities in the cerebral cortex and basal forebrain. *Am. J. Psychiatry* **2001**, *158*, 1058–1066. [CrossRef] [PubMed]

55. Schredl, M.; Weber, B.; Leins, M.L.; Heuser, I. Donepezil-induced REM sleep augmentation enhances memory performance in elderly, healthy persons. *Exp. Gerontol.* **2001**, *36*, 353–361. [CrossRef]

56. Moraes Wdos, S.; Poyares, D.R.; Guilleminault, C.; Ramos, L.R.; Bertolucci, P.H.; Tufik, S. The effect of donepezil on sleep and REM sleep EEG in patients with Alzheimer disease: A double-blind placebo-controlled study. *Sleep* **2006**, *29*, 199–205. [CrossRef] [PubMed]

57. Thirumalai, S.S.; Shubin, R.A.; Robinson, R. Rapid eye movement sleep behavior disorder in children with autism. *J. Child Neurol.* **2002**, *17*, 173–178. [CrossRef] [PubMed]

58. Ravassard, P.; Pachoud, B.; Comte, J.C.; Mejia-Perez, C.; Scote-Blachon, C.; Gay, N.; Claustrat, B.; Touret, M.; Luppi, P.H.; Salin, P.A. Paradoxical (REM) sleep deprivation causes a large and rapidly reversible decrease in long-term potentiation, synaptic transmission, glutamate receptor protein levels, and ERK/MAPK activation in the dorsal hippocampus. *Sleep* **2009**, *32*, 227–240. [CrossRef] [PubMed]

59. Buckley, A.W.; Sassower, K.; Rodriguez, A.J.; Jennison, K.; Wingert, K.; Buckley, J.; Thurm, A.; Sato, S.; Swedo, S. An open label trial of donepezil for enhancement of rapid eye movement sleep in young children with autism spectrum disorders. *J. Child Adolesc. Psychopharmacol.* **2011**, *21*, 353–357. [CrossRef] [PubMed]

60. Hernandez, R.K.; Farwell, W.; Cantor, M.D.; Lawler, E.V. Cholinesterase Inhibitors and Incidence of Bradycardia in Patients with Dementia in the Veterans Affairs New England Healthcare System. *J. Am. Geriatr. Soc.* **2009**, *57*, 1997–2003. [CrossRef] [PubMed]

61. Rossi, P.G.; Posar, A.; Parmeggiani, A.; Pipitone, E.; D'Agata, M. Niaprazine in the treatment of autistic disorder. *J. Child Neurol.* **1999**, *14*, 547–550. [CrossRef] [PubMed]

62. Griffin, C.E., 3rd; Kaye, A.M.; Bueno, F.R.; Kaye, A.D. Benzodiazepine pharmacology and central nervous system-mediated effects. *Ochsner J.* **2013**, *13*, 214–223. [PubMed]

63. Olsen, L.G. Hypnotic hazards: Adverse effects of zolpidem and other z-drugs. *Aust. Prescr.* **2008**, *31*, 146–149. [CrossRef]

64. Trotti, L.M.; Bhadriraju, S.; Becker, L.A. Iron for restless legs syndrome. *Cochrane Database Syst. Rev.* **2012**, Cd007834. [CrossRef] [PubMed]

65. Dosman, C.F.; Brian, J.A.; Drmic, I.E.; Senthilselvan, A.; Harford, M.M.; Smith, R.W.; Sharieff, W.; Zlotkin, S.H.; Moldofsky, H.; Roberts, S.W. Children with autism: Effect of iron supplementation on sleep and ferritin. *Pediatr. Neurol.* **2007**, *36*, 152–158. [CrossRef] [PubMed]

66. Cancelo-Hidalgo, M.J.; Castelo-Branco, C.; Palacios, S.; Haya-Palazuelos, J.; Ciria-Recasens, M.; Manasanch, J.; Perez-Edo, L. Tolerability of different oral iron supplements: A systematic review. *Curr. Med. Res. Opin.* **2013**, *29*, 291–303. [CrossRef] [PubMed]

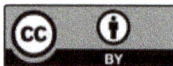

*medical
sciences*

MDPI

Review

Sleep and Delirium in Pediatric Critical Illness: What Is the Relationship?

Amy Calandriello [1], Joanna C. Tylka [1] and Pallavi P. Patwari [1,2,*]

[1] Pediatric Critical Care Medicine, Rush Children's Hospital, Rush University Medical Center, 1750 W. Harrison Street, Chicago, IL 606012, USA; Amy_E_Calandriello@rush.edu (A.C.); Joanna_C_Tylka@rush.edu (J.C.T.)

[2] Pediatric Sleep Medicine, Rush Children's Hospital, Rush University Medical Center, 1750 W. Harrison Street, Chicago, IL 606012, USA

* Correspondence: Pallavi_Patwari@rush.edu

Received: 7 August 2018; Accepted: 3 October 2018; Published: 10 October 2018

Abstract: With growing recognition of pediatric delirium in pediatric critical illness there has also been increased investigation into improving recognition and determining potential risk factors. Disturbed sleep has been assumed to be one of the key risk factors leading to delirium and is commonplace in the pediatric critical care setting as the nature of intensive care requires frequent and invasive monitoring and interventions. However, this relationship between sleep and delirium in pediatric critical illness has not been definitively established and may, instead, reflect significant overlap in risk factors and consequences of underlying neurologic dysfunction. We aim to review the existing tools for evaluation of sleep and delirium in the pediatric critical care setting and review findings from recent investigations with application of these measures in the pediatric intensive care unit.

Keywords: Acute illness; children; circadian disturbance; mechanical ventilation; melatonin; non-pharmacologic management; pediatric intensive care unit; screening; sedation

1. Introduction

Both disturbed sleep and delirium are notoriously difficult to recognize in the pediatric population and recognition becomes more challenging in the pediatric intensive care unit (PICU) when the underlying disease process and the administered medications contribute to alterations in level of consciousness. Further, during the acute phase of illness, primary goals for maintaining patient stability and safety focus on level of sedation rather than promoting sleep. There have been recent improvements in recognizing delirium in the hospitalized pediatric patient, particularly with validated screening tools, and increased attention to promoting sleep in the PICU setting. However, delirium screening and sleep promotion by pediatric intensivists are not widely applied internationally [1]. Despite advances to promote natural/physiologic sleep to prevent or treat delirium, the cause-effect relationship of sleep and delirium has yet to be clearly established. It may be that both dysregulated sleep and delirium are "sister" disorders that indicate underlying neurologic dysfunction.

2. Defining Delirium

The key feature of delirium is an alteration in both cognition and arousal that can have hypoactive or hyperactive subtypes. The American Psychiatric Association's Diagnostic and Statistical Manual of Mental Disorders, Fifth Edition (DSM-5) defines delirium as a noticeable change in the patient's neurocognitive baseline with an acute disturbance in attention, awareness, and cognition, and is thought to be a direct result of another medical condition rather than due to an established/evolving neurocognitive disorder [2] Additionally, clinical presentations of delirium can vary among pediatric patients and present in three different subtypes: Hyperactive, hypoactive, and mixed. Hyperactive delirium is characterized as agitation and aggression [3]. Hypoactive delirium is identified as a decrease in mental status and lethargy [3]. Mixed delirium, commonly referred to as emerging delirium, will manifest with both clinical signs of hyperactive and hypoactive delirium [3]. Pediatric patients in the critical care setting are predisposed to metabolic and environmental risk factors for delirium such as infection, withdrawal, disturbed sleep, immobility, noise disturbances, and sensory overload [4]. Delirium is a severe complication of pediatric critical illness associated with negative patient outcomes such as mortality, morbidity, and increased medical costs up to fourfold as a result of increased length of hospitalization [4,5].

3. Introduction of Validated Pediatric Delirium Screening Tools

Early detection of delirium can decrease long-term consequences related to neurocognitive impairment, inattentiveness, post-traumatic stress disorder, and spatial or verbal memory disturbances [3]. This has led to a recognition of the importance of screening for, diagnosing, and treating delirium including the creation of guidelines. The American College of Critical Care Medicine published guidelines for adult patients recommend routine monitoring of delirium in intensive care unit (ICU) patients [6]. Additionally, The European Society of Paediatric and Neonatal Intensive Care (ESPNIC) recommends that delirium be assessed and documented every 8–12 h [7]. However, as of the time of this publication, there are no guidelines for diagnosing delirium in pediatric intensive care units in the Unites States.

There are many challenges to detecting and diagnosing delirium in the PICU. First, diagnosis requires knowledge and a high index of suspicion by providers [8]. Second, the fluctuating nature of delirium can make it very difficult for providers that only spend short periods of time with the patient. Next, it can be difficult to differentiate between delirium, iatrogenic withdrawal syndrome, pain, and under-sedation as many of the symptoms overlap. Finally, the vast differences in neurocognitive development in infants and children make detecting delirium in young and developmentally delayed patients particularly challenging [9]. Recognition of delirium can be increased through use of a screening tool. An ideal screening tool for delirium would detect all three subtypes of delirium in patients of all ages and all developmental levels; accounting for the wide range of developmental milestones that occur and the severity of illness. Additionally, it would need to be quick, reliable, sensitive and specific. Multiple screening tools have been developed and validated to assist in identifying delirium in the pediatric intensive care population each with advantages and drawbacks as seen in Table 1.

4. Delirium Screening Tools

The Delirium Rating Scale (DRS) is one of the first screening tools for delirium to be developed [10]. It was designed to be used by psychiatrists and is labor intensive. However, in addition to detecting delirium, it can be used to determine delirium severity and follow severity over time. Though designed for adult patients, a retrospective study in PICU patients found the scale to be applicable [11]. The first tool specifically designed for the pediatric population, the Pediatric Anesthesia Emergence Delirium (PAED) scale was designed to detect emergence delirium following anesthesia [12]. While not developed for the PICU population, it has been applied in this population with notably poor sensitivity [13]. This is likely due to the fact that the questions focus on symptoms of the hyperactive subtype and thus may under detect the mixed and hypoactive subtypes. The Cornell Assessment of Pediatric Delirium (CAP-D) was developed from the PAED [14]. It is the tool recommended by the ESPNIC as it is simple, quick, and requires minimal training prior to implementation [7]. Another advantage of the CAP-D tool is that it has identified subtle clinical signs of hypoactive delirium which has been associated with worse clinical outcomes in pediatric critical care [15]. However, while sensitivity was retained in the developmentally delayed population the specificity decreased significantly.

Table 1. Advantages and Limitations of Pediatric Delirium Screening Tools.

Tool	How It Works	Validation Study *	Population	Sensitivity **	Specificity **	Interrater Reliability (κ)***	Observation Time for Score	Sleep Assessment	Pros	Cons
Cornell Assessment of Pediatric Delirium (CAP-D) [14]	8 questions rated on a scale of 0–4 based on interactions with patient over shift	111 patients Prospective	0–21 years + Intubated patients + Develop-mentally delayed RASS score –3 or greater	94%	79%	0.94	Once per shift	1 question assesses restlessness	Takes less than 2 minutes to complete	Decreased specificity in develop-mentally delayed children
Pediatric Confusion Assessment Method (pCAM-ICU) [16]	4 step screen with 2 steps requiring patient interaction squeezing hand, nodding or answering yes/no	68 patients Prospective	5 years and older + Intubated patients RASS score –3 or greater	83%	99%	0.96	None specified	None	Screen identifies if patients have required (DSM) delirium features	Must have cognitive development of 5 years of greater May require tools (cards/pictures)
Severity scale for the Pediatric Confusion Assessment Method for the ICU (sspCAM-ICU) [13]	Adds a point system to the pCAM-ICU	64 patients Prospective	5 years and older + Intubated patients	85%	98%	Not assessed	None specified	None	Performed better than pCAM-ICU in direct testing	Complex scoring system
Preschool Confusion Assessment Method for the ICU (psCAM-ICU) [17]	4 step screen with 1 step requiring patient to look at picture/cards	300 patients Prospective	6 months–5 years + Intubated patients	91%	75%	0.79	None specified	1 step assesses sleep-wake cycle	Screen identifies if patients have required DSM delirium features	Requires tools (cards/pictures) Not able to be used on develop-mentally delayed children of children with visual/audi-tory impairments

Table 1. Cont.

Tool	How It Works	Validation Study *	Population	Sensitivity **	Specificity **	Interrater Reliability (κ) ***	Observation Time for Score	Sleep Assessment	Pros	Cons
Delirium Rating Scale (DRS) [11]	10 items scored on a scale from 0 to 4	84 patients Retrospective #	6 months–19 years	N/A	N/A	N/A	24 h	1 of the 10 items assess sleep-wake cycle	Scale has been validated in adults [10]	Unable to assess sensitivity, specificity or interrater reliability due to retrospective design
Sophia Observation withdrawal Symptoms-Paediatric Delirium scale (SOS-PD) [18]	22 item yes or no check list based on at least 4 h with patient	146 patients	3 months to 16 years +Intubated patients COMFORT scale ≥ 11	97%	92%	0.9	Once per shift (minimum of 4 h with patient)	1 question assesses the length of sleep	Also detects withdrawal	Only patients with positive SOS-PD screens were seen by psychiatrist (may miss patients)
Pediatric Anesthesia Emergence Delirium (PAED) scale [12]	5 items rated on a scale of 1–4	64 patients [13] Prospective	5 years and older +Intubated patients	69%	98%	0.8	None specified for pediatric intensive care unit (PICU) setting	1 question assesses restlessness	Simplest screening tool with just 5 questions	Designed for post-anesthesia emergence delirium

* All validation studies were single center studies in PICUs; ** Compared with diagnosis of delirium by a psychiatrist using Diagnostic and Statistical Manual of Mental Disorders (DSM; version DSM-III-R or DSM-IV depending on time); *** Cohen's κ coefficient; # Retrospective study of patients diagnosed with delirium; PICU: pediatric intensive care unit.

The Pediatric Confusion Assessment Method (pCAM-ICU) was adapted from the most widely used adult delirium screen for children 5 years and older [16]. It can be completed by any provider as it does not require a prolonged interaction time with the patient, making it ideal for screening patients frequently or when suspicions arise. However, it requires patients to have the cognitive development of a 5-year-old and be cooperate with the screening, which limits utility. The pCAM-ICU also requires more extensive training of the provider than other screening tools. The Severity Scale for the Pediatric Confusion Assessment Method for the ICU (sspCAM-ICU) took the pCAM-ICU and added a scoring system [13]. This increases the sensitivity of the original screen, but also makes it more difficult to implement. Finally, The Preschool Confusion Assessment Method for the ICU (psCAM-ICU) is an adaptation of the pCAM-ICU for patients six months to five years of age [17]. It has many of the same advantages and disadvantages of the pCAM-ICU, however it does allow for assessment of some patients with developmental delays.

Recognizing that withdrawal symptoms overlap with delirium, Ista et al. developed the Sophia Observation withdrawal Symptoms-Paediatric Delirium scale (SOS-PD) [18]. The SOS-PD is designed to be completed by the bedside nurse after a minimum of 4 h of interaction with the patient and is quick to complete and easy to implement. However, its greatest advantage is its ability to detect both delirium and withdrawal due to overlap of in symptoms such as anxiety, agitation, irritability, and disturbed sleep.

At this time no screening tool has emerged as superior. Validation studies have all been single center, small to medium sized with differences in designs that make it difficult to compare the screening tools. More research is warranted on screening tools. In particular, research that compares these tools across multiple centers and accounts for baseline developmental stage, withdrawal symptoms, and sleep disturbances [9]. Further, the existing pediatric delirium tools have limited evaluation of sleep disturbance and include a single perspective such as sleep-wake cycle [11,17], sleep duration [18], or restlessness [12,14].

5. Delirium in Pediatric Intensive Care Unit Patients

Within the last few years, there has been a robust increase in publications focused on pediatric delirium, as seen in Table 2. Studies included in this review were found through searching the electronic databases, PubMed and Scopus, using the key words: pediatric, delirium, and critical care. Criteria for inclusion was primary research focused on delirium with a primary cohort in the PICU or pediatric cardiac intensive care unit (CICU). Finally, further articles were found based on references from the primary searches. These studies have yielded a large amount of information on associations of patient characteristics, treatment modalities, and outcomes with delirium in the critically ill pediatric population.

Many studies have assessed associations between patient characteristics such as age, gender, severity of illness, reason for admission, and developmental delay in order to identify risk factors for development of delirium with varying results. Nine studies looked for associations between delirium and age with eight studies finding an association [5,15,19–25]. However, two found that delirium was associated with older age (>12 years) [19,20], while the other six found that delirium was associated with associated with younger age (<2, <5, or 2–5 years) [5,15,21–24]. Interestingly, the two studies that found associations with older age used exams by a psychiatrist to diagnose delirium while the other studies used screening tools (CAP-D or psCAM-ICU). These differences in the methods of diagnosing delirium may contribute to the inconsistent results and underscores the need for a consistent tool to screen and diagnose delirium in the PICU.

Gender has been investigated in multiple studies; four studies found no association [5,20–22], with one study noting an association between the male gender and delirium [25]. Results have also been inconsistent with respect to severity of illness and delirium; three studies noted an association [23,24,26], but two found no association [25,27]. Pertaining to reason for admission, two studies found no association between reason for admission and delirium [5,20], while a study focusing on post-operative patients found a much higher incidence of delirium (66%) indicating that the post-operative status may be a risk factor for developing delirium [22]. Finally, developmental delay has been associated with delirium. Both Traube et al. [24] and Silver et al. [21] found on multivariate analysis that those with developmental delay had over 3 times the odds of developing delirium as those with normal development (odds ratio (OR) 3.31 and 3.45 respectively).

Many treatment modalities also have been found to have associations with delirium including extracorporeal membrane oxygenation (ECMO), red blood cell (RBC) transfusions, anticholinergic medications, antiepileptic medications, benzodiazepine administration, and mechanical ventilation. Other treatment modalities have either been found to not have an association or have an unclear association with delirium including opioid medications, vasopressor medications, cyanotic heart disease, and cardiopulmonary bypass time. A study by Patel et al. [28] of pediatric patients requiring ECMO found that all eight patients developed delirium during their course. While this study is small, the 100% incidence must certainly add ECMO to the list of risk factors for delirium. Another treatment that has been associated with risk for delirium is RBC transfusions. Nellis et al. [29] found that children who received RBC transfusions had more than twice the incidence of delirium as children who were never transfused. Medications that have been associated with delirium in the PICU setting on multivariate analysis include anticholinergics [24], antiepileptics [5], and benzodiazepines.

Benzodiazepines are routinely used in pediatric critical illness with the intention to alleviate anxiety and ensure safety with invasive interventions. Recent studies have found higher frequency of delirium with benzodiazepine exposure in this population [5,23,24,30]. Traube et al. used the CAP-D tool and found that delirium was significantly more likely with benzodiazepine exposure from both a point prevalence study and a prospective longitudinal study [5,24]. Using the CAP-D tool, Mody et al. also found benzodiazepine exposure (but not opiates) to be an independent risk factor for development of delirium with more than a fourfold increase in transitioning from a normal mental status to a delirious state [30]. This association has been more closely evaluated in a narrower pediatric age group (0.5–5 years old) using the psCAM-ICU with findings of a non-linear increase in delirium frequency the day after benzodiazepine exposure and greater duration of delirium [23].

Respiratory failure requiring intubation and mechanical ventilator support is another risk factor for delirium independent of benzodiazepine exposure [5,15,20,21,24,25,30]. Traube et al. found that of 29% of 642 patients that ever required mechanical ventilation developed delirium as compared to 9% of 905 patients with delirium who never received mechanical ventilation [24]. Interestingly, in a pediatric CICU, the authors found no statistically significant differences in frequency of delirium based on type of respiratory support even comparing those who were ever mechanically ventilated (64% with delirium) to never mechanically ventilated (42% with delirium) during the admission, but found a statistically significant association between delirium and length of mechanical ventilator support [15]. This cohort of 99 patients in a pediatric CICU had a high incidence of delirium (57%) compared to general PICU cohorts and with a subgroup analysis found delirium to be more likely in children with cyanotic heart disease (26 of 36 patients with delirium) as compared to non-hypoxic cardiac defects (26 of 52 patients) [15].

Opioid medications on the other hand have mostly been found to not be a risk factor for delirium, which is based on multivariate analysis from three different studies [23,24,30]. Traube et al. [5], however, did find that patients with opioid exposure had twice the odds of delirium as those children without opioid exposure. Vasopressor medications have been found to be both associated with [5] and not associated with delirium [24]. While apparently contradictory results, it may be that vasopressor medications are used as a marker for disease severity rather than independently being a risk factor. Finally, both cardiopulmonary bypass time [15] and cyanotic heart disease [23] have been found not to be risk factors for delirium in single studies, contradicting the findings of Alverez et al. [15].

Table 2. Delirium in Pediatric Intensive Care Unit Patients.

Authors (year)	Study Design	Age (yrs)	Number of Patients	Delirium Frequency	Measurement/Tool Used	Risk Factors Associated with Delirium *	Risk Factors NOT Associated with Delirium *	Outcomes
Schieveld et al. (2007) [19] and Schieveld et al. (2008) [26] **	Single center, Prospective, descriptive study	0–18	877; 61 with possible delirium	5% of total population; 66% of suspected population (n = 40)	Exam by a pediatric neuropsychiatrist using Diagnostic and Statistical Manual of Mental Disorders, Fourth Edition, (DSM-IV) criteria	Older Age (>12 years); Severity of illness (Pediatric Index of Mortality and Pediatric Risk of Mortality scores)	N/A	All patients fully recovered from delirium
Smeets et al. (2010) [20]	Single center, Prospective, descriptive study	1–18	49 diagnosed with delirium; 98 randomly selected patients without delirium	N/A	Exam by a neuropsychiatrist using DSM-IV criteria.	Older Age; Mechanical Ventilation	Gender; Reason for admission	Delirium was associated with increased length of hospitalization and medical costs.
Silver et al. (2015) [21]	Single center, Prospective observational study	0–21	99	21%	Cornell Assessment of Pediatric Delirium (CAP-D) twice daily	Developmental delay; Mechanical ventilation; Preschool age (2–5 years)	Severity of illness (Pediatric Index of Mortality 2); Gender	N/A
Traube et al. (2016) [31]	Single center, Prospective observational study	0–21	464	16% (n = 74)	CAP-D twice daily	N/A	N/A	After controlling confounding factors, delirium was associated with an 85% increase in PICU costs
Meyburg et al. (2017) [22]	Single center, prospective, observational study	0–17	93 post elective surgical patients	66% (n = 61)	CAP-D twice daily	Postoperative state; Younger age	Gender	Delirium was found to be a predictor of increased hospital length of stay.

Table 2. *Cont.*

Authors (year)	Study Design	Age (yrs)	Number of Patients	Delirium Frequency	Measurement/Tool Used	Risk Factors Associated with Delirium *	Risk Factors NOT Associated with Delirium *	Outcomes
Patel et al. (2017) [28]	Single center, Prospective observational longitudinal cohort study	0.6–16	8 patients requiring ECMO	100% (n = 8)	CAP-D daily	Extracorporeal membrane oxygenation (ECMO)	N/A	Only 13% of days on ECMO were delirium and coma free Delirium screening was successfully completed on 97% of ECMO days
Simone et al. (2017) [25]	Single center, Prospective observational study	0–21	1875	17% (n = 140)	CAP-D	Male Gender Mechanical Ventilation	Severity of illness (Pediatric Index of Mortality 2) Age	PICU length of stay, hospital length of stay, and duration of mechanical ventilation were significantly longer in patients with delirium than without
Smith et al. (2017) [23]	Single center, Prospective observational study	0.5–5	300	41% (n = 124)	psCAM-ICU	Benzodiazepine exposure Younger age (<2 years) Severity of illness (Pediatric Risk of Mortality Score at admission)	Cyanotic Heart disease Opioid exposure Mechanical Ventilation Lowest Oxygen saturation	Delirium increased length of hospitalization in pre-school aged patients.
Traube et al. (2017) [24]	Single center, Prospective, longitudinal cohort study	0–21	1547	17% (n = 267)	CAP-D twice daily	Younger age (<2 years) Developmental delay (Pediatric Cerebral Performance Category 4) Severity of illness (Pediatric Index of Mortality-3 score) Mechanical ventilation Benzodiazepine exposure Anticholinergic exposure	Opioid exposure Corticosteroid exposure Vasopressor medication exposure	PICU length of stay was increased in children with delirium Delirium was a strong and independent predictor of mortality

Table 2. *Cont.*

Authors (year)	Study Design	Age (yrs)	Number of Patients	Delirium Frequency	Measurement/Tool Used	Risk Factors Associated with Delirium *	Risk Factors NOT Associated with Delirium *	Outcomes
Traube et al. (2017) [5]	Multi institutional, international point-prevalence study	0–21	835 (developmentally delayed children excluded)	25%	CAP-D	Younger age (<2 years) Mechanical ventilation Benzodiazepine exposure Opioid exposure Antiepileptic exposure Vasopressor medication exposure	Reason for admission Gender Ethnicity	Delirium was associated with a prolonged length of stay (>5 days)
Alvarez et al. (2018) [15]	Single center, Prospective observational cohort study	0–21	99 total patients screened after admission to cardiac intensive care unit (CICU) >12 h	57% (n = 56)	CAP-D twice daily	Younger age Mechanical ventilation Benzodiazepine exposure	Cardiopulmonary bypass time	Delirium is associated with increased length of mechanical ventilation and increased length of hospital stay.
Barnes et al. (2018) [32]	Single center, Retrospective chart review	2–20	50 patients who received child psychiatry consult	32% (n = 16)	Exam by a pediatric psychiatrist using DSM-IV criteria	N/A	N/A	81% (n = 13) of the patients with delirium were prescribed an antipsychotic.
Meyburg et al. (2018) [33]	Single center point prevalence study	1–16	47 patients diagnosed with delirium	N/A	CAP-D twice daily	N/A	N/A	No association between pediatric delirium and long-term cognition or behavior.
Mody et al. (2018) [30]	Single center, Retrospective observational study	0–18	580	23% (n = 131)	CAP-D daily	Benzodiazepine exposure Mechanical ventilation	Opioid exposure	The strongest predictor of delirium was being delirious on the day prior
Nellis et al. (2018) [29]	Single center, Nested retrospective cohort study within prospective cohort study	0–21	1547 total 166 patients who received RBC transfusion	17% (n = 267)	CAP-D twice daily	Transfusion of RBCs	Anemia (nadir hemoglobin) Age of blood transfused	N/A

* Associations based on multivariate analysis if completed; ** Both studies were completed on the same group of patients.

Delirium in the PICU population has been associated with several negative outcomes. A large number of studies have found an association with delirium and increased length of stay [5,15,20,22–25]. Additionally, delirium has been associated with increased duration of mechanical ventilation in two studies [15,25]. Smeets et al. [20] found an increase in direct medical costs of 1.5% due to pediatric delirium. Similarly, Traube et al. [31] noted that the median total PICU costs were significantly higher in patients with delirium than in patients who were never delirious. Further, after controlling for confounding factors (age, gender, severity of illness, and PICU length of stay), delirium was associated with an 85% increase in PICU costs. Finally, Traube et al. [24] found a significant increase in in-hospital mortality for children with delirium (5.24% vs. 0.94%). This persisted even after controlling for probability of mortality at admission (using the Pediatric Index of Mortality-3 score); the odds of mortality for those ever delirious was 4 times that of the never delirious group (OR = 4.39).

Less is known about the longer-term outcomes of the pediatric critical care population however a few studies have been published with encouraging results. Schieveld et al. [19] noted that delirium resolved in all study patients and that 38 of the 40 patients (95%) were successfully treated with antipsychotic medications. Similarly, Barnes et al. [32] found that 81% of patients diagnosed with delirium were prescribed antipsychotic medications, with only 23% (3 of 13) being discharged on these medications. Meyburg et al. [33] found no association between delirium in the PICU and long-term cognition or behavior based on follow-up questionnaires and exams preformed 12 to 24 months after the delirium event.

6. Sleep in Pediatric Intensive Care Patients

Patients in the intensive care unit are at increased risk for significant disturbance in sleep quality and quantity and for alteration of the sleep-wake pattern, which is generally accepted as unavoidable. Exogenous influences upon sleep in the PICU include environmental factors (light, noise, intrusive monitoring and intervention) and medications. Endogenous influences can be attributed to the underlying disease process such as hypoxia, respiratory failure, sepsis/inflammation, central nervous system injury including traumatic brain injury, and pain. Short-term sleep deprivation is known to affect behavior and chronic long-term sleep disturbances affect neurocognitive development in children—both important factors to consider for improving short and long term outcomes during recovery from critical illness. For this review, "sleep disturbance" is a non-specific term that refers to changes from baseline of total sleep time, sleep architecture, and circadian rhythm. In other words, sleep disturbance includes inadequate total sleep time, sleep fragmentation (frequent arousals), variance in the quantity and distribution of sleep stages (particularly slow wave sleep and rapid eye movement (REM) sleep), and circadian rhythm disturbance (or circadian misalignment). Underlying or pre-existing primary sleep disorders such as obstructive sleep apnea or hypoventilation (sleep related breathing disorders), narcolepsy (hypersomnolence disorders), and sleep related movement disorders are not included in the scope of this review.

The most challenging issue is defining and measuring sleep disturbance in critical illness, which is complicated by variable neurocognitive baseline, distinguishing sedated state from normal sleep stages, constant physiologic changes over a 24 h period, and determining the correct timing for evaluation. Polysomnography (PSG), the gold-standard for measuring sleep, is not a reasonable tool for prolonged monitoring; Alternative, objective measures of sleep are limited in accuracy and usefulness in the PICU. For example, actigraphy is not reliable in patients who are heavily sedated or paralyzed, serial melatonin levels would be impractical and difficult to interpret, limited montage electroencephalogram (EEG) is also cumbersome and time-intensive, and bispectral index monitoring cannot distinguish normal sleep from sedated state.

The number of studies that have evaluated sleep in pediatric critical illness have variable methodology, variable aims, and with only a few studies that utilized limited montage EEG assessment of sleep [34], which limits broad application of findings. Further, bedside evaluation of sleep is not reliable. Armour et al. closely compared observer assessment and PSG data in 40 pediatric burn patients and found that patient sleep is often falsely over-estimated with 56.3% false-positive rate and 96.5% true-positive rate [35]. In day-to-day practice, evaluation of sleep in the PICU setting is based on bedside nursing assessment since the gold-standard for objective evaluation of sleep with polysomnography (PSG) is cumbersome, expensive, and of limited utility with non-24 hour recording.

Two studies in the pediatric critical care setting found fragmented sleep and absence of diurnal variation [36,37]. Carno evaluated sleep via PSG recording in 2 mechanically ventilated children under neuromuscular blockade and found that sleep was fragmented, demonstrated variance in sleep stage distribution as compared to published normal values, and that a large proportion of sleep occurred during the day. Further, sleep was variable from day-to-night and from day-to-day indicating significant circadian disruption. Marseglia et al. [38] also found altered circadian rhythm in mechanically ventilated children based on repeated measures of serum melatonin.

Only one study directly evaluated sleep with polysomnogram and medication intervention. The authors evaluated sleep and hormone response to zolpidem or haloperidol in pediatric burn victims and found that both medications improve sleep continuity; zolpidem increased stage N3 (slow wave) sleep and REM sleep and haloperidol increased total sleep time and stage N2 sleep [39].

7. Sleep and Delirium Relationship in the Intensive Care Unit

A direct relationship of sleep disturbance and delirium has not been evaluated in pediatric critical illness. What we can glean from studies in adult patients is that the evidence that sleep disturbance leads to delirium is not clearly established. With the specific aim of determining if improving sleep is associated with reduction in delirium, Flannery et al. [40] performed a systematic review and found 6 of 10 studies reported statistically significant reduction in adult ICU delirium with sleep promotion, but only 3 of these 6 studies included a sleep assessment. Of the 10 studies, sleep assessment was included in only 4 studies which were based on patient report, which would not be feasible in a patient with delirium who would be dependent on bedside observations of sleep [40]. Patel et al. [41] were the only authors who found a decrease in delirium along with improvement in sleep measures in adult patients in the ICU setting; the intervention group was given non-pharmacologic treatment with reduction in light, noise, and disturbance during the night and found clinically and statistically significant reduction in delirium incidence from 33% (55 of 167 patients) prior to intervention to 14% (24 of 171 patients) after intervention. A recent Cochrane review regarding sleep promotion in adult ICU settings looked specifically at non-pharmacologic interventions and found low quality evidence for an effect on objective and subjective sleep measures (including patient satisfaction), delirium risk, length of ICU stay, and adverse events; Though, meta-analysis from two studies demonstrated a lower incidence of delirium and improved total sleep time based on nurse observation with use of earplugs and eye masks [42].

Both sleep disturbance and delirium have similar risks and management in the ICU setting, as seen in Figure 1. Risks includes hypoxia, mechanical ventilation, infection/inflammation, central nervous system (CNS) injury, pain, exposure to sedative medications, and withdrawal. Regarding sleep disturbance, frequent interventions, intubation with mechanical ventilation, and pain can contribute to inadequate sleep time, sleep fragmentation, and disrupt the normal progression of sleep states. Sedative medications will affect the quantity and distribution of sleep stages such that slow wave sleep and REM sleep are significantly reduced (opioids are known to reduce slow wave sleep; benzodiazepines are known to suppress REM sleep). Further, systemic infection and inflammation such as sepsis can lead to circadian rhythm disturbance. Mentioned previously, risk factors for delirium have significant overlap to these risk factors for sleep disturbance. Further, due to the complex nature of critical illness, dissecting out the specific cause of acute change in neurocognition and awareness is extremely difficult.

Both delirium and sleep involve a change in mental state—one is pathologic and the latter is physiologic. Evaluation of changes in mental state are challenging in critically ill children. Extrapolating from adult studies and applying to pediatric patients has limitations that include increase use of sedation (younger children cannot safely tolerate intubation or other invasive intervention without significant anxiety and high risk for self-harm), inability for accurate self-report of sleep quantity and quality, and significant changes in sleep characteristics in the first decade of life (duration, pattern, sleep stage distribution). Even with these limitations, non-pharmacologic strategies to improve sleep are reasonable based on low risk and possible benefit. While not easily measured in the PICU, the underlying justification for sleep promotion is that sleep is inherently restorative (particularly slow wave and REM sleep), improving "sleep" can potentially reduce the amount of sedative required, and can improve pain tolerance [43].

Relationship of Sleep Disturbance and Delirium in Pediatric Critical Illness

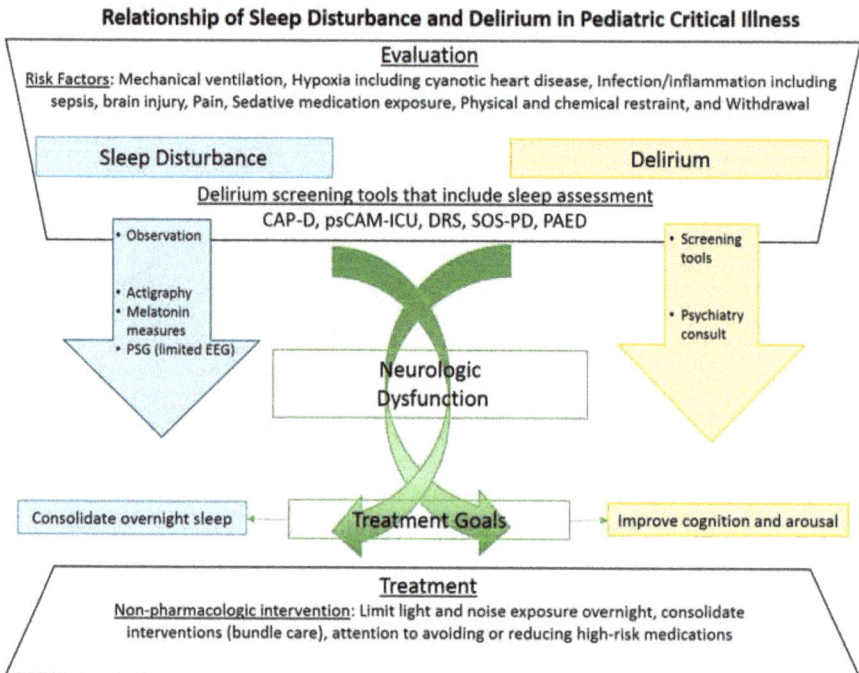

Figure 1. The first step in evaluating sleep disturbance and delirium are recognizing the similar risk factors. Next, identification of sleep disturbance and delirium are distinct except for a few delirium screening tools. Distinct measurements for sleep disturbance and delirium are noted by the large arrows with associated treatment goals noted by the corresponding color boxes. Finally, noted at the bottom, non-pharmacologic intervention for both sleep disturbance and delirium are the same. Abbreviations: polysomnogram (PSG) with limited electroencephalogram (EEG).

8. Treatment

Strategies to prevent both sleep disruption and delirium should be the first step in management. This includes non-pharmacologic interventions to reduce noise and light exposure overnight and bundled nursing interventions to limit sleep fragmentation. Other strategies would include attention to medications that affect sleep (through changes in sleep stage distribution or circadian rhythm) and pose higher risk for development of delirium; this includes benzodiazepines, opioids, steroids, beta-blockers, dopamine, and norepinephrine. Lastly, routinely used medications for sleep promotion in pediatric patients is limited to melatonin, while pharmacologic agents for delirium include antipsychotic agents.

There have been many studies in the adult ICU population on non-pharmacologic strategies for the prevention of delirium. Prominent among them is a multicomponent program known as the Hospital Elder Life Program (HELP) which has shown great success in reducing delirium in the elderly population [44]. This program prioritizes regular cognitive orientation, therapeutic activities, sleep enhancement, early mobilization, vision and hearing adaptations, fluid repletion, and feeding assistance. A recent meta-analysis of this program found that 14 studies demonstrated significant reductions in delirium incidence (OR 0.47) [44]. Unfortunately, while these strategies hold great promise, they have yet to be shown to be effective outside of the elderly population. The adult guidelines recommend early mobilization of patients as a delirium prevention strategy, but make no further recommendations on either pharmacological or non-pharmacological methods [6]. In the PICU population, Simone et al. [25] implemented a multidisciplinary bundle that included establishing daily routines, encouraging parental involvement, orientation, creating a familiar environment, reducing restraint use, and creating an uninterrupted sleep environment between 11 p.m. and 4 a.m. This bundle's implementation was associated with a reduction in delirium from 19.3% to 11.8% [25]; encouraging results that underscore the need for further studies.

The primary role of intrinsic melatonin is to regulate the circadian rhythm (sleep-wake timing), but other potential effects including, but not limited to, neuroprotective and anti-inflammatory roles are particularly relevant to critical illness. Investigation of exogenous melatonin use in pediatric critical illness has not been completed, but non-standardized administration of melatonin is common during the recovery period in PICU to facilitate sleep onset. A recent Cochrane review evaluated the effect of melatonin on sleep in adult ICU patients and included 4 studies that met sufficient criteria for inclusion. Of these, the authors found no significant effect on subjective and objective report of sleep quality and quantity, no significant difference in anxiety, mortality, or length of stay.

Pharmacologic agents used to treat pediatric delirium include typical and atypical antipsychotics. Haloperidol has been used successfully in the PICU on agitated and delirious patients [45], however, given its side effect profile it has been largely superseded by other options with lower risks. Atypical antipsychotics that have been used in the treatment of pediatric delirium include olanzapine, risperidone, and quetiapine. Turkel at al. [46] found a comparable response between these three medications in a retrospective review of 110 patients with delirium. Additionally, mean DRS (revised-98) scores were significantly decreased with treatment [46]. Further, quetiapine was found to be safe for short term use in this population in a retrospective review of 50 patients [47]. A final area that should be considered when treating PICU patients with delirium is choice of sedation medications. Benzodiazepines in particular should be reduced or discontinued. Dexmedetomidine is recommended over benzodiazepines for sedation infusions in the adult guidelines based on results of two randomized controlled trials [6]. While studies in the pediatric population are lacking, this approach may be helpful in treating pediatric delirium.

9. Conclusions

Both delirium and sleep disturbance are problems in the PICU population that have been increasingly recognized in recent years. Delirium has been associated with a number of adverse outcomes including increased length of stay [5,15,20,22–25], increased duration of mechanical ventilation [15,25], increased medical costs [20,31] and increased in-hospital mortality [24]. Non-pharmacologic interventions for promoting sleep and reducing delirium in the PICU setting has low risk, low cost, and potential benefit and should be the initial focus for all children at risk for delirium. Overall, there is no evidence of a direct cause-effect relationship between sleep disturbances and delirium in children, and it may be that improvement in sleep occurs in parallel with reduction in delirium. Therefore, attention to both improving sleep and preventing delirium are equally important in pediatric critical illness.

Regarding management strategies, we recommend the following actions to prevent, diagnose and treat delirium in the PICU. The first step in reducing and treating delirium is early recognition, thus screening all PICU patients with a validated delirium screening tool should be completed every 8–12 h. We recommend implementing environmental strategies to promote sleep and decreased delirium that include establishing a daily routine with attention to sleep and wake time, reducing light and noise exposure during sleep times (by encouraging reduced room lighting and eliminating electronic media exposure), encouraging parental involvement and attention to having familiar items in the environment, reducing arousals and awakenings with bundled-care during sleep time, frequent age-appropriate re-orientation for the child, reducing restraint use, and early mobilization. Medications should be reviewed to reduce those associated with delirium (if appropriate and feasible), particularly benzodiazepine use. While, it is not yet clear if melatonin administration leads to meaningful and/or positive outcomes, it should be considered when circadian misalignment (sleep wake disturbance) is suspected. We recommend the use of melatonin in patients with positive delirium screen and suspected sleep disturbance as it is a relatively benign medication with potential benefit. After early recognition of delirium based on screening tools, collaboration and support from pediatric psychiatry should be encouraged for guiding pharmacotherapy in the critically ill child; particularly confirmation of diagnosis and support in deciding if antipsychotic medications would be helpful as pediatric intensivists have less experience with use of antipsychotic medications.

For future directions, given that research on sleep and delirium in the PICU population is far behind what has been done in the adult population, more investigation is needed. The first step is establishing a standardized, accurate, and simplified tool to detect both sleep disturbance and delirium. Significant progress has been made with the emergence of validated delirium screening tools for use in pediatric patients; however, multicenter studies and comparison studies are needed to establish which screening tool best serves the pediatric population with critical illness and account for the broad developmental spectrum. Objective, cost-effective measures for sleep has been the greatest limiting step for progress with understanding causes and consequences of sleep disturbance (quality, quantity, and pattern) in the ICU setting, and thus requires future attention to accurately characterize sleep as well as delineate the relationship between sleep and delirium. Further, it would be ideal to determine which interventions have the greatest impact on improving both sleep and reducing delirium. Use of melatonin supplementation is theoretically promising but use in pediatric critical illness still needs to be clarified regarding who, when, and how long administration would be needed. Finally, it is imperative to have future investigations with focus on treatments, both pharmacologic and non-pharmacologic, as well as short and long term outcomes. To our knowledge, this is the first review to address the parallel between sleep disturbance and delirium in pediatric patients affected by critical illness and to emphasize the entwined roles rather than a cause-effect relationship.

Funding: This research received no external funding.

Conflicts of Interest: The authors declare no conflicts of interest.

References

1. Kudchadkar, S.R.; Yaster, M.; Punjabi, N.M. Sedation, Sleep Promotion, and Delirium Screening Practices in the Care of Mechanically Ventilated Children: A Wake-up Call for the Pediatric Critical Care Community. *Crit. Care Med.* **2014**, *42*, 1592–1600. [CrossRef] [PubMed]
2. American Psychiatric Association. *Diagnostic and Statistical Manual of Mental Disorders*; American Psychiatric Association: Washington, DC, USA, 2013.
3. Smith, H.A.B.; Brink, E.; Fuchs, D.C.; Ely, E.W.; Pandharipande, P.P. Pediatric Delirium. Monitoring and Management in the Pediatric Intensive Care Unit. *Pediatr. Clin. N. Am.* **2013**, *60*, 742–760.
4. Schieveld, J.N.M.; Van Zwieten, J.J. On Risk Factors for Pediatric Delirium at Noon. *Pediatr. Crit. Care Med.* **2015**, *16*, 375–376. [CrossRef] [PubMed]
5. Traube, C.; Silver, G.; Reeder, R.W.; Doyle, H.; Hegel, E.; Wolfe, H.A.; Schneller, C.; Chung, M.G.; Dervan, L.A.; Digennaro, J.L.; et al. Delirium in Critically Ill Children: An International Point Prevalence Study. *Crit. Care Med.* **2017**, *45*, 584–590. [CrossRef] [PubMed]
6. Barr, J.; Fraser, G.L.; Puntillo, K.; Ely, E.W.; Gélinas, C.; Dasta, J.F.; Davidson, J.E.; Devlin, J.W.; Kress, J.P.; Jofe, A.M.; et al. Clinical Practice Guidelines for the Management of Pain, Agitation, and Delirium in Adult Patients in the Intensive Care Unit: Executive Summary. *Am. J. Health Pharm.* **2013**, *70*, 53–58. [CrossRef] [PubMed]

7. Harris, J.; Ramelet, A.S.; van Dijk, M.; Pokorna, P.; Wielenga, J.; Tume, L.; Tibboel, D.; Ista, E. Clinical Recommendations for Pain, Sedation, Withdrawal and Delirium Assessment in Critically Ill Infants and Children: An ESPNIC Position Statement for Healthcare Professionals. *Intensive Care Med.* **2016**, *42*, 972–986. [CrossRef] [PubMed]

8. Flaigle, M.C.; Ascenzi, J.; Kudchadkar, S.R. Identifying Barriers to Delirium Screening and Prevention in the Pediatric ICU: Evaluation of PICU Staff Knowledge. *J. Pediatr. Nurs.* **2016**, *31*, 81–84. [CrossRef] [PubMed]

9. Schieveld, J.N.M.; Leentjens, A.F.G.; Jellinck, M.S. Delirium in Severely Ill Young Children in the Pediatric Intensive Care Unit (PICU). *J. Am. Acad. Child Adolesc. Psychiatry* **2005**, *44*, 392–394. [CrossRef] [PubMed]

10. Trzepacz, P.T.; Baker, R.W.; Greenhouse, J. A Symptom Rating Scale for Delirium. *Psychiatry Res.* **1988**, *23*, 89–97. [CrossRef]

11. Turkel, S.B.; Braslow, K.; Tavaré, C.J.; Trzepacz, P.T. The Delirium Rating Scale in Children and Adolescents. *Psychosomatics* **2003**, *44*, 126–129. [CrossRef] [PubMed]

12. Sikich, N.; Lerman, J. Development and Psychometric Evaluation of the Pediatric Anesthesia Emergence Delirium Scale. *J. Am. Soc. Anesthesiol.* **2004**, *100*, 1138–1145. [CrossRef]

13. Luetz, A.; Gensel, D.; Müller, J.; Weiss, B.; Martiny, V.; Heinz, A.; Wernecke, K.D.; Spies, C. Validity of Different Delirium Assessment Tools for Critically Ill Children: Covariates Matter. *Crit. Care Med.* **2016**, *44*, 2060–2069. [CrossRef] [PubMed]

14. Traube, C.; Silver, G.; Kearney, J.; Patel, A.; Atkinson, T.M.; Yoon, M.J.; Halpert, S.; Augenstein, J.; Sickles, L.E.; Li, C.; et al. Cornell Assessment of Pediatric Delirium: A Valid, Rapid, Observational Tool for Screening Delirium in the PICU. *Crit. Care Med.* **2014**, *42*, 656–663. [CrossRef] [PubMed]

15. Alvarez, R.V.; Palmer, C.; Czaja, A.S.; Peyton, C.; Silver, G.; Traube, C.; Mourani, P.M.; Kaufman, J. Delirium Is a Common and Early Finding in Patients in the Pediatric Cardiac Intensive Care Unit. *J. Pediatr.* **2018**, *195*, 206–212. [CrossRef] [PubMed]

16. Smith, H.A.B.; Boyd, J.; Fuchs, D.C.; Melvin, K.; Berry, P.; Shintani, A.; Eden, S.K.; Terrell, M.K.; Boswell, T.; Wolfram, K.; et al. Diagnosing Delirium in Critically Ill Children: Validity and Reliability of the Pediatric Confusion Assessment Method for the Intensive Care Unit. *Crit. Care Med.* **2011**, *39*, 150–157. [CrossRef] [PubMed]

17. Smith, H.A.B.; Gangopadhyay, M.; Goben, C.M.; Jacobowski, N.L.; Chestnut, M.H.; Savage, S.; Rutherford, M.T.; Denton, D.; Thompson, J.L.; Chandrasekhar, R.; et al. The Preschool Confusion Assessment Method for the ICU: Valid and Reliable Delirium Monitoring for Critically Ill Infants and Children. *Crit. Care Med.* **2016**, *44*, 592–600. [CrossRef] [PubMed]

18. Ista, E.; te Beest, H.; van Rosmalen, J.; de Hoog, M.; Tibboel, D.; van Beusekom, B.; van Dijk, M. Sophia Observation Withdrawal Symptoms-Paediatric Delirium Scale: A Tool for Early Screening of Delirium in the PICU. *Aust. Crit. Care* **2017**, *31*, 266–273. [CrossRef] [PubMed]

19. Schieveld, J.N.M.; Leroy, P.L.J.M.; van Os, J.; Nicolai, J.; Vos, G.D.; Leentjens, A.F.G. Pediatric Delirium in Critical Illness: Phenomenology, Clinical Correlates and Treatment Response in 40 Cases in the Pediatric Intensive Care Unit. *Intensive Care Med.* **2007**, *33*, 1033–1040. [CrossRef] [PubMed]

20. Smeets, I.A.P.; Tan, E.Y.L.; Vossen, H.G.M.; Leroy, P.L.J.M.; Lousberg, R.H.B.; Van Os, J.; Schieveld, J.N.M. Prolonged Stay at the Paediatric Intensive Care Unit Associated with Paediatric Delirium. *Eur. Child Adolesc. Psychiatry* **2010**, *19*, 389–393. [CrossRef] [PubMed]

21. Silver, G.; Traube, C.; Gerber, L.M.; Sun, X.; Kearney, J.; Patel, A.; Greenwald, B. Pediatric Delirium and Associated Risk Factors: A Single-Center Prospective Observational Study. *Pediatr. Crit. Care Med.* **2015**, *16*, 303–309. [CrossRef] [PubMed]

22. Meyburg, J.; Dill, M.L.; Traube, C.; Silver, G.; Von Haken, R. Patterns of Postoperative Delirium in Children. *Pediatr. Crit. Care Med.* **2017**, *18*, 128–133. [CrossRef] [PubMed]

23. Smith, H.A.B.; Gangopadhyay, M.; Goben, C.M.; Jacobowski, N.L.; Chestnut, M.H.; Thompson, J.L.; Chandrasekhar, R.; Williams, S.R.; Griffith, K.; Ely, E.W.; et al. Delirium and Benzodiazepines Associated with Prolonged ICU Stay in Critically Ill Infants and Young Children. *Crit. Care Med.* **2017**, *45*, 1427–1435. [CrossRef] [PubMed]

24. Traube, C.; Silver, G.; Gerber, L.M.; Kaur, S.; Mauer, E.A.; Kerson, A.; Joyce, C.; Greenwald, B.M. Delirium and Mortality in Critically Ill Children: Epidemiology and Outcomes of Pediatric Delirium. *Crit. Care Med.* **2017**, *45*, 891–898. [CrossRef] [PubMed]

25. Simone, S.; Edwards, S.; Lardieri, A.; Walker, L.K.; Graciano, A.L.; Kishk, O.A.; Custer, J.W. Implementation of an ICU Bundle: An Interprofessional Quality Improvement Project to Enhance Delirium Management and Monitor Delirium Prevalence in a Single PICU. *Pediatr. Crit. Care Med.* **2017**, *18*, 531–540. [CrossRef] [PubMed]

26. Schieveld, J.N.M.; Lousberg, R.; Berghmans, E.; Smeets, I.; Leroy, P.L.J.M.; Vos, G.D.; Nicolai, J.; Leentjens, A.F.G.; van Os, J. Pediatric Illness Severity Measures Predict Delirium in a Pediatric Intensive Care Unit. *Crit. Care Med.* **2008**, *36*, 1933–1936. [CrossRef] [PubMed]

27. Silver, G.; Traube, C.; Kearney, J.; Kelly, D.; Yoon, M.J.; Nash Moyal, W.; Gangopadhyay, M.; Shao, H.; Ward, M.J. Detecting Pediatric Delirium: Development of a Rapid Observational Assessment Tool. *Intensive Care Med.* **2012**, *38*, 1025–1031. [CrossRef] [PubMed]

28. Patel, A.K.; Biagas, K.V.; Clark, E.C.; Traube, C. Delirium in the Pediatric Cardiac Extracorporeal Membrane Oxygenation Patient Population: A Case Series. *Pediatr. Crit. Care Med.* **2017**, *18*, e621–e624. [CrossRef] [PubMed]

29. Nellis, M.E.; Goel, R.; Feinstein, S.; Shahbaz, S.; Kaur, S.; Traube, C. Association Between Transfusion of RBCs and Subsequent Development of Delirium in Critically Ill Children. *Pediatr. Crit. Care Med.* **2018**, *19*, 925–929. [CrossRef] [PubMed]

30. Mody, K.; Kaur, S.; Mauer, E.A.; Gerber, L.M.; Greenwald, B.M.; Silver, G.; Traube, C. Benzodiazepines and Development of Delirium in Critically Ill Children. *Crit. Care Med.* **2018**, *46*, 1486–1491. [CrossRef] [PubMed]

31. Traube, C.; Mauer, E.A.; Gerber, L.M.; Kaur, S.; Joyce, C.; Kerson, A.; Carlo, C.; Notterman, D.; Worgall, S.; Silver, G.; et al. Cost Associated with Pediatric Delirium in the ICU. *Crit. Care Med.* **2016**, *44*, e1175–e1179. [CrossRef] [PubMed]

32. Barnes, S.S.; Grados, M.A.; Kudchadkar, S.R. Child Psychiatry Engagement in the Management of Delirium in Critically Ill Children. *Crit. Care Res. Pract.* **2018**, *2018*, 9135618. [CrossRef] [PubMed]

33. Meyburg, J.; Ries, M.; Zielonka, M.; Koch, K.; Sander, A.; von Haken, R.; Reuner, G. Cognitive and Behavioral Consequences of Pediatric Delirium. *Pediatr. Crit. Care Med.* **2018**, *19*, e531–e537. [PubMed]

34. Kudchadkar, S.R.; Aljohani, O.A.; Punjabi, N.M. Sleep of Critically Ill Children in the Pediatric Intensive Care Unit: A Systematic Review. *Sleep Med. Rev.* **2014**, *18*, 103–110. [CrossRef] [PubMed]

35. Armour, A.D.; Khoury, J.C.; Kagan, R.J.; Gottschlich, M.M. Clinical Assessment of Sleep Among Pediatric Burn Patients Does Not Correlate with Polysomnography. *J. Burn Care Res.* **2011**, *32*, 529–534. [CrossRef] [PubMed]

36. Carno, M.A.; Hoffman, L.A.; Henker, R.; Carcillo, J.; Sanders, M.H. Sleep Monitoring in Children during Neuromuscular Blockade in the Pediatric Intensive Care Unit: A Pilot Study. *Pediatr. Crit. Care Med.* **2004**, *5*, 224–229. [CrossRef] [PubMed]

37. Al-Samsam, R.H.; Cullen, P. Sleep and Adverse Environmental Factors in Sedated Mechanically Ventilated Pediatric Intensive Care Patients. *Pediatr. Crit. Care Med.* **2005**, *6*, 562–567. [CrossRef] [PubMed]

38. Marseglia, L.; Aversa, S.; Barberi, I.; Salpietro, C.D.; Cusumano, E.; Speciale, A.; Saija, A.; Romeo, C.; Trimarchi, G.; Reiter, R.J.; et al. High Endogenous Melatonin Levels in Critically Ill Children: A Pilot Study. *J. Pediatr.* **2013**, *162*, 357–360. [CrossRef] [PubMed]

39. Gottschlich, M.M.; Khoury, J.; Warden, G.D.; Kagan, R.J. Review: An Evaluation of the Neuroendocrine Response to Sleep in Pediatric Burn Patients. *J. Parenter. Enter. Nutr.* **2009**, *33*, 317–326. [CrossRef] [PubMed]

40. Flannery, A.H.; Oyler, D.R.; Weinhouse, G.L. The Impact of Interventions to Improve Sleep on Delirium in the ICU: A Systematic Review and Research Framework. *Crit. Care Med.* **2016**, *44*, 2231–2240. [CrossRef] [PubMed]

41. Patel, J.; Baldwin, J.; Bunting, P.; Laha, S. The Effect of a Multicomponent Multidisciplinary Bundle of Interventions on Sleep and Delirium in Medical and Surgical Intensive Care Patients. *Anaesthesia* **2014**, *69*, 540–549. [CrossRef] [PubMed]

42. Hu, R.-F.; Jiang, X.; Chen, J.; Zeng, Z.; Chen, X.; Li, Y.; Huining, X.; Evans, J. Non-Pharmacological Interventions for Sleep Promotion in the Intensive Care Unit. *Cochrane Database Syst. Rev.* **2015**. [CrossRef] [PubMed]

43. Valrie, C.R.; Bromberg, M.H.; Palermo, T.; Schanberg, L.E. A Systematic Review of Sleep in Pediatric Pain Populations. *J. Dev. Behav. Pediatr.* **2013**, *34*, 120–128. [CrossRef] [PubMed]

44. Hshieh, T.T.; Yang, T.; Gartaganis, S.L.; Yue, J.; Inouye, S.K. Hospital Elder Life Program: Systematic Review and Meta-Analysis of Effectiveness. *Am. J. Geriatr. Psychiatry* **2018**, *26*, 1015–1033. [CrossRef] [PubMed]

45. Harrison, A.M.; Lugo, R.A.; Lee, W.E.; Davis, S.J.; McHugh, M.J.; Weise, K.L. The Use of Haloperidol in Agitated Critically Ill Children. *Clin. Pediatr.* **2002**, *41*, 51–54. [CrossRef] [PubMed]

46. Turkel, S.B.; Hanft, A. The Pharmacologic Management of Delirium in Children and Adolescents. *Pediatr. Drugs* **2014**, *16*, 267–274. [CrossRef] [PubMed]
47. Joyce, C.; Witcher, R.; Herrup, E.; Kaur, S.; Mendez-Rico, E.; Silver, G.; Greenwald, B.M.; Traube, C. Evaluation of the Safety of Quetiapine in Treating Delirium in Critically Ill Children: A Retrospective Review. *J. Child Adolesc. Psychopharmacol.* **2015**, *25*, 666–670. [CrossRef] [PubMed]

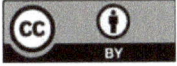

medical
sciences

MDPI

Review

It Takes a Village: Multidisciplinary Approach to Screening and Prevention of Pediatric Sleep Issues

Jessica R. Sevecke * and Tawnya J. Meadows

Department of Psychiatry, Geisinger Health System, 100 North Academy Avenue, Danville, PA 17821, USA; tjmeadows@geisinger.edu
* Correspondence: jsevecke@geisinger.edu; Tel.: +1-570-271-6516

Received: 31 July 2018; Accepted: 10 September 2018; Published: 14 September 2018

Abstract: Sleep is essential to human development. Poor sleep can have significant effects on cognition, learning and memory, physical and behavioral health, and social-emotional well-being. This paper highlights the prevalence of common pediatric sleep problems and posits that a multidisciplinary approach to the assessment and intervention of sleep problems is ideal. Primary care providers are often the first professionals to discuss sleep issues with youth and families. However, dentists, otolaryngologists, childcare providers, school personnel, and behavioral health providers have a vital role in screening and prevention, providing intervention, and monitoring the progress of daily functioning. The strengths of this approach include better provider-to-provider and provider-to-family communication, streamlined assessment and intervention, earlier identification of sleep issues with more efficient referral, and longer-term monitoring of progress and impact on daily functioning. Barriers to this approach include difficulty initiating and maintaining collaboration among providers, limited provider time to obtain the necessary patient permission to collaborate among all multidisciplinary providers, lack of financial support for consultation and collaboration outside of seeing patients face-to-face, geographic location, and limited resources within communities. Research investigating the utility of this model and the overall impact on pediatric patient sleep issues is warranted and strongly encouraged.

Keywords: multidisciplinary; pediatric sleep; anticipatory guidance

1. Introduction

Sleep is essential to human development across all life stages. Adequate sleep is important for physical growth, cognitive development, learning and memory, physical health, social-emotional well-being, and mental and behavioral health. If an individual obtains inadequate sleep, significant implications across these domains could occur [1–4]. Among adult US citizens, about 50 to 70 million report experiencing a sleep disorder [5]. Because sleep issues often present in childhood and may continue to have impact into adulthood, early identification of medical sleep disorders and behaviorally based sleep problems is essential to prevent future problems such as persistent insomnia or death secondary to issues such as driving while drowsy [5]. Among children, sleep is crucial to ensure that developmental milestones are met and that children thrive academically, socially, and behaviorally across the systems and environments in which they function. The prevalence of sleep issues among infants, children, and adolescents varies according to type of sleep concern and age. Medically based sleep disorders include diagnoses such as obstructive sleep apnea (OSA), bruxism, restless leg syndrome (RLS), and periodic limb movement disorder (PLMD). Medically based sleep disorders are less common than behaviorally based sleep problems, with about 5% of children and adolescents experiencing a medically-based sleep disorder [6] and up to about 40% of children experiencing a behaviorally based sleep problem sometime during childhood [6]. Behaviorally based sleep problems include night wakings, bedtime issues, inadequate sleep, and poor sleep hygiene. In one study, about 20% of 4- to 12-year-old children experienced a behaviorally based sleep problem at least one night per week [7]. Children who rated higher on parasomnias were also more likely to experience falls and exhibit pica symptoms [7]. Despite this level of prevalence, less than half of the parents in this study discussed sleep issues with their primary care provider [7]. Another study suggests that low prevalence rates of sleep issues (3.7%) within primary care compared to epidemiological studies may be due to primary care providers not asking families about sleep problems [6].

2. Pediatric Sleep Across Disciplines

2.1. Primary Care Providers

Commonly, a child's primary care provider is the first person to discuss sleep issues and short- and long-term implications of sleep problems during a well-child visit. Anticipatory guidance is a process whereby primary care providers discuss issues with families in anticipation of their emergence [8]. Mindell and Owens [9] highlight when to introduce and discuss issues across infancy, childhood, and adolescence in conjunction with scheduled medical well-child visits. This is an expansion on anticipatory guidance recommendations provided by the American Academy of Pediatrics (AAP) [8]. Discussions around sleep can and should take place prior to the birth of a child during the mother's prenatal visits. During this time, age-appropriate sleep expectations, sleeping arrangements, and safe sleep practices should be discussed [9].

2.2. Behavioral Health Providers and Psychiatrists

The role of the behavioral health provider (i.e., a person with graduate or medical school training who has a master of social work (MSW) degree, is a licensed clinical social worker (LCSW) or licensed professional counselor (LPC), or a master's-level psychologist, doctoral-level psychologist, or psychiatric nurse practitioner or psychiatrist) is to offer psychoeducation and empirically supported interventions to address common sleep problems. Topics that may be addressed by a behavioral health provider include, but are not limited to, behavior management for bedtime refusal behaviors; establishment and implementation of a bedtime routine; strategies to improve independent sleep onset and management of night wakings, to decrease nighttime feeds, or to decrease parasomnia concerns such as sleepwalking and sleep talking; and intervention to address circadian rhythm disorders in adolescents and teenagers. Due to the high rate of occurrence of these issues, it is advised that all behavioral health providers screen all patients for sleep difficulties. Adherence strategies to improve the use of medical interventions for sleep disorders (e.g., adherence to a continuous positive airway pressure (CPAP) machine for OSA) may also be addressed.

Behavioral health providers may provide services within an integrated primary care setting or work collaboratively with pediatricians in the community to help assess and treat behaviorally based sleep issues. Behavioral health providers in primary care practice can implement the Sleep Checkup, a clinical tool designed to prevent, identify, and manage pediatric sleep difficulties [10]. Behavioral health providers are also encouraged to coordinate with school personnel to help them understand the functional impact of sleep on behavior, academic performance, and emotional regulation. Behavioral health providers may also be involved in the assessment of attention-deficit hyperactivity disorder (ADHD), which requires getting feedback from teachers. It is estimated that 25–50% of youth with ADHD have difficulty initiating and maintaining sleep, with sleep issues occurring in two to three times more youth with ADHD than those without ADHD [9]. Behavioral health providers should screen for sleep concerns to help ensure appropriate diagnosis when comorbidities are present between behavioral issues, poor emotional regulation, anxiety, depression, and other psychiatric concerns. Considering the presence of sleep issues and their impact on emotional and behavioral regulation is crucial to prevent misdiagnosis and inappropriate medication management. Screening should include timing of sleep onset, night wakings, restless sleep, snoring, sleep regularity and duration, and daytime sleepiness [9]. Similarly, with ADHD, behavioral health providers should consider sleep issues when screening for and treating anxiety and depression. It is estimated that 40–50% of children with emotional regulation issues have comorbid sleep concerns [9]. Behavioral health providers can also offer practical recommendations to parents on managing sleep problems and work collaboratively with school systems in the US on incorporating sleep recommendations and school-based accommodations through either a 504 Plan or individualized education plans (IEPs). Periodic screening of sleep concerns should also be employed as a means of monitoring progress and the impact on daytime functioning [9].

2.3. Childcare Providers and School Personnel

Childcare professionals and school personnel such as teachers, nurses, social workers, and school psychologists can play an essential role in identifying daytime sleepiness and participating in intervention and monitoring of the impact of sleep issues on academic performance, emotional regulation, and daytime behavior. Among school-age youth, poor sleep has implications such as decreased academic performance, truancy, behavior problems, increased internalized symptoms consistent with anxiety and depression, memory and attention difficulties, and safety concerns [11]. Knowing the possible impact of poor sleep on daytime functioning, it is important that school personnel screen for sleep problems when assessing for learning problems and designing IEPs or school-based accommodations [12]. Without considering these factors, youth may be misdiagnosed or inappropriately classified as having ADHD or emotional disturbance (ED), or meet special education criteria for learning problems when also experiencing sleep issues.

In addition to early identification of sleep issues, strategies to help prevent and treat sleep problems can be provided by school personnel. Psychoeducation and tips for prevention and intervention of sleep problems can be incorporated into the general curriculum and in health classes as well as group lessons for parents and teachers. Wilson and colleagues [13] evaluated the impact of preschool-based sleep education targeting parents and teachers across a two-week period. Results demonstrated an increase in parents' knowledge, attitudes, self-efficacy, and beliefs around sleep as well as increased weeknight sleep for children compared to a group who did not attend the training. Another school-based family intervention found improved sleep habits for first-grade students over a 12-month period after families received a brief consultation around sleep concerns [14]. Among older adolescents, similar improvements in sleep habits and knowledge were found following school-based sleep intervention [15,16].

Schools can also implement system-wide changes to help decrease sleep problems among children and adolescents. In one study, delaying school start time by one hour resulted in increased sleep duration, decreased attempts to "make up" sleep on the weekends, and decreased motor vehicle accidents [17]. In another study, start times were delayed by 30 min, resulting in an increase in total sleep duration and an overall decrease in daytime sleepiness among students [18]. Similar results were found in a larger longitudinal study among students in China [19]. The AAP [20] has expressed strong support for school administrations considering changing to later start times. Other recommendations include schools educating parents and students on optimal sleep durations for adolescents and teenagers, health care providers within schools serving as advisors to help schools be more aware of youth sleep needs, supporting schools that provide educational interventions for youth and parents, and educating the general community on potential risks of chronic sleep loss in adolescents.

2.4. Dentists and Otolaryngologists

Obstructive sleep apnea is a prevalent sleep disorder that has significant implications for pediatric patients if left untreated, including behavioral, academic, social-emotional, and medical. Within the discipline of pediatric dentistry, there has been increased attention on pediatric dentists screening for problems and referring patients for consultation with providers outside of dentistry if sleep problems are suspected. In 2016, the American Academy of Pediatric Dentistry (AAPD) adopted a policy strongly encouraging dentists to screen for possible OSA, snoring, and other sleep-disordered breathing concerns, assess for tonsillar hypertrophy, assess tongue positioning for possible obstruction, recognize that obesity can contribute to the prevalence of OSA, refer to an appropriate professional if OSA is suspected (e.g., otolaryngologist, sleep medicine physician, pulmonologist), and consider nonsurgical oral appliances only after "complete orthodontic/craniofacial assessment of the patient's growth and development as part of a multidisciplinary approach" [21]. The AAPD's recommendations support an interdisciplinary approach to identification and treatment of pediatric sleep concerns and can help in early detection of sleep concerns. The AAPD recommends that children first see a dentist once their first tooth erupts or by their first birthday. It is recommended that children see a dentist about every six months thereafter [22]. Thus, if a child is seeing a dentist at regular intervals, the dentist will have an important role in early identification of sleep-disordered breathing and tonsillar hypertrophy, recognizing abnormal craniofacial growth patterns, and screening for sleep-disordered breathing concerns [23]. Obstructive sleep apnea screening is also essential before recommending sedation for a pediatric patient, as children may be more susceptible to airway collapse during a procedure and recovery if they also meet the criteria for OSA [24]. The modified STOP-BANG questionnaire (snoring (S), tonsillar hypertrophy (T), obstruction (O), daytime tiredness, behavior problems or daytime irritability (P), BMI (B), age (A), Neuromuscular Disorder (N), Genetic/Congenital Disorder (G)) for pediatrics is one screening tool that has shown potential utility among dentists in screening for OSA risk factors [25]. Aside from OSA and other sleep-disordered breathing concerns, bruxism is a highly prevalent sleep disorder among pediatric patients, which can increase sleep arousals and impact daytime functioning [26]. In fact, in a small sample of pediatric patients aged 5 to 18, there was a statistically significant difference in the arousal index with bruxism compared to age- and sex-matched controls [26].

Aside from primary care physicians and dentists, otolaryngologists are the medical professionals children are most likely to encounter. Otitis media with effusion (OME) commonly presents in children, especially between the ages of 1 and 3 years, with a prevalence of 10–30% and a cumulative incidence of 80% by age 4 [27]. Myringotomy with insertion of tympanostomy tubes is the most common operation among children in the United States [28]. The high incidence of ear infections and frequent need for tubes result in a relatively high percentage of children who are seen in otolaryngology clinics. Otolaryngologists can play a role in the screening and treatment of medically related sleep disorders. Of the nearly 500,000 pediatric tonsillectomies and adenoidectomies (T&As) performed each year, the majority are to treat sleep-disordered breathing. Otolaryngologists, who are specialists in upper airway anatomy, physiology, and surgery, are uniquely qualified to treat patients with OSA. Enlarged tonsils and adenoids are a common cause of sleep-disordered breathing. As such, surgical removal of the tonsils and adenoids is the primary treatment. In the pediatric population, resolution of OSA occurs in 82% of patients who are treated with T&A [29]. A recent study estimated that the prevalence of OSA among obese children and adolescents was as high as 60% [30]. Obstructive sleep apnea may be more severe in obese children and adolescents compared to age-matched nonobese children and adolescents [31].

3. Multidisciplinary Sleep Model

Infants, children, and adolescents function across a variety of systems, and poor sleep can affect more than one area of a child's life. For example, a child who does not get enough sleep at night may experience daytime drowsiness at school, impacting academic performance, as well as irritability during after-school sports practice, impairing social relationships. This paper posits that the various professionals within these systems should screen for and intervene on sleep-related concerns to positively impact the health and well-being of all children and should work to communicate with children and families as well as across disciplines to provide coordinated care to identify, screen for, and assist in the treatment of pediatric sleep problems (Figure 1).

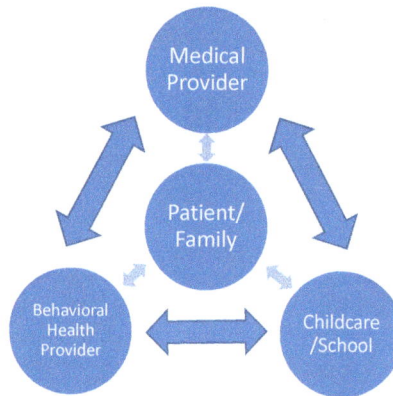

Figure 1. Multidisciplinary approach to the assessment and intervention of sleep problems with emphasis on communication between patients/families and providers as well as across providers.

A medical provider such as a primary care provider or pediatrician routinely monitors a child's sleep starting at the mother's prenatal visits by educating the mother on expectations and establishing the sleep environment, continuing over the life of the child during well-child visits. Other medical providers such as dentists, orthodontists, and otolaryngologists can screen for possible obstructive sleep apnea or bruxism. Childcare and education professionals can help by informing caregivers of a child's level of daytime alertness and mood. Given the significant implications of sleep on behavior and learning, it is appropriate and necessary that these professionals provide interprofessional care. Unfortunately, there is limited research and discussion on a coordinated, multidisciplinary approach to the assessment and treatment of sleep issues.

4. Discussion

A multidisciplinary approach to screening and prevention can help with early identification of and intervention for sleep problems. Table 1 outlines anticipatory guidance for sleep-related topics across ages that can be introduced and discussed with patients/families by the team of providers. Sleep issues may also arise at ages other than what is presented in this table. Therefore, multidisciplinary providers are encouraged to use this as a guide and consistently gather relevant information as issues arise outside of the context of regular anticipatory guidance.

Table 1. Multidisciplinary anticipatory guidance recommendations [9,10,21–26].

	Sleep Anticipatory Guidance: Infants
Primary Care Provider	<u>1 to 6 Months</u> - Encourage parents to get plenty of sleep and sleep when infant is sleeping - Help baby wake for feedings by light patting, changing the diaper, or undressing - Continue to offer feeds during the night every 3 h - Put infant to sleep on his/her back; choose a crib with slats 2 ⅜ inches apart; do not use loose, soft bedding - Put baby to sleep drowsy but awake - Pay attention to infant's cues for sleep - Develop a schedule for naps and nighttime sleep - Infant should sleep in crib in caregiver's room - Do not but baby in crib with a bottle - Create daily routine for naps and bedtime for baby - Choose mesh playpen with weave less than ¼ inches <u>7 to 12 Months</u> - Discuss changing sleep pattern - Discuss limit setting and positive discipline - Nighttime feeds not necessary

Table 1. *Cont.*

	Sleep Anticipatory Guidance: Infants
Behavioral Health Provider	1 to 6 Months - Provide coping skill recommendations to caregivers to help with transition of having a newborn at home and impact on parental sleep and stress level - Help family set a consistent schedule and routine for sleep - Provide psychoeducation on sleep-onset associations - Discuss routine for feeds - Provide psychoeducation on daytime disruptive behavior management (i.e., differential attention) 7 to 12 Months - Help family gradually reduce nighttime feeds - Further discuss limit-setting techniques and positive discipline
Childcare/School	1 to 6 Months - Maintain regular sleep and feeding schedules - Maintain safety recommendations - Put baby to sleep drowsy but awake - Implement consistent routine for sleep - Provide feedback to caregivers on daytime sleep habits - Support independent sleep onset and reduce feedings during naps 7 to 12 Months - Provide family with feedback on helpful behavioral strategies and positive discipline techniques used at daycare - Monitor sleepiness outside of daily sleep schedule - Monitor developmental performance (i.e., cognitive, oral, and motor development)
Dentist/Otolaryngologist	- First visit with a dentist by the time of eruption of first tooth or first birthday - Screen for breathing concerns, oral and craniofacial abnormalities, and obstructions
	Sleep Anticipatory Guidance: Toddlers (1 to 3 Years)
Primary Care Provider	- Continue one nap per day - Follow nightly bedtime routine - Encourage quiet time such as reading, singing, and a favorite toy before bed - Maintain consistent bedtime routines and sleep times - Discuss night awakenings: parents should reassure briefly, give a preferred object (blanket or stuffed animal), and put back to bed - Do not put TV, computer, or digital device in bedroom - No bottle in bed - Use methods other than TV or digital media when tired to improve calming behavior
Behavioral Health Provider	- Discuss nap schedule so as to not disrupt nighttime sleep - Discuss use of transitional object for sleep and how to decrease maladaptive sleep onset associations - Discuss limit setting around electronics and digital media for sleep
Childcare/School	- Maintain consistent naptime earlier in the afternoon to avoid impact on nighttime sleep - Use transitional object at naptime - Continue to monitor developmental gains and recommend early intervention services or developmental assessment as indicated - Assess for sleep concerns if developmental delays appear evident
Dentist/Otolaryngologist	- Encourage regular dental visits (i.e., every 6 months) - Dentist discusses incorporating nightly oral hygiene habits into bedtime routine - Dentist screens for consumption of sugary and caffeinated drinks and provide education on impact of dental health and sleep - Screen for tonsillar hypertrophy, oral and craniofacial abnormalities, and nighttime breathing concerns and mouth breathing; may use pediatric-adapted screening tools such as STOP-BANG [25] - Dentist assesses for and provide psychoeducation about bruxism - Dentist discusses use of positional therapy to reduce snoring or bruxism - Otolaryngologist screens for obstructive sleep apnea (OSA)

Table 1. *Cont.*

	Sleep Anticipatory Guidance: School-Aged Children
Primary Care Provider	- Create and maintain a calm bedtime routine - Limit TV to no more than 1 h a day, no TV in bedroom - Monitor school performance and consider impact of poor sleep on tardiness, daytime behavior - Consider implementing a family media plan to balance needs of physical activity, sleep, school, and quiet time without media (www.healthychildren.org/mediauseplan) - Maintain consistent sleep routine (even on weekends) to obtain adequate sleep - Do not operate machinery, especially motor vehicles, when drowsy - Discuss maintaining a sleep routine in light of other activities, work, school, exercise, extracurricular activities, free time - Provide psychoeducation around proper use of melatonin if used
Behavioral Health Provider	- Help family establish a consistent bedtime routine that is not too long (e.g., bath, brush teeth, PJs, story, lights out) - Encourage daytime exercise and limit electronics use; eliminate TV and other screens at least 1 h before bed - Introduce Cognitive Behavioral Therapy (CBT) strategies for older children to help calm bedtime fears, anxiety, and mood concerns - Help family implement behavioral strategies for bedtime refusal, night awakenings, and parasomnias - Discuss daily schedule to maintain balance between school, friends, homework, and work - Discuss setting limits around driving a vehicle if sleep deprived
School	- Monitor drowsiness in school, report episodes of sleep during school day to caregivers - Monitor academic and behavioral performance; assess sleep difficulties when evaluating concerns - Introduce psychoeducation on sleep during class time and to parents during parent-teacher meetings and back-to-school night - Monitor tardiness, school attendance, and changes in mood or anxiety levels - Encourage regular exercise (e.g., PE classes) - Consider changing school start times - Provide psychoeducation on the impact of poor sleep on driving behavior and safety - Manage school schedules so extracurricular activities do not occur too early in the morning or too late at night
Dentist/Otolaryngologist	- Dentist assesses for tooth wear and screen for bruxism if wear is evident - Otolaryngologist screens for and monitors tonsillar hypertrophy and sleep-disordered breathing concerns; screens for OSA before sedating a child for oral surgery - Otolaryngologist discusses impact of obesity on breathing-related sleep disorders - Otolaryngologist discusses impact of decongestants and corticosteroids on sleep - Otolaryngologist screens for nocturnal enuresis in patients who snore - Discuss nonsurgical appliances to help correct oral abnormalities that may impact sleep-disordered breathing

Consequently, implications of poor sleep such as daytime sleepiness, academic difficulties, poor social-emotional regulation, and behavior difficulties can be mitigated. Other prospective strengths of this model include collaboration among providers, which can streamline treatment approaches and enhance coordination of care for the patient. Streamlined prevention and treatment strategies can result in more consistent and clear messages to families, increasing the likelihood of implementation. Barriers to this approach include difficulties sharing health information, as providers across systems often do not have integrated medical records unless they are within the same health agency. Without integrated health records, providers require release of information forms to be completed by families to allow coordinated communication among providers. This can be difficult to complete if it is not a regular procedure among providers. Additionally, time is a barrier to this multidisciplinary approach. True coordinated care among providers to address sleep issues requires communication via electronic health record, fax, secure email, or phone. Each mode of communication has different procedures, and using these procedures impacts a medical provider's day differently.

Often providers do not have time built into their schedule for consultation and collaboration, and often there is no additional financial compensation for the time required to execute these activities well. An additional barrier to the use of this approach is not having enough providers or having many multidisciplinary providers within a given geographic area, making it difficult to establish and potentially maintain collaboration. Geographic locations that require providers to be significant distances apart can also present a barrier, because patient follow-through for appointments may be difficult due to transportation difficulties. Integrated approaches that have a collocated or preexisting coordinated (i.e., interdisciplinary clinic) structure can help in navigating this barrier [32].

At this time, there is limited empirical evidence supporting a multidisciplinary approach for the assessment and treatment of sleep problems. While some professional associations have established best practice guidelines (e.g., pediatrics, dentistry) regarding assessment of sleep difficulties in pediatric patients, not all relevant specialties have established guidelines, and certainly no guidelines have taken into consideration coordination of care across environments. It is also important to note that specialty providers, including neurologists, endocrinologists, and geneticists, can play a role in the screening and prevention of childhood sleep problems. This review does not discuss their role, as the general pediatric population is less likely to encounter these professionals in routine care. To explore the utility of a multidisciplinary approach, empirical research studies should be employed evaluating the process as well as clinical outcomes data measuring the impact on patient care. Data examining whether a multidisciplinary approach allows patient access to services sooner may further support this model as well as attenuate the severity of symptoms. Research should also explore possible solutions to the aforementioned barriers and propose strategies to help improve the limited widespread nature of this approach.

Author Contributions: Both authors contributed to the conceptualization, writing—original draft preparation, and writing—review and editing of this work.

Funding: The authors received no external funding to complete this work.

Conflicts of Interest: The authors declare no conflict of interest.

References

1. Baum, K.T.; Desai, A.; Field, J.; Miller, L.E.; Rausch, J.; Beebe, D.W. Sleep restriction worsens mood and emotional regulation in adolescents. *J. Child Psychol. Psychiatry* **2014**, *55*, 180–190. [CrossRef] [PubMed]
2. Beebe, D.W. Cognitive, behavioral, and functional consequences of inadequate sleep in children and adolescents. *Pediatr. Clin. N. Am.* **2011**, *58*, 649–665. [CrossRef] [PubMed]
3. Beebe, D.W.; Simon, S.; Summer, S.; Hemmer, S.; Strotman, D.; Dolan, L.M. Dietary intake following experimentally restricted sleep in adolescents. *Sleep* **2013**, *36*, 827–834. [CrossRef] [PubMed]
4. Garetz, S.L.; Mitchell, R.B.; Partker, P.D.; Moore, R.H.; Rosen, C.L.; Giordani, B.; Redline, S. Quality of life and obstructive sleep apnea symptoms after pediatric adenotonsillectomy. *Pediatrics* **2015**, *135*, e477–e486. [CrossRef] [PubMed]
5. *Sleep and Sleep Disorder Statistics*; American Sleep Association: Lititz, PA, USA, 2018; Available online: www.sleepassociation.org/about-sleep/sleep-statistics (accessed on 28 August 2018).
6. Meltzer, L.J.; Johnson, C.; Crosetter, J.; Ramos, M.; Mindell, J.A. Prevalence of diagnoses sleep disorders in pediatric primary care practices. *Pediatrics* **2010**, *125*, 1410–1418. [CrossRef] [PubMed]
7. Stein, M.A.; Mendelsohn, J.; Obermeyer, W.H.; Amromin, J.; Benca, R. Sleep and behavior problems in school-aged children. *Pediatrics* **2001**, *107*, 1–9. [CrossRef]
8. Hagan, J.F.; Shaw, J.S.; Duncan, P.M. (Eds.) Guidelines for health supervision of infants, children, and adolescents. In *Bright Futures*, 4th ed.; American Psychological Association: Worcester, MA, USA, 2017.
9. Mindell, J.A.; Owens, J.A. *A Clinical Guide to Pediatric Sleep: Diagnosis and Management of Sleep Problems*, 3rd ed.; Lippincott Williams & Williams: Philadelphia, PA, USA, 2015; ISBN 978-1451193008.

10. Honaker, S.M.; Saunders, T. The Sleep Checkup: Sleep screening, guidance, and management in pediatric primary care. *Clin. Pract. Pediatr. Psychol.* **2018**, *6*, 201–210. [CrossRef]
11. Dahl, R.E. Biological, developmental, and neurobehavioral factors relevant to adolescent driving risks. *Am. J. Prev. Med.* **2008**, *35*, S278–S284. [CrossRef] [PubMed]
12. Taras, H.; Potts-Datema, W. Sleep and student performance at school. *J. School Health* **2005**, *75*, 248–254. [CrossRef] [PubMed]
13. Wilson, K.E.; Miller, A.L.; Bonuck, K.; Lumeng, J.C.; Chervin, R.D. Evaluation of a sleep education program for low-income preschool children and their families. *Sleep* **2014**, *37*, 1117–1125. [CrossRef] [PubMed]
14. Quach, J.; Hisock, H.; Ukoumunne, O.C.; Wake, M. A brief sleep intervention improves outcomes in the school entry year: A randomized control trial. *Pediatrics* **2011**, *128*, 692–701. [CrossRef] [PubMed]
15. Moseley, L.; Gradisar, M. Evaluation of school-based intervention for adolescent sleep problems. *Sleep* **2009**, *32*, 334–341. [CrossRef] [PubMed]
16. Cain, N.; Gradisar, M.; Moseley, L. A motivational school-based intervention for adolescent sleep problems. *Sleep Med.* **2011**, *12*, 246–251. [CrossRef] [PubMed]
17. Danner, F.; Philips, B. Adolescent sleep, school start times, and teen motor vehicle crashes. *J. Clin. Sleep Med.* **2008**, *4*, 533–535. [PubMed]
18. Owens, J.A.; Belon, K.; Moss, P. Impact of delaying school start time an adolescent sleep, mood, and behavior. *Arch. Pediatr. Adolesc. Med.* **2010**, *164*, 608–614. [CrossRef] [PubMed]
19. Li, S.; Arguelles, L.; Jiang, F.; Chen, W.; Jin, X.; Yan, C.; Tian, Y.; Hong, X.; Qian, C.; Zhang, J.; et al. Sleep, school performance, and a school-based intervention among school-aged children: A sleep series study in China. *PLoS ONE* **2013**, *8*, e67928. [CrossRef] [PubMed]
20. American Academy of Pediatrics. Policy statement: School start times and adolescents. *Pediatrics* **2014**, 642–649. [CrossRef]
21. American Academy of Pediatric Dentistry. Policy on Obstructive Sleep Apnea. *Oral Health Policies* **2016**, *39*, 96–98.
22. Ask Your Doctor about Regular Dental Visits. *Am. Acad. Pediatr. Dent.* **2011**. Available online: www.aapd.org (accessed on 30 July 2018).
23. Major, M.P.; El-Hakim, H.; Witmans, M.; Major, P.W.; Flores-Mir, C. Adenoid hypertrophy in pediatric sleep disordered breathing and craniofacial growth: The emerging role of dentistry. *J. Dent. Sleep Med.* **2014**, *1*, 83–87. [CrossRef]
24. Brown, K. Pediatric consideration in sedation for patients with obstructive sleep apnea syndrome. *Semin. Anesth. Perioper. Med. Pain* **2007**, *26*, 94–102. [CrossRef]
25. Chiang, H.K.; Cronly, J.K.; Best, A.M.; Brickhouse, T.H.; Leszczyszyn, D.J. Development of a simplified pediatric obstructive sleep apnea (OSA) screening tool. *J. Dental Sleep Med.* **2015**, *2*, 163–173. [CrossRef]
26. Herrera, M.; Valencia, I.; Grant, M.; Metroka, D.; Chialastri, A.; Kothare, S.V. Bruxism in children: Effect on sleep architecture and daytime cognitive performance and behavior. *Sleep* **2006**, *29*, 1143–1148. [CrossRef] [PubMed]
27. Lous, J.; Burton, M.J.; Felding, J.U.; Ovesen, T.; Rovers, M.M.; Williamson, I. Grommets (ventilation tubes) for hearing loss associated with otitis media with effusion in children. *Cochrane Database Syst. Rev.* **2005**, *1*, 1–46. [CrossRef]
28. Paradise, J.L.; Feldman, H.M.; Campbell, T.F.; Dollaghan, C.A.; Colborn, D.K.; Bernard, B.S.; Rockette, H.E.; Janosky, J.E.; Pitcairn, D.L.; Sabo, D.L.; et al. Effect of early or delayed insertion of tympanostomy tubes for persistent otitis media on developmental outcomes at the age of three years. *N. Engl. J. Med.* **2001**, *344*, 1179–1187. [CrossRef] [PubMed]
29. Brietzke, S.; Gallagher, D. The effectiveness of tonsillectomy and adenoidectomy in the treatment of pediatric obstructive sleep apnea/hypopnea syndrome: A meta-analysis. *Otolaryngol. Head Neck Surg.* **2006**, *136*, 979–984. [CrossRef] [PubMed]

30. Ali, N.J.; Pitson, D.J.; Stradling, J.R. Snoring, sleep disturbance, and behaviour in 4–5-year olds. *Arch. Dis. Child.* **1993**, *68*, 360–366. [CrossRef] [PubMed]
31. Redline, S.; Tishle, P.V.; Schluchter, M.; Aylor, J.; Clark, K.; Graham, G. Risk factors for sleep-disordered breathing in children. Associations with obesity, race, and respiratory problems. *Am. J. Respir. Crit. Care Med.* **1999**, *159*, 1527–1532. [CrossRef] [PubMed]
32. Meltzer, L.J.; Moore, M.; Mindell, J.A. The need for interdisciplinary pediatric sleep clinics. *Behav. Sleep Med.* **2008**, *6*, 266–282. [CrossRef] [PubMed]

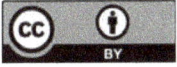

medical sciences

MDPI

Review

Relationship between Sleep and Psychosis in the Pediatric Population: A Brief Review

Meelie Bordoloi [1] and Ujjwal Ramtekkar [2,*]

[1] Department of Psychiatry, University of Missouri, Columbia, MO 65212, USA;
    bordoloim@health.missouri.edu
[2] Department of Psychiatry, Nationwide Children's Hospital, Columbus, OH 43025, USA
*   Correspondence: ujjwal.ramtekkar@nationwidechildrens.org

Received: 19 August 2018; Accepted: 10 September 2018; Published: 14 September 2018

Abstract: Sleep disorders are common in several psychiatric disorders, including schizophrenia. In the pediatric population, the relationship between sleep and psychosis is not completely understood due to limited research studies investigating the link. Insomnia is noted to be a predictor of psychosis, especially in ultrahigh risk adolescents. Sleep difficulties are also associated with a two to three-fold increase in paranoid thinking. Biological factors, such as decrease in thalamic volume, have been observed in children with schizophrenia and ultrahigh risk adolescents with associated sleep impairment. Objective studies have indicated possible actigraphy base measures to be the predictor of psychosis after a one year follow-up. The studies using polysomnography have rare and inconsistent results. In this brief review, we provide an overview of existing literature. We also posit that future research will be beneficial in understanding the initiation, course and progression of sleep disturbance in the high risk pediatric population with the goal of implementing interventions to alter the development of psychosis.

Keywords: sleep disturbance; psychosis; schizophrenia; pediatric sleep

1. Introduction

Sleep disturbance is considered an important transdiagnostic factor implicated in the development and maintenance of a range of psychiatric disorders [1]. As early as age 4, sleep disturbances, such as difficulty falling asleep, sleep walking, and restless sleep, lead to increased externalizing problems [2]. In adolescents, sleep disorders, such as insomnia, are generally coexistent with internalizing problems like depression and may even predict suicidality [3]. It has been hypothesized that the association between sleep and psychiatric symptoms is often bidirectional and co-occurring sleep or psychiatric disorder impacts the severity of other comorbid disorders [4]. Psychotic disorders are relatively uncommon, yet are some of the most debilitating psychopathologies with onset in late adolescence [5]. The well-formed psychotic disorder, schizophrenia, is characterized by positive symptoms including hallucinations, delusions, disorganization and negative symptoms such as cognitive impairment, apathy, affective flattening, and social withdrawal. There are both objective and subjective studies indicating that a variety of sleep problems ranging from insomnia to parasomnias are associated with psychosis in adults. Certain sleep disorders like insomnia, periodic limb movement disorder, obstructive sleep apnea, and restless leg syndrome are frequently seen in adults with schizophrenia. Presence of significant insomnia has often been observed as a preceding symptom before a psychotic episode and is also shown to impact the prognosis when it continues during the course of illness [5]. There is growing evidence indicating the importance of sleep disorders as potential markers for emergence of psychotic symptoms as well as prognosis of psychotic disorders in adults. However, in the pediatric population, the association between sleep and psychosis is far less researched and not well understood, largely because of the rare prevalence and diagnostic challenges related to ill-defined presentation, convergence of symptom presentation with developmental stages, and difficulty in obtaining reliable chronological history. The purpose of this brief review is to present an overview of the existing literature on the relationship between sleep and psychosis in the pediatric population.

2. Methods

A literature search was conducted in PubMed and Medline databases for original research using search terms "psychosis in children", "childhood sleep disturbances", "sleep and psychosis", "sleep as a predictor of psychosis", and "insomnia and children" limited to pediatric age range (0–18 years). Both objective and subjective studies published to date in English were included. The titles and abstracts were screened for relevance and the case reports and articles not specifically related to sleep and psychosis in children were excluded.

3. Results

3.1. Subjective Studies in Sleep and Psychosis in Children

A multicenter longitudinal study was conducted in North America aimed to identify predictors of psychosis in youth with high psychosis risk [6]. The study results indicated that five features assessed at baseline contributed uniquely to the prediction of psychosis: a genetic risk for schizophrenia with recent deterioration in functioning, higher levels of unusual thought content, higher levels of suspicion/paranoia, greater social impairment, and a history of substance abuse. Sleep disturbance was included in the category of general symptoms, but it did not significantly contribute as a predictor of psychosis. The authors concluded that sleep disturbance accounted for "general symptoms" but did not have any significant predictability factor for psychosis.

A population-based study in United Kingdom that was an offshoot from the second British National survey of Psychiatric morbidity investigated the effect of insomnia [7]. The results determined that sleep difficulties and paranoid fears maintained each other in a circular relationship. Whether the difficulty in falling or staying asleep was mild or severe, the association with paranoia remained; likewise, whether the paranoid thought was of mild or severe content, the association with insomnia was maintained. The results indicated that insomnia was associated with an approximately two to threefold increase in paranoid thinking. The authors concluded that insomnia was a significant contributor to the development and maintenance of paranoid fears.

A similar UK-based large scale epidemiological study was conducted aiming to investigate the association between specific parasomnias (nightmares, night terrors, and sleepwalking) in childhood and later adolescent psychotic experiences [8] The subjects were recruited from The Avon Longitudinal Study of Parents and Children (ALSPAC) which is a birth cohort study set in the UK. The strength of this study was certainly the sample size which was 4720 individuals. Experience of nightmares, night terrors, and sleepwalking were assessed using a semi-structured interview at age 12. Psychotic experiences were assessed at ages 12 and 18 using a semi-structured clinical interview-Pliksi (Psychosis-Like Symptoms semi-structured interview). Results demonstrated that there was a significant association between the presence of nightmares at age 12 and psychotic experiences at 18 when adjusted for possible confounders and psychotic experiences at 12. As proposed in the study, patients experiencing psychosis may have blurred boundaries between the sleep and awake state and may have brief moments of oscillating between the two, even during the awake state. Nightmares which occur in rapid eye movement (REM) sleep may thus be experienced as hallucinations during the day. Conversely, one could transition into the awake state while asleep, resulting in sleep terrors and sleepwalking in a non-rapid eye movement (NREM) stage.

A study by Lee et al. investigated the relationship between psychotic-like experiences (PLEs) and sleep disturbances in adolescents [9]. The authors reported that insomnia and excessive daytime sleepiness were found to predict psychotic-like experiences in adolescents independent of depression. The study results indicated that all three types of insomnia (sleep onset, maintenance, and terminal insomnia) predicted high risk of clinical psychosis. Of note, excessive daytime sleepiness was considered to be an independent predictor of PLEs, after controlling for antipsychotic medication, which itself caused sedation.

On similar lines, Taylor et al. tested the hypothesis that shared genetic or environmental influences underlined sleep disturbances and vulnerability to PLEs (psychotic-like experiences) [10]. The study included about 4800 pairs of 16-year-old twins participating in the Twins Early Development Study (TEDS) as part of the Longitudinal Experiences and Perceptions (LEAP) project. The authors concluded that their hypothesis was correct. Three positive symptoms, namely paranoia, hallucinations, and grandiosity, and two negative symptoms of anhedonia and parent -rated negative symptoms were among the PLEs that shared genetic and environmental influences, along with sleep disturbances and cognitive disorganization. This was the only twin study included in our literature search.

Another study examined sleep dysfunction in adolescents at ultrahigh-risk (UHR) for psychosis, relationships between sleep disturbances and psychosis symptoms, volume of an integral sleep-structure (thalamus), and associations between thalamic abnormalities and sleep impairment in UHR youth [11]. In the study, UHR was defined by moderate levels of positive symptoms (unusual thought content/delusional idea, suspicious persecutory ideas, grandiose ideas, perceptual abnormalities/hallucinations, disorganized communication) and/or a decline in global functioning accompanying the presence of schizotypal personality disorder and/or a family history of psychosis [11]. Subjects fulfilling this criterion were included. Conclusively, increased latency to sleep onset and disrupted continuity of sleep were the sleep disturbances observed in UHR adolescents along with decreased bilateral thalamus volume. Interestingly, sleep disturbances in the subjects were associated with greater negative symptom severity as compared to positive symptoms. These findings of specific sleep deficits in UHR youth possibly indicated a likely role for domains of sleep dysfunction (latency, continuity) in the etiology of psychosis. Second, evidence of thalamic reductions in the UHR sample suggested that a critical brain structure supporting sleep function was compromised in adolescents at risk of psychosis. As these abnormalities were present prior to onset, those findings indicated that reductions in sleep-related structures might play a potential role in schizophrenia pathophysiology.

3.2. Objective Studies of Sleep and Psychosis

There has been a very limited number of studies investigating sleep and psychosis using objective measures such as polysomnography and actigraphy in the pediatric age group. A study conducted in 1969 attempted to explore sleep patterns in normal and psychotic children [12]. Considering previous evidence that there was marked decrease in stage 4 sleep in chronic schizophrenic patients, all-night sleep electroencephalograms and power-density configurations were obtained and studied for a group of psychotic and normal prepubertal children. Singular attention was focused on whether stage-4 sleep was affected in the psychotic population who were clearly manifesting thought disorders. Authors reported that there was no significant difference in stage 4 sleep in psychotic versus normal prepubertal children. The authors also concluded that the mean difference of 1 h 37 min in total sleep time between the psychotic and normal children largely reflected the differences in daytime activities between the groups.

More recently, a pilot study was conducted to investigate REM disturbances in children with major depressive disorder (MDD) and schizophrenia [13]. The study concluded that although there was significant REM latency in MDD, it was not seen in children with schizophrenia. However, pronounced impairment of sleep continuity was noted in schizophrenic patients.

In an extension of the above-mentioned subjective study by Lunsford-Avery et al. the authors also obtained the data from actigraphy at baseline and after one year in relation to the psychotic symptoms of ultra-high risk group. The results indicated that the specific sleep measures of actigraphy; reduced duration of sleep, reduced efficiency of sleep, and wake time after sleep onset (WASO), were predictive of the worsening of positive symptoms after a year after controlling for baseline psychosis symptoms [14].

4. Discussion

The relationship between sleep disturbance as a predictor of psychosis is not extensively studied in the pediatric population. Sleep research is challenging due to reliability of subjective reports and cognitive abilities affecting self-awareness during different developmental stages in children and adolescents. On the other hand, psychotic disorders are very rare in children and phenomenology can be complex due to the multi-factorial nature of PLEs in that age group, ranging from trauma, mood disorders, maladaptive coping mechanisms to stress, and underlying medical etiologies.

In the study by Lee et al. [9], the authors concluded that adolescent insomnia was a predictor of PLEs. In contrast, the longitudinal study by Cannon et al. [6], did not support the findings but acknowledged that sleep disturbance is merely a general symptom in youth with risk of psychosis. Although the results of these studies are contradictory, sleep disturbance may have indirectly led to higher levels of unusual thought content or higher levels of suspicion/paranoia in the former study which were considered as predictors of psychosis. It is also important to note that although one study found insomnia to be a predictor of PLE, all PLEs may not eventually progress to psychosis. An interesting finding of the former study is that EDS (excessive day time sleepiness) is an independent predictor for PLE. The authors made an interesting point that narcolepsy having ill-defined boundaries between sleep and wakefulness, as characterized by sleep paralysis and hypnopompic and hypnogogic hallucinations, might be considered as a differential diagnosis of adolescent psychosis and vice versa.

In the study by Lunsford-Avery et al. [11], the authors stated that problematic sleep might represent a core feature of psychosis, over and above concurrent mood symptoms. However, the offshoot of the same study that used actigraphy measures demonstrated that specific objective parameters at baseline were associated with positive symptoms of psychosis at one year follow-up [14]. On similar lines, the British national survey data indicated specific parasomnias being associated with development of PLEs in future [7]. The authors did attribute the daytime PLEs to the brief lapse into REM sleep. However, while few studies have found poor sleep/wake boundaries among individuals with psychotic symptoms, there is little evidence of intrusions of REM sleep into waking states in patients with schizophrenia experiencing hallucinations.

The twin study by Taylor [10] and study of structural thalamic abnormalities by Lunsford-Avery [11] indicate genetic and biological underpinnings to the association between sleep abnormalities and psychosis. However, the evidence is only limited to association, without any identified direction of effect or causality.

One of the proposed models to provide a plausible explanation for the bidirectional nature of sleep and psychosis is the neurodevelopmental diathesis-stress model [15]. According to this model, there are shared genetic and environmental factors that affect development of psychosis as well as sleep dysfunction. Additionally, the stress related to psychosocial and biological changes intertwined with neuromaturational factors across developmental stages in children result in the interplay between sleep and cognitive deficits resulting in psychosis like symptoms. While the conceptualization is untested, it draws upon the traditional stress-diathesis model for schizophrenia and also supports the biological underpinnings of sleep and psychiatric disorders.

Regarding objective studies, the topic has received scant attention and there are very few studies investigating the relationship between objective sleep measures and psychosis. Of the studies described above, only the actigraphy study was longitudinal and reported specific measures to predict psychosis after one year follow-up. However, the rest were mostly limited due to small sample size, different diagnostic criteria, and variability in age groups. Interestingly, the literature in adults indicated that different studies reached different conclusions regarding the objective measures associated with or predicting psychosis.

5. Conclusions

Despite increasing evidence that sleep problems are clinically significant in patients with psychosis and may function as predictors of development of psychosis in individuals with high risk, robust research in this area is lacking. The available literature posits a biological and psychosocial model for explaining the association between sleep dysfunction and psychosis. Large, longitudinal, and objective studies specifically investigating the sleep–psychosis relationship are needed. Further studies should consider replicating some of the findings in adult literature and also investigate the differences between pediatric and adult age groups, thereby providing insights into developmental aspects of psychopathology. It would also be valuable to explore the interventions specific to sleep and cognition as possible ways to alter the development or alleviate dysfunction resulting from psychosis. Finally, it would be important to include sleep symptom assessments in clinical practice as an integral part of assessment and treatment planning for youth presenting with psychosis-like experiences.

Funding: This research did not receive any funding.

Conflicts of Interest: The authors declare no conflict of interest.

References

1. Dolsen, M.R.; Asarnow, L.D.; Harvey, A.G. Insomnia as a Transdiagnostic Process in Psychiatric Disorders. *Curr. Psychiatry Rep.* **2015**, *16*, 471. [CrossRef] [PubMed]
2. Quach, J.; Nguyen, C.; Williams, K.; Sciberras, E. Bidirectional Associations Between Child Sleep Problems and Internalizing and Externalizing Difficulties From Preschool to Early Adolescence. *JAMA Pediatr.* **2018**, *172*, e174363. [CrossRef] [PubMed]
3. De Zambotti, M.; Goldstone, A.; Colrain, I.M.; Baker, F.C. Insomnia disorder in adolescence: Diagnosis, impact, and treatment. *Sleep Med. Rev.* **2018**, *39*, 12–24. [CrossRef] [PubMed]
4. Ramtekkar, U.; Ivanenko, A. Sleep in Children With Psychiatric Disorders. *Semin. Pediatr. Neurol.* **2015**, *22*, 148–155. [CrossRef] [PubMed]
5. American Psychiatric Association. *Diagnostic and Statistical Manual of Mental Disorders*, 5th ed.; American Psychiatric Publishing: Arlington, VA, USA, 2013.
6. Cannon, T.D.; Cadenhead, K.; Cornblatt, B.; Woods, S.W.; Addington, J.; Walker, E.; Seidman, L.J.; Perkins, D.; Tsuang, M.; McGlashan, T.; et al. Prediction of psychosis in youth at high clinical risk: A multisite longitudinal study in North America. *Arch. Gen. Psychiatry* **2008**, *65*, 28–37. [CrossRef] [PubMed]
7. Freeman, D.; Brugha, T.; Meltzer, H.; Jenkins, R.; Stahl, D.; Bebbington, P. Persecutory ideation and insomnia: Findings from the second British National Survey Of Psychiatric Morbidity. *J. Psychiatr. Res.* **2010**, *44*, 1021–1026. [CrossRef] [PubMed]
8. Thompson, A.; Lereya, S.T.; Lewis, G.; Zammit, S.; Fisher, H.L.; Wolke, D. Childhood sleep disturbance and risk of psychotic experiences at 18: UK birth cohort. *Br. J. Psychiatry* **2015**, *207*, 23–29. [CrossRef] [PubMed]
9. Lee, Y.J.; Cho, S.J.; Cho, I.H.; Jang, J.H.; Kim, S.J. The relationship between psychotic-like experiences and sleep disturbances in adolescents. *Sleep Med.* **2012**, *13*, 1021–1027. [CrossRef] [PubMed]
10. Taylor, M.J.; Gregory, A.M.; Freeman, D.; Ronald, A. Do sleep disturbances and psychotic-like experiences in adolescence share genetic and environmental influences? *J. Abnorm. Psychol.* **2015**, *124*, 674–684. [CrossRef] [PubMed]
11. Lunsford-Avery, J.R.; Orr, J.M.; Gupta, T.; Pelletier-Baldelli, A.; Dean, D.J.; Watts, A.K.; Bernard, J.; Millman, Z.B.; Mittal, V.A. Sleep dysfunction and thalamic abnormalities in adolescents at ultra high-risk for psychosis. *Schizophr. Res.* **2013**, *151*, 148–153. [CrossRef] [PubMed]
12. Caldwell, D.F.; Brane, A.J.; Beckett, P.G.S. Sleep Patterns in Normal and Psychotic Children. *Arch. Gen. Psychiatry* **1970**, *22*, 500–503. [CrossRef] [PubMed]
13. Riemann, D.; Kammerer, J.; Low, H.; Schmidt, M.H. Sleep in adolescents with primary major depression and schizophrenia: A pilot study. *J. Child Psychol. Psychiatry Allied Discip.* **1995**, *36*, 313–326. [CrossRef]

14. Lunsford-Avery, J.R.; LeBourgeois, M.K.; Gupta, T.; Mittal, V.A. Actigraphic-measured sleep disturbance predicts increased positive symptoms in adolescents at ultra high-risk for psychosis: A longitudinal study. *Schizophr. Res.* **2015**, *164*, 15–20. [CrossRef] [PubMed]
15. Lunsford-Avery, J.R.; Mittal, V.A. Sleep dysfunction prior to the onset of schizophrenia: A review and neurodevelopmental diathesis-stress conceptualization. *Clin. Psychol. Sci. Pract.* **2013**, *20*, 291–320. [CrossRef]

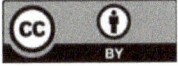

*medical
sciences*

MDPI

Review

Insomnia in Adolescence

Innessa Donskoy * [ID] **and Darius Loghmanee**

Advocate Children's Hospital, Park Ridge, IL 60068, USA; Darius.Loghmanee@advocatehealth.com
* Correspondence: Innessa.Donskoy@advocatehealth.com; Tel.: +1-847-723-9070

Received: 3 August 2018; Accepted: 29 August 2018; Published: 1 September 2018

Abstract: Adolescent insomnia is a common condition that negatively impacts a developing young adult's mental and physical health. While the treatment of adult insomnia has been standardized, the treatment of pediatric insomnia is very practitioner-dependent and few large-scale studies are available to determine a standard recommended practice. There is great hope that as the adolescent medicine and sleep medicine fields flourish, larger cohort analyses will be performed to determine the prevalence and precipitating factors of adolescent insomnia, allowing for standardized treatment recommendations and systematic efforts to make these recommendations available to all adolescents.

Keywords: insomnia; adolescents; adolescence; teenagers; delayed sleep phase; cognitive behavioral therapy for insomnia (CBT-I)

1. Introduction

Insomnia is a nocturnal disorder that profoundly impacts an individual's performance during waking hours, taking away the restorative physical and cognitive properties that sleep provides [1,2]. Rather, insomnia fills this void with impatience, anxiety, and ultimately leads to maladaptive behaviors; these often involve utilization of screens, providing stimulation and light exposure, which is correlated with even later sleep onset [3]. Adolescence encompasses a wide time range which includes early (11–13 years), middle (14–18 years) and late periods (19–21 years old or through college age) [4]. Within this timeframe most individuals will go through the pubertal process, move from more logical thought to abstract thinking with problem-solving abilities, and experience a peak in impulsivity that gradually dissipates into behaviors such as self-regulation and planning [3]. This is also a time during which the adolescent will distance him or herself from the family unit and develop stronger relationships with peer groups, romantic interests, and ultimately physically separate to live independently and pursue goals such as further education or employment. This separation includes decreased sharing of medical information, even in cases of pain [5], due to embarrassment and a desire for independence. These factors do not bode well for the trend of increased issues with sleep in adolescence [6]. The amount of recommended sleep during the adolescent period is greater than expected, with the National Sleep Foundation recommending 9–11 h of sleep for children 6–13 years old and 8–10 h per night for individuals aged 14–17 years old [7]. In today's world of increased demands on adolescents for afterschool activities to compete for limited spots in universities [8], increased exposure to screens even in their own bedrooms [7], early start times for schools [9], and a physiologic sleep/wake delay [10], there are a multitude of reasons that adolescents do not reach the critical amount of sleep they need. In fact, the National Sleep Foundation poll of 12th graders (17–18 years old) reported that 75% slept less than 8 h per night [11]; this is even more striking when considered in light of the fact that self-report of sleep by adolescents is often overestimated [12]. These adolescents are not getting adequate sleep, affecting performance during formative years [13,14], and not seeking help for it. In the setting of any underlying physiological or psychological conditions, this is often exacerbated [15–17]. In adults, the standard of care for insomnia has moved away from medication in recent years to more cognitive behavioral therapy for insomnia (CBT-I) [18] and while benefit has been seen in adolescents undergoing CBT-I [19–21] there is still limited access for those who are seeking providers of this specific technique [22]. While insomnia in the adolescent is challenging due to its multifactorial nature, it is a topic that deserves specific attention.

2. Epidemiology

As early as infancy, insomnia can be found disrupting schedules, family life, and the ability for a child to have adequate daytime alertness and energy to reach their developmental goals [22]. Behavioral insomnia of infancy is a condition largely influenced by environmental factors and caregiver choices. It also provides a breeding ground for maladaptive behaviors; sleep onset associations, inappropriate limit setting, and mistiming of sleep onset time can all linger and become part of an older child's sleep related issues. It is estimated that insomnia can be as common as 36% in preschool (3–5 year old) children and approximately 20% in school age (5–10 year old) children [23]. The prevalence of insomnia in adolescents remains in the same approximate range, as high as 23.8% [24]. This suggests that it is the most common sleep disorder in this age group. These values arise from the use of the fourth edition of the Diagnostic and Statistical Manual of Mental Disorders (DSM-IV) criteria for diagnosis of primary insomnia which is defined as at least one month of symptoms including difficulties with sleep onset, maintenance, or a sensation of unrefreshing sleep [25]. This is in contrast to fifth edition of the Diagnostic and Statistical Manual of Mental Disorders (DSM-V) which has stricter criteria for insomnia diagnosis, requiring a chronicity of 3 months [26]. In the sleep field, insomnia is diagnosed according to the third edition of the International Classification of Sleep Disorders (ICSD-3); it is described as a sleep onset or maintenance problem in the setting of an adequate opportunity to sleep, with some reported daytime impairment [27]. The causes of insomnia are multifactorial, with genetic, biologic, environmental and social factors playing some role [28]. To be considered chronic, it should last at least three months with symptoms at least three times per week; this is purposely very close to the DSM-V diagnosis. While this unified change is more restrictive than the previous DSM-IV diagnosis and limits the amount of diagnoses that can be made, it also highlights the often long-standing nature of the disorder. Unspoken in the diagnostic criteria are the many maladaptive behaviors that a person may develop in reaction to their insomnia which continue to perpetuate the issue, such as anxiety about sleep itself or nocturnal behaviors during periods of inability to sleep [27]. It is just as important to address these responses as to treat the underlying disorder as they often persist long after the precipitating incident that initially triggered the insomnia has passed.

In one of the few larger studies of adolescents with insomnia, the onset of symptoms occurred at a median age of 11 years with no difference between prepubescent boys and girls [29]. However, after puberty there is a notable uptick in the incidence of insomnia in girls, specifically a 2.75-fold increase after menarche [29], the culmination of puberty in females. Interestingly, as these young women mature into older women, while they may objectively sleep better than their male counterparts, they also report more sleep-related complaints [30]. As these women age and pass menopause, they seem to have an objective worsening of sleep architecture [30]. However, in the adolescent period alone (especially in later adolescence), there is an increase in the prevalence of insomnia in females [24].

3. Circadian Confounder

A crucial point to mention in the epidemiology of adolescent insomnia is the potential confounding diagnosis of delayed sleep wake phase disorder (DSWPD). DSWPD is characterized by a delay in the phase of the "major sleep period" with normal sleep duration and non-rapid eye movement/rapid eye movement (NREM/REM) cycling, according to the ICSD-2 classification system [31]. In the ICSD-3 criteria, these symptoms need to be ongoing for at least 3 months with objective data (e.g., sleep logs or actigraphy supported by a delayed melatonin onset) demonstrating the delay in sleep onset by more than 2 h compared to what is socially accepted or desired by the individual [27]. There also needs to be a delay in wake onset, with a significant daytime impact, again defined by the individual [27]. The ICSD-2 acknowledges the common predisposition of adolescents towards developing this syndrome [31]. No definite prevalence has been agreed upon, but between 1% and 16% of adolescents are diagnosed with DSWPD [30,32]. While behaviorally induced delayed sleep onset for reasons such as school work, employment, extracurricular activities, screen time, and parental influences [10] may certainly contribute to the development of this condition, at least one specific polymorphism has been associated with the development of DSWPD so far, and more research in this area is ongoing [33,34]. Across international studies, a consistent pattern of shifting sleep onset times has been demonstrated in adolescents, with a 1–2 h delay in weekend versus weekday bedtime [10]. This coincides with a significantly earlier school start time [10] and truncated sleep due to the lack of opportunity to sleep until the natural end of the sleep-wake phase. This leads to sleep inertia, described as an overwhelming difficulty rising upon awakening to be ready for school, work, etc.

Sleep is driven by two main processes. Process C is the circadian system, governed by the central clock, the suprachiasmatic nucleus in the hypothalamus, which dictates when in the 24 h day an individual is most likely to sleep or wake naturally [35]. Process S is the homeostatic drive for sleep, which is governed by how long an individual has been awake. This accounts for how much "sleep debt" they have accumulated [35]. These two processes partner to determine when an individual will actually fall asleep. Given the often unmet increased requirement for sleep in this age [7], there is an increased sleep debt and heightened homeostatic drive for sleep at earlier evening hours than the delayed circadian phase of the adolescent would dictate. This ability to fall asleep at these earlier times can make elucidating the diagnosis of DSWPD difficult. Since falling asleep earlier than one's circadian time may not ensure a stable period of continuous sleep, adolescents often report intermittent difficulty with sleep onset and even maintenance, symptoms often attributed to insomnia. The treatment of insomnia (as discussed later in this article) is different than the entrainment necessary to shift one's delayed sleep/wake phase to earlier hours [36–38]. Given the high prevalence of this circadian rhythm disorder, it is important to make sure it is ruled out prior to initiating a treatment for insomnia. The timing of sleep onset, wake time and quality of sleep during weekends and prolonged holidays are important to ascertain when evaluating adolescents. When permitted to sleep on a schedule that feels most "natural", an adolescent with delayed sleep wake phase disorder will likely not experience any decrease in sleep quality, issues with sleep maintenance, or sleep inertia. An adolescent who has no issues with their sleep when following their own circadian rhythm must either find work or school schedules that accommodate their natural sleep/wake cycle or make efforts to entrain their circadian rhythm to match the requirements of their social situations. Adolescents who continue to have difficulty initiating and maintaining sleep despite sleeping according to their circadian sleep phase should undergo further evaluation for insomnia.

4. Impact

Insomnia is not without physiologic effects. In the adult, studies looking at "short sleepers" and "long sleepers" ($\leq$6 h per night and >8 h per night, respectively) have shown an association with an increased risk in all-cause mortality [2]. In a large cohort study of over 3000 aging individuals with sleep time that was either too short or too long, there was a significant elevation in markers of inflammation such as interleukin-6 (IL-6) and tumor necrosis factor-alpha (TNF-α) as well as an increase in mortality in both groups compared to the mean [2]. Other studies have demonstrated decreased sleep duration being associated with obesity, metabolic syndrome, diabetes, hypertension, coronary artery disease and increased all-cause mortality in the adult population [39]. In the adolescent, fewer large cohort analyses have been performed looking at systemic consequences of decreased duration or quality of sleep. Some studies, however, have suggested an associated increase in overweight status and obesity [40,41] and an increased risk of prehypertension and hypertension independent of obesity [41,42] putting these children at risk for long term cardiovascular morbidity. Interestingly, there is no clear increased risk of sleeping too long seen in children/adolescents [41] as seen in adults.

In the adolescent suffering from sleep issues, decreased sleep quality has many deleterious effects on neurological and psychological outcomes. Along with poor performance the next day [13,14], there is also an increased risk of anxiety and depression [15], including an increased risk of suicidal ideation [16,17]. Even more frightening is that these are also young adults who are less willing to confide in a parent or seek out medical care on their own [43], allowing their sleep pathology to go unchecked. In adults, decreased sleep efficiency as well as decreased overall satisfaction with sleep have been shown to be correlated with an increased incidence of depression [39]. In teenagers, there is a strong correlation with insomnia, anxiety and depression but determining causality is challenging [44]. Although some studies have suggested that the presence of insomnia more commonly precedes the development of anxiety and depression [45,46], the consensus is that they are likely mutually influencing conditions which have many of the same underlying etiologies and that treatment of one should most certainly include addressing the others.

A large cohort of adolescents with self-described difficulty with sleep had reported daytime symptoms of chronic tiredness/fatigue and had objectively worse school performance [14]. The converse is also true, with decreased symptoms of insomnia correlating with higher grades in non-foreign language studies as well as mathematics in both boys and girls [14]. Even outside of school performance, the presence of insomnia significantly predicts school absenteeism [47]. This is likely multifactorial in that these adolescents are trying to make up for little or non-restorative sleep at night, by sleeping longer in the morning. They are either still in bed missing school or physically present in the classroom but having microsleeps when awake, similar to a drowsy driver [48]. While this latter example is extreme, it highlights a very tangible disruption in daytime alertness, when an adolescent's main task is to stay awake in the classroom to learn.

While beyond the scope of this review, it is important to note that adolescence is a time that teenagers are getting behind the wheel, learning to drive and doing so independently for the first time. Any decrease in alertness can increase the risk of serious bodily harm, especially in the novice driver [48]. In an effort to keep adolescents safe, in school, and with the highest chance of academic success, there has been a very strong push for delaying school start times [49,50]. While this will not necessarily address every cause of sleepiness in adolescents, aligning school time with ideal periods of physiologic wakefulness in adolescents is an important step towards mitigating the risks associated with suboptimal sleep health in this population. The American Academy of Pediatrics (AAP) and American Academy of Sleep Medicine (AASM) have both put forward emphatic formal statements identifying early school start time as a key modifiable contributor to insufficient sleep in the adolescent population and suggesting that 8:30 am should be the very earliest that schools begin [49,50]. Having these recommendations from major professional organizations for the pediatric and sleep fields respectively demonstrates how vast of an issue delaying school start times has become, and will hopefully encourage more efforts at identifying and endorsing policy changes that will support cultural shifts in our society that prioritize sleep health in adolescents.

5. Contributing Factors & Comorbidities

Certain populations of adolescents are more vulnerable to developing insomnia than others. As previously discussed, psychopathologies such as depression and anxiety are highly correlated with insomnia. Additionally, up to 73% of children with Attention-Deficit/Hyperactivity Disorder (ADHD) endorse sleep issues pertaining to initiating and maintaining sleep [51,52]. A recent randomized controlled trial aiming to provide behavioral tools to manage sleep symptoms demonstrated improvement in the severity of the ADHD symptoms while the subjects were still taking a stimulant medication as a first line therapy [51]. There is no current data to suggest that behavioral interventions alone are as effective for ADHD as in combination with medication [45], but this remains an area to be further investigated. It has been shown that in children with ADHD, there is an increase in cortical hyperarousal, ascertained by an increase in beta frequency EEG waves resembling wake throughout the night [53]. This was seen even during the deepest stages of sleep, which should have a predominance of much slower frequencies [53]. This suggests that there is much more to be explored regarding the underlying pathophysiology of ADHD and how great of a role sleep may play in it.

Adolescents with neurodevelopmental disorders other than ADHD are also at risk for sleep difficulties [54,55]. This includes Autism Spectrum Disorders, Cerebral Palsy, Fetal Alcohol Syndrome, Down Syndrome, and other conditions manifesting early in childhood with significant cognitive and emotional/behavioral difficulties. A very recent comprehensive review on this subject reported that among children with neurodevelopmental disorders compared to typically developing controls there is an increased incidence of bedtime resistance, anxiety, difficulty settling down to sleep, delayed sleep onset, sleep maintenance issues, and overall restless sleep [54]. There are currently no specific guidelines for managing insomnia in the neurodevelopmental disability group. Likely due to this lack of guidelines, behavioral interventions for insomnia being more thoroughly studied in the typically developing cohort [56], and few pediatric patients having access to these therapies [57], an impressive majority (81%) of neurodevelopmentally impacted children has been prescribed a medication to treat insomnia in the last year [58]. Much more research is needed on the complexity of insomnia in the neurodevelopmental disability group and clarifying first line therapies and a step-wise approach to treatment.

Other populations at risk for insomnia include children with chronic illnesses [59–61] and in difficult social situations such as poverty and food scarcity [62] and in turbulent home environments due to an array of issues as severe as exposure to violence [62,63]. Many of these insomnia symptoms are inextricable from the PTSD, depression and anxiety that these adolescents also face [55,62].

Having another underlying sleep disorder may lead to difficulties with sleep onset and sleep maintenance. While delayed sleep wake phase disorder has a great deal of overlap with insomnia, other circadian disorders such as Irregular Sleep Wake Rhythm Disorder and Non-24 Sleep Wake Rhythm Disorder can lead to the development of similar symptoms. Although difficulties with sleep latency are not commonly seen [52], adolescents with obstructive sleep apnea (OSA) may have sleepiness during the day [64] and difficulties with sleep maintenance due to intermittent obstructive respiratory events and hypoxia [65]. Adolescents with OSA are often overweight and have difficulty maintaining attention in the classroom [65,66] symptoms that are difficult to differentiate from the adolescent with insomnia. Therefore, any concern for possible obstructive sleep apnea should be pursued with polysomnography (PSG) before attributing sleep issues to insomnia alone.

Restless legs syndrome is a disorder described by an urge to move the legs which is most prominent at rest, relieved by movement, and often presents in a circadian pattern of peak symptoms in the evening, which can greatly impact sleep onset and sleep maintenance [67]. This is a clinical diagnosis that should be inquired about when investigating complaints of insomnia, as the associated discomfort can cause a prolonged sleep onset latency. A related disorder, Periodic Limb Movement Disorder (PLMD) [27] can cause daytime sleepiness due to sleep disruption throughout the night without obvious symptoms prior to sleep onset. This diagnosis requires a polysomnogram to rule out, similar to OSA.

Finally, while narcolepsy is a disorder of central hypersomnolence, individuals suffering from this condition do report difficulties with sleep consolidation and maintenance [27]. These adolescents often present with sleep paralysis, hypnagogic/hypnapompic hallucinations and excessive daytime sleepiness, but these can be seen due to sleep deprivation from insomnia as well. Very vivid dreams and dream enactment can be seen in narcolepsy, leading to reports of difficulties staying asleep. If a suspicion for narcolepsy arises during an adolescent's report of insomnia, it should be more thoroughly investigated and a PSG followed by a multiple sleep latency test should be considered.

6. Treatment

The treatment of insomnia in adults has been standardized to promote cognitive behavioral therapy for insomnia (CBT-I) as an effective and recommended initial treatment option [68]. This was reaffirmed by the American Academy of Sleep Medicine in a recent position statement on pharmacologic treatment of insomnia, as well, emphasizing that behavioral techniques need to be a standard of treatment [69]. CBT-I is comprised of a short course (4–8 weeks) of weekly visits with a trained professional to learn, implement, and follow up on techniques such as stimulus control, sleep restriction, relaxation and relapse prevention, as well as further sleep education [70]. While alone these techniques are very effective, they have shown to be more efficacious and longer lasting when put into action together with a close relationship with a CBT-I provider [70,71]. This has been found to be as efficacious and more long lasting than medication alone [71]. In the adolescent population, CBT-I delivered in person one-on-one [72] as well as in a group setting and through specific internet-based programing has been shown to be effective for the treatment of insomnia [73]. The treatment of adolescent insomnia with CBT-I was shown to decrease somatic complaints as well as anxiety, oppositional behavior, and ADHD symptoms [74]. However, similar to the adult population [70] there are currently not enough trained providers available to deliver these services to children and adolescents [75]. Until more providers become available, consideration should be given to continuing to trial group based CBT-I as well as validated internet-based CBT-I, as these are now proving to be effective for adolescents [21].

Outside of providing behavioral interventions, medications are frequently used in the pediatric population to treat insomnia, even surpassing the rates seen in the adult population [58]. In younger children, more sedating medications are used, such as off-label use of antihistamines (e.g., hydroxyzine and diphenhydramine) or supraphysiologic doses of melatonin [58]. The efficacy of melatonin may suggest that a there is a circadian misalignment contributing to/causing difficulty initiating sleep [36,37]. Interestingly, in specifically the ADHD population as well as children with neurodevelopmental disabilities, high (5 mg and above) doses of melatonin were shown to improve sleep as well as daytime behavior [76,77]. The mechanism behind this improvement is still not completely understood, other than that these children are able to get more quality hours of sleep. Fortunately, as further research continues, long term use of melatonin even at high doses has been shown to be without adverse effects [78]. Melatonin agonists (namely Ramelteon) have been approved for adolescents over 18 years old, and have been effective in small case reports with off-label use for younger children [79].

In the ADHD population, clonidine (an alpha-2 agonist) has been used as a short-acting sedating medication, to help with sleep onset in these challenging children and adolescents [80]. However, it is not without risk given its antihypertensive properties, and can cause hypotension during use and rebound hypertension after discontinuation.

While benzodiazepines were commonly used in adults for sleep onset insomnia, due to the high risk of overdose, dependency, and abuse, they are no longer commonly used [69]. An exception to this is for the treatment of parasomnias, but this is beyond the scope of this review.

The available benzodiazepine receptor agonist medications (BzRA) or "Z" drugs (Zolpidem, Zaleplon, and Eszopiclone) are medications only approved for use in patients above 18 years of age, as well. They are non-benzodiazepine medications, and augment gamma-aminobutyric acid (GABA) activity at the receptor only if GABA is present, unlike benzodiazepines which act directly at the place of the receptor even in the absence of endogenous GABA. This theoretically provides for a better safety profile [81]. Zaleplon is the shortest acting of the three, with a half-life of one hour, compared to 1.4–4.5 h for Zolpidem and 6 h for Eszopiclone [82]. In the adult population, all three have been shown to be effective in the short term for treating sleep onset and maintenance insomnia, but long-term data is lacking, with some suggestion the behavioral techniques are even more effective [71,82]. Zolpidem has been shown to have potential side effects of complex behaviors at night as well as next day "hangover" effects on driving, memory and motor ability, risks that often outweigh its benefits [83,84]. Zaleplon and Eszopiclone have been implicated in complex sleep behaviors as well, but only in limited case reports [84,85]. Zaleplon and Eszopiclone have not been studied in the pediatric population. Zolpidem has been studied in an open label trial in pediatric patients and from a pharmacokinetic perspective was shown to be well tolerated at a dose of 0.25 mg/kg [86]. However, in studies using Zolpidem off-label for sleep augmentation in specific populations such as pediatric burn victims [86] and children with ADHD [87], it was not effective for reducing sleep latency on polysomnography. There is also an increased risk of Zolpidem misuse in the adolescent population [88] given their increased propensity for impulsivity and risk-taking behavior [3]. In light of the risk profile and lack of efficacy, BzRA medications cannot be reasonably recommended for children and younger adolescents with insomnia.

Small trials of reversible orexin receptor antagonists (Suvorexant) have been shown to be relatively safe in adolescents (with abnormal dreams and daytime sleepiness as the most prominent side effects) [89]. More studies need to be performed to determine efficacy in this population.

An exciting newer medication available for adults with insomnia is a low dose of an old tricyclic antidepressant, Doxepin. In very low doses (3 mg or 6 mg) it can help with sleep maintenance and ensuring a quality duration of sleep, though not necessarily with sleep onset [90]. It has not been studied in pediatrics, but given its safety profile, consideration should be given to further studies of Doxepin in the adolescent population.

Gabapentin is an antiepileptic medication that is often utilized for the treatment of restless legs syndrome and periodic limb movement disorder when iron supplementation is not sufficient to control symptoms [67]. Aside from being sedating, it has been shown that Gabapentin also has an enhancing effect on slow wave sleep, the "deep sleep" so often sought after [91]. For this reason, it is also utilized for insomnia in that it can improve sleep maintenance [91]. In children with neurodevelopmental disorders, use of Gabapentin for insomnia (5 mg/kg to 15 mg/kg) has been shown to be effective in improving sleep based on parental report [92]. More studies are needed regarding Gabapentin use in typically developing children and adolescents, given its demonstrated efficacy and low risk profile [92].

Given the ability of antidepressant (Doxepin) and anticonvulsants (Gabapentin) medications to serve secondary roles of augmenting sleep, if a child is already on a medication for his or her psychological or physiological comorbidity, consideration should be given to examining the possible side effects of these medications, and assessing if they could be utilized to help promote better sleep.

Finally, while Trazodone is an antidepressant that has been used in the past for treating sleep difficulty in ill or neurodevelopmentally devastated children and adolescents [93,94], there is very little data on the efficacy or safety of this medication.

7. Conclusions & Call to Action

Adolescence is a transformative time, typified by great intellectual, physiologic, psychologic, and social changes. Insomnia deprives adolescents of the attention and cognition required to play an active role in these exciting and demanding processes. Other sleep disorders such as obstructive sleep apnea, restless legs syndrome, circadian rhythm disorders, and narcolepsy impact sleep negatively, but insomnia is more common than each of these conditions, multifactorial, and more complicated to treat [24]. Short sleep duration in the adolescent has a multitude of negative somatic, neurodevelopmental and psychological outcomes, similar to that of the adult cohorts [13,14,39]. While clear recommendations exist for treating adult insomnia with CBT-I and medication if necessary [69], treating children and adolescents is much more complex. Behavioral therapies are challenging from many angles, including gauging maturity level, respecting autonomy in patients while acknowledging parental responsibilities for decision making, as well as the paucity of sleep psychologists trained and available to provide CBT-I in younger patients [70,75]. Another layer of complexity is that a larger proportion of adolescents with physiological, psychological and developmental comorbidities report insomnia compared to the general population, and their treatment plans need to be even more individually tailored. The recent growth in the adolescent medicine and sleep medicine fields [95,96] presents an incredible opportunity to collaborate and conduct large scale analysis of adolescent sleep health, hopefully allowing us to demonstrate prevalence of insomnia among adolescents and to further analyze the predisposing, precipitating, and perpetuating factors of adolescent insomnia [70]. Perhaps the demonstration of confirmed prevalence across multiple centers, with a more rigorous exploration of the impact of poor sleep may strengthen the argument for implementation of policies such as delaying school start times. Perhaps it may simply publicize this issue and encourage more adolescents to come forward and seek treatment, or give educators/coaches/employers more credibility in suggesting to families that an adolescent may benefit from additional help. Perhaps applying systematic treatment regimens to adolescents with insomnia will allow us to standardize behavioral and pharmaceutical approaches and move towards the establishment of guidelines. One thing is clear: given the far-reaching impact of adolescent insomnia, all health practitioners who care for adolescents should remain vigilant about this important issue while making efforts to optimize their growth and development. Their future, and ours, depends on it.

Funding: This research received no external funding.

Conflicts of Interest: The authors declare no conflicts of interest.

References

1. Rasch, B.; Born, J. About sleep's role in memory. *Physiol. Rev.* **2013**, *93*, 681–766. [CrossRef] [PubMed]
2. Hall, M.H.; Smagula, S.F.; Boudreau, R.M.; Ayonayon, H.N.; Goldman, S.E.; Harris, T.B.; Naydeck, B.L.; Rubin, S.M.; Samuelsson, L.; Satterfield, S.; et al. Association between sleep duration and mortality is mediated by markers of inflammation and health in older adults: The Health, Aging and Body Composition Study. *Sleep* **2015**, *38*, 189–195. [CrossRef] [PubMed]
3. Foley, L.S.; Maddison, R.; Jiang, Y.; Marsh, S.; Olds, T.; Ridley, K. Presleep activities and time of sleep onset in children. *Pediatrics* **2013**, *131*, 276–282. [CrossRef] [PubMed]
4. Chulani, V.L.; Gordon, L.P. Adolescent growth and development. *Prim. Care* **2014**, *41*, 465–487. [CrossRef] [PubMed]
5. Henderson, E.M.; Keogh, E.; Eccleston, C. Why go online when you have pain? A qualitative analysis of teenagers' use of the Internet for pain management advice. *Child Care Health Dev.* **2014**, *40*, 572–579. [CrossRef] [PubMed]
6. Owens, J. Adolescent Sleep Working Group, Committee on Adolescence. Insufficient sleep in adolescents and young adults: An update on causes and consequences. *Pediatrics* **2014**, *134*, e921e32. [CrossRef] [PubMed]
7. Hirshkowitz, M.; Whiton, K.; Albert, S.M.; Alessi, C.; Bruni, O.; DonCarlos, L.; Hazen, N.; Herman, J.; Katz, E.S.; Kheirandish-Gozal, L.; et al. National Sleep Foundation's sleep time duration recommendations: Methodology and results summary. *Sleep Health* **2015**, *1*, 40–43. [CrossRef] [PubMed]
8. Haveman, R.; Smeeding, T. The role of higher education in social mobility. *Future Child.* **2006**, *16*, 125–150. [CrossRef] [PubMed]
9. Boergers, J.; Gable, C.J.; Owens, J.A. Later school start time is associated with improved sleep and daytime functioning in adolescents. *J. Dev. Behav. Pediatr.* **2014**, *35*, 11–17. [CrossRef] [PubMed]
10. Crowley, S.J.; Acebo, C.; Carskadon, M.A. Sleep, circadian rhythms, and delayed phase in adolescence. *Sleep Med.* **2007**, *8*, 602–612. [CrossRef] [PubMed]
11. National Sleep Foundation. *Teens and Sleep. Sleep in America Polls*; National Sleep Foundation: Washington, DC, USA, 2006; Available online: www.sleepfoundation.org/article/sleep-america-polls/2006-teens-and-sleep (accessed on 2 July 2018).
12. Arora, T.; Broglia, E.; Pushpakumar, D.; Lodhi, T.; Taheri, S. An investigation into the strength of the association and agreement levels between subjective and objective sleep duration in adolescents. *PLoS ONE* **2013**, *8*, e72406. [CrossRef] [PubMed]
13. Dewald, J.F.; Meijer, A.M.; Oort, F.J.; Kerkhof, G.A.; Bogels, S.M. The influence of sleep quality, sleep duration and sleepiness on school performance in children and adolescents: A meta-analytic review. *Sleep Med. Rev.* **2010**, *14*, 179–189. [CrossRef] [PubMed]

14. Kronholm, E.; Puusniekka, R.; Jokela, J.; Villberg, J.; Urrila, A.S.; Paunio, T.; Välimaa, R.; Tynjälä, J. Trends in self-reported sleep problems, tiredness and related school performance among Finnish adolescents from 1984 to 2011. *J. Sleep Res.* **2015**, *24*, 3–10. [CrossRef] [PubMed]

15. Siomos, K.E.; Avagianou, P.A.; Floros, G.D.; Skenteris, N.; Mouzas, O.D.; Theodorou, K.; Angelopoulos, N.V. Psychosocial correlates of insomnia in an adolescent population. *Child Psychiatry Hum. Dev.* **2010**, *41*, 262–273. [CrossRef] [PubMed]

16. Wong, M.M.; Brower, K.J.; Zucker, R.A. Sleep problems, suicidal ideation, and self-harm behaviors in adolescence. *J. Psychiatr. Res.* **2011**, *45*, 505–511. [CrossRef] [PubMed]

17. Hysing, M.; Sivertsen, B.; Stormark, K.M.; O'Connor, R.C. Sleep problems and self-harm in adolescence. *Br. J. Psychiatry* **2015**. [CrossRef] [PubMed]

18. Dautovich, N.D.; Mcnamara, J.; Williams, J.M.; Cross, N.J.; Mccrae, C.S. Tackling sleeplessness: Psychological treatment options for insomnia. *Nat. Sci. Sleep* **2010**, *2*, 23–37. [PubMed]

19. Taylor, D.J.; Zimmerman, M.R.; Gardner, C.E.; Williams, J.M.; Grieser, E.A.; Tatum, J.I.; Bramoweth, A.D.; Francetich, J.M.; Ruggero, C. A pilot randomized controlled trial of the effects of cognitive-behavioral therapy for insomnia on sleep and daytime functioning in college students. *Behav. Ther.* **2014**, *45*, 376–389. [CrossRef] [PubMed]

20. De bruin, E.J.; Oort, F.J.; Bögels, S.M.; Meijer, A.M. Efficacy of internet and group-administered cognitive behavioral therapy for insomnia in adolescents: A pilot study. *Behav. Sleep Med.* **2014**, *12*, 235–254. [CrossRef] [PubMed]

21. De bruin, E.J.; Bögels, S.M.; Oort, F.J.; Meijer, A.M. Efficacy of Cognitive Behavioral Therapy for Insomnia in Adolescents: A Randomized Controlled Trial with Internet Therapy, Group Therapy and a Waiting List Condition. *Sleep* **2015**, *38*, 1913–1926. [CrossRef] [PubMed]

22. Maski, K.P.; Kothare, S.V. Sleep deprivation and neurobehavioral functioning in children. *Int. J. Psychophysiol.* **2013**, *89*, 259–264. [CrossRef] [PubMed]

23. Combs, D.; Goodwin, J.L.; Quan, S.F.; Morgan, W.J.; Shetty, S.; Parthasarathy, S. Insomnia, Health-Related Quality of Life and Health Outcomes in Children: A Seven Year Longitudinal Cohort. *Sci. Rep.* **2016**, *6*, 27921. [CrossRef] [PubMed]

24. Hysing, M.; Pallesen, S.; Stormark, K.; Lundervold, A.; Sivertsen, B. Sleep patterns and insomnia among adolescents: A population-based study. *J. Sleep Res.* **2013**, *22*, 549–556. [CrossRef] [PubMed]

25. American Psychiatric Association. *Diagnostic and Statistical Manual of Mental Disorders*, 4th ed.; American Psychiatric Association: Washington, DC, USA, 1994.

26. American Psychiatric Association. *Diagnostic and Statistical Manual of Mental Disorders*, 5th ed.; American Psychiatric Association: Washington, DC, USA, 2013.

27. Sateia, M.J. International classification of sleep disorders-third edition: Highlights and modifications. *Chest* **2014**, *146*, 1387–1394. [CrossRef] [PubMed]

28. De zambotti, M.; Goldstone, A.; Colrain, I.M.; Baker, F.C. Insomnia disorder in adolescence: Diagnosis, impact, and treatment. *Sleep Med. Rev.* **2018**, *39*, 12–24. [CrossRef] [PubMed]

29. Krishnan, V.; Collop, N.A. Gender differences in sleep disorders. *Curr. Opin. Pulm. Med.* **2006**, *12*, 383–389. [CrossRef] [PubMed]

30. Magee, M.; Marbas, E.M.; Wright, K.P.; Rajaratnam, S.M.; Broussard, J.L. Diagnosis, Cause, and Treatment Approaches for Delayed Sleep-Wake Phase Disorder. *Sleep Med. Clin.* **2016**, *11*, 389–401. [CrossRef] [PubMed]

31. Thorpy, M.J. Classification of sleep disorders. *Neurotherapeutics* **2012**, *9*, 687–701. [CrossRef] [PubMed]

32. Gradisar, M.; Crowley, S.J. Delayed sleep phase disorder in youth. *Curr. Opin. Psychiatry* **2013**, *26*, 580–585. [CrossRef] [PubMed]

33. Patke, A.; Murphy, P.J.; Onat, O.E.; Krieger, A.C.; Özçelik, T.; Campbell, S.S.; Young, M.W. Mutation of the Human Circadian Clock Gene CRY1 in Familial Delayed Sleep Phase Disorder. *Cell* **2017**, *169*, 203–215. [CrossRef] [PubMed]

34. Von Schantz, M. Natural Variation in Human Clocks. *Adv. Genet.* **2017**, *99*, 73–96. [PubMed]

35. Borbély, A.A.; Daan, S.; Wirz-justice, A.; Deboer, T. The two-process model of sleep regulation: A reappraisal. *J. Sleep Res.* **2016**, *25*, 131–143. [CrossRef] [PubMed]

36. Richardson, C.; Cain, N.; Bartel, K.; Micic, G.; Maddock, B.; Gradisar, M. A randomised controlled trial of bright light therapy and morning activity for adolescents and young adults with Delayed Sleep-Wake Phase Disorder. *Sleep Med.* **2018**, *45*, 114–123. [CrossRef] [PubMed]

37. Sletten, T.L.; Magee, M.; Murray, J.M.; Gordon, C.J.; Lovato, N.; Kennaway, D.J.; Gwini, S.M.; Bartlett, D.J.; Lockley, S.W.; Lack, L.C.; et al. Efficacy of melatonin with behavioural sleep-wake scheduling for delayed sleep-wake phase disorder: A. double-blind, randomised clinical trial. *PLoS Med.* **2018**, *15*, e1002587. [CrossRef] [PubMed]

38. Castro-faúndez, J.; Díaz, J.; Ocampo-garcés, A. Temporal Organization of the Sleep-Wake Cycle under Food Entrainment in the Rat. *Sleep* **2016**, *39*, 1451–1465. [CrossRef] [PubMed]

39. Buysse, D.J. Sleep health: Can we define it? Does it matter? *Sleep* **2014**, *37*, 9–17. [CrossRef] [PubMed]

40. Fatima, Y.; Doi, S.A.; Mamun, A.A. Longitudinal impact of sleep on overweight and obesity in children and adolescents: A systematic review and bias-adjusted meta-analysis. *Obes. Rev.* **2015**, *16*, 137–149. [CrossRef] [PubMed]

41. Navarro-Solera, M.; Carrasco-Luna, J.; Pin-Arboledas, G.; González-Carrascosa, R.; Soriano, J.M.; Codoñer-Franch, P. Short Sleep Duration Is Related to Emerging Cardiovascular Risk Factors in Obese Children. *J. Pediatr. Gastroenterol. Nutr.* **2015**, *61*, 571–576. [CrossRef] [PubMed]

42. Kuciene, R.; Dulskiene, V. Associations of short sleep duration with prehypertension and hypertension among Lithuanian children and adolescents: A cross-sectional study. *BMC Public Health* **2014**, *14*, 255. [CrossRef] [PubMed]

43. Mmari, K.; Marshall, B.; Hsu, T.; Shon, J.W.; Eguavoen, A. A mixed methods study to examine the influence of the neighborhood social context on adolescent health service utilization. *BMC Health Serv. Res.* **2016**, *16*, 433. [CrossRef] [PubMed]

44. Blake, M.J.; Trinder, J.A.; Allen, N.B. Mechanisms underlying the association between insomnia, anxiety, and depression in adolescence: Implications for behavioral sleep interventions. *Clin. Psychol. Rev.* **2018**, *63*, 25–40. [CrossRef] [PubMed]

45. Lovato, N.; Gradisar, M.; Short, M.; Dohnt, H.; Micic, G. Delayed sleep phase disorder in an Australian school-based sample of adolescents. *J. Clin. Sleep Med.* **2013**, *9*, 939–944. [CrossRef] [PubMed]

46. McMakin, D.L.; Alfano, C.A. Sleep and anxiety in late childhood and early adolescence. *Curr. Opin. Psychiatry* **2015**, *28*, 483–489. [CrossRef] [PubMed]

47. Bauducco, S.V.; Tillfors, M.; Özdemir, M.; Flink, I.K.; Linton, S.J. Too tired for school? The effects of insomnia on absenteeism in adolescence. *Sleep Health* **2015**, *1*, 205–210. [CrossRef] [PubMed]

48. Liang, Y.; Horrey, W.J.; Howard, M.E.; Lee, M.L.; Anderson, C.; Shreeve, M.S.; O'Brien, C.S.; Czeisler, C.A. Prediction of drowsiness events in night shift workers during morning driving. *Accid. Anal. Prev.* **2017**. [CrossRef] [PubMed]

49. Adolescent Sleep Working Group; Committee on Adolescence; Council on School Health. School start times for adolescents. *Pediatrics* **2014**, *134*, 642–649. [CrossRef] [PubMed]

50. Watson, N.F.; Martin, J.L.; Wise, M.S.; Carden, K.A.; Kirsch, D.B.; Kristo, D.A.; Malhotra, R.K.; Olson, E.J.; Ramar, K.; Rosen, I.M.; et al. Delaying Middle School and High School Start Times Promotes Student Health and Performance: An American Academy of Sleep Medicine Position Statement. *J. Clin. Sleep Med.* **2017**, *13*, 623–625. [CrossRef] [PubMed]

51. Hiscock, H.; Sciberras, E.; Mensah, F.; Gerner, B.; Efron, D.; Khano, S.; Oberklaid, F. Impact of a behavioural sleep intervention on symptoms and sleep in children with attention deficit hyperactivity disorder, and parental mental health: Randomised controlled trial. *BMJ* **2015**, *350*, 1–14. [CrossRef] [PubMed]

52. Lichstein, K.L.; Justin Thomas, S.; Woosley, J.A.; Geyer, J.D. Co-occurring insomnia and obstructive sleep apnea. *Sleep Med.* **2013**, *14*, 824–829. [CrossRef] [PubMed]

53. Fernandez-Mendoza, J.; Li, Y.; Vgontzas, A.N.; Fang, J.; Gaines, J.; Calhoun, S.L.; Liao, D.; Bixler, E.O. Insomnia is associated with cortical hyperarousal as early as adolescence. *Sleep* **2016**, *39*, 1029–1036. [CrossRef] [PubMed]

54. Rigney, G.; Ali, N.S.; Corkum, P.V.; Brown, C.A.; Constantin, E.; Godbout, R.; Hanlon-Dearman, A.; Ipsiroglu, O.; Reid, G.J.; Shea, S.; et al. A systematic review to explore the feasibility of a behavioural sleep intervention for insomnia in children with neurodevelopmental disorders: A transdiagnostic approach. *Sleep Med. Rev.* **2018**. [CrossRef] [PubMed]

55. Wang, Y.; Raffeld, M.R.; Slopen, N.; Hale, L.; Dunn, E.C. Childhood adversity and insomnia in adolescence. *Sleep Med.* **2016**, *21*, 12–18. [CrossRef] [PubMed]

56. Meltzer, L.J.; Mindell, J.A. Systematic review and meta-analysis of behavioral interventions for pediatric insomnia. *J. Pediatr. Psychol.* **2014**, *39*, 932–948. [CrossRef] [PubMed]

57. Stojanovski, S.D.; Rasu, R.S.; Balkrishnan, R.; Nahata, M.C. Trends in medication prescribing for pediatric sleep difficulties in US outpatient settings. *Sleep* **2007**, *30*, 1013–1017. [CrossRef] [PubMed]

58. Pelayo, R.; Yuen, K. Pediatric sleep pharmacology. *Child Adolesc. Psychiatr. Clin. N. Am.* **2012**, *21*, 861–883. [CrossRef] [PubMed]

59. Kanstrup, M.; Holmström, L.; Ringström, R.; Wicksell, R.K. Insomnia in paediatric chronic pain and its impact on depression and functional disability. *Eur. J. Pain* **2014**, *18*, 1094–1102. [CrossRef] [PubMed]

60. Zhou, E.S.; Recklitis, C.J. Insomnia in adult survivors of childhood cancer: A report from project REACH. *Support. Care Cancer* **2014**, *22*, 3061–3069. [CrossRef] [PubMed]

61. Hankins, J.S.; Verevkina, N.I.; Smeltzer, M.P.; Wu, S.; Aygun, B.; Clarke, D.F. Assessment of sleep-related disorders in children with sickle cell disease. *Hemoglobin* **2014**, *38*, 244–251. [CrossRef] [PubMed]

62. Umlauf, M.G.; Bolland, A.C.; Bolland, K.A.; Tomek, S.; Bolland, J.M. The effects of age, gender, hopelessness, and exposure to violence on sleep disorder symptoms and daytime sleepiness among adolescents in impoverished neighborhoods. *J. Youth Adolesc.* **2015**, *44*, 518–542. [CrossRef] [PubMed]

63. Arns, M.; Conners, C.K.; Kraemer, H.C. A decade of EEG Theta/Beta Ratio Research in ADHD: A meta-analysis. *J. Atten. Disord.* **2013**, *17*, 374–383. [CrossRef] [PubMed]

64. Corlateanu, A.; Pylchenko, S.; Sircu, V.; Botnaru, V. Predictors of daytime sleepiness in patients with obstructive sleep apnea. *Pneumologia* **2015**, *64*, 21–25. [PubMed]

65. Schwengel, D.A.; Dalesio, N.M.; Stierer, T.L. Pediatric obstructive sleep apnea. *Anesthesiol. Clin.* **2014**, *32*, 237–261. [CrossRef] [PubMed]

66. Barnes, M.E.; Gozal, D.; Molfese, D.L. Attention in children with obstructive sleep apnoea: An event-related potentials study. *Sleep Med.* **2012**, *13*, 368–377. [CrossRef] [PubMed]

67. Venkateshiah, S.B.; Ioachimescu, O.C. Restless legs syndrome. *Crit. Care Clin.* **2015**, *31*, 459–472. [CrossRef] [PubMed]

68. Morgenthaler, T.; Kramer, M.; Alessi, C.; Friedman, L.; Boehlecke, B.; Brown, T.; Coleman, J.; Kapur, V.; Lee-Chiong, T.; Owens, J.; et al. Practice parameters for the psychological and behavioral treatment of insomnia: An update. An American academy of sleep medicine report. *Sleep* **2006**, *29*, 1415–1419. [PubMed]

69. Sateia, M.J.; Buysse, D.J.; Krystal, A.D.; Neubauer, D.N.; Heald, J.L. Clinical Practice Guideline for the Pharmacologic Treatment of Chronic Insomnia in Adults: An American Academy of Sleep Medicine Clinical Practice Guideline. *J. Clin. Sleep Med.* **2017**, *13*, 307–349. [CrossRef] [PubMed]

70. Williams, J.; Roth, A.; Vatthauer, K.; Mccrae, C.S. Cognitive behavioral treatment of insomnia. *Chest* **2013**, *143*, 554–565. [CrossRef] [PubMed]

71. Mitchell, M.D.; Gehrman, P.; Perlis, M.; Umscheid, C.A. Comparative effectiveness of cognitive behavioral therapy for insomnia: A systematic review. *BMC Fam. Pract.* **2012**, *13*, 40. [CrossRef] [PubMed]

72. Ma, Z.R.; Shi, L.J.; Deng, M.H. Efficacy of cognitive behavioral therapy in children and adolescents with insomnia: A systematic review and meta-analysis. *Braz. J. Med. Biol. Res.* **2018**, *51*, e7070. [CrossRef] [PubMed]

73. Blake, M.J.; Sheeber, L.B.; Youssef, G.J.; Raniti, M.B.; Allen, N.B. Systematic Review and Meta-analysis of Adolescent Cognitive-Behavioral Sleep Interventions. *Clin. Child Fam. Psychol. Rev.* **2017**, *20*, 227–249. [CrossRef] [PubMed]

74. De bruin, E.J.; Bögels, S.M.; Oort, F.J.; Meijer, A.M. Improvements of adolescent psychopathology after insomnia treatment: Results from a randomized controlled trial over 1 year. *J. Child Psychol. Psychiatry* **2018**, *59*, 509–522. [CrossRef] [PubMed]

75. Gradisar, M.; Richardson, C. CBT-I Cannot Rest Until the Sleepy Teen Can. *Sleep* **2015**, *38*, 1841–1842. [CrossRef] [PubMed]

76. Van der Heijden, K.B.; Smits, M.G.; Van Someren, E.J.; Ridderinkhof, K.R.; Gunning, W.B. Effect of melatonin on sleep, behavior, and cognition in ADHD and chronic sleep-onset insomnia. *J. Am. Acad. Child Adolesc. Psychiatry* **2007**, *46*, 233–241. [CrossRef] [PubMed]

77. Wrojanan, J.; Jacquemont, S.; Diaz, R.; Bacalman, S.; Anders, T.F.; Hagerman, R.J.; Goodlin-Jones, B.L. The efficacy of melatonin for sleep problems in children with autism, fragile X syndrome, or autism and fragile X syndrome. *J. Clin. Sleep Med.* **2009**, *5*, 145–150.

78. Hoebert, M.; van der Heijden, K.B.; van Geijlswijk, I.M.; Smits, M.G. Long-term follow-up of melatonin treatment in children with ADHD and chronic sleep onset insomnia. *J. Pineal. Res.* **2009**, *47*, 1–7. [CrossRef] [PubMed]

79. Stigler, K.A.; Posey, D.J.; McDougle, C.J. Ramelteon for insomnia in two youths with autistic disorder. *J. Child Adolesc. Psychopharmacol.* **2006**, *16*, 631–636. [CrossRef] [PubMed]

80. Efron, D.; Lycett, K.; Sciberras, E. Use of sleep medication in children with ADHD. *Sleep Med.* **2014**, *15*, 472–475. [CrossRef] [PubMed]

81. Levy, H.B. Non-benzodiazepine hypnotics and older adults: What are we learning about zolpidem? *Expert Rev. Clin. Pharmacol.* **2014**, *7*, 5–8. [CrossRef] [PubMed]

82. Roehrs, T.; Roth, T. Insomnia pharmacotherapy. *Neurotherapeutics* **2012**, *9*, 728–738. [CrossRef] [PubMed]

83. Macfarlane, J.; Morin, C.M.; Montplaisir, J. Hypnotics in insomnia: The experience of zolpidem. *Clin. Ther.* **2014**, *36*, 1676–1701. [CrossRef] [PubMed]

84. Chen, Y.W.; Tseng, P.T.; Wu, C.K.; Chen, C.C. Zaleplon-induced Anemsic Somnambulism with Eating Behaviors under Once Dose. *Acta Neurol. Taiwan* **2014**, *23*, 143–145. [PubMed]

85. Pennington, J.G.; Guina, J. Eszopiclone-induced Parasomnia with Suicide Attempt: A Case Report. *Innov. Clin. Neurosci.* **2016**, *13*, 44–48. [PubMed]

86. Stockmann, C.; Gottschlich, M.M.; Healy, D.; Khoury, J.C.; Mayes, T.; Sherwin, C.M.; Spigarelli, M.G.; Kagan, R.J. Relationship between zolpidem concentrations and sleep parameters in pediatric burn patients. *J. Burn. Care Res.* **2015**, *36*, 137–144. [CrossRef] [PubMed]

87. Blumer, J.L.; Findling, R.L.; Shih, W.J.; Soubrane, C.; Reed, M.D. Controlled clinical trial of zolpidem for the treatment of insomnia associated with attention-deficit/hyperactivity disorder in children 6 to 17 years of age. *Pediatrics* **2009**, *123*, e770–e776. [CrossRef] [PubMed]

88. Ford, J.A.; Mccutcheon, J. The misuse of Ambien among adolescents: Prevalence and correlates in a national sample. *Addict. Behav.* **2012**, *37*, 1389–1394. [CrossRef] [PubMed]

89. Kawabe, K.; Horiuchi, F.; Ochi, M.; Nishimoto, K.; Ueno, S.I.; Oka, Y. Suvorexant for the Treatment of Insomnia in Adolescents. *J. Child Adolesc. Psychopharmacol.* **2017**, *27*, 792–795. [CrossRef] [PubMed]

90. Yeung, W.F.; Chung, K.F.; Yung, K.P.; Ng, T.H. Doxepin for insomnia: A systematic review of randomized placebo-controlled trials. *Sleep Med. Rev.* **2015**, *19*, 75–83. [CrossRef] [PubMed]

91. Lo, H.S.; Yang, C.M.; Lo, H.G.; Lee, C.Y.; Ting, H.; Tzang, B.S. Treatment effects of gabapentin for primary insomnia. *Clin. Neuropharmacol.* **2010**, *33*, 84–90. [CrossRef] [PubMed]

92. Robinson, A.A.; Malow, B.A. Gabapentin shows promise in treating refractory insomnia in children. *J. Child Neurol.* **2013**, *28*, 1618–1621. [CrossRef] [PubMed]

93. Bursch, B.; Forgey, M. Psychopharmacology for medically ill adolescents. *Curr. Psychiatry Rep.* **2013**, *15*, 395. [CrossRef] [PubMed]

94. Owens, J.A.; Rosen, C.L.; Mindell, J.A.; Kirchner, H.L. Use of pharmacotherapy for insomnia in child psychiatry practice: A national survey. *Sleep Med.* **2010**, *11*, 692–700. [CrossRef] [PubMed]

95. Hergenroeder, A.C.; Benson, P.A.; Britto, M.T.; Catallozzi, M.; D'Angelo, L.J.; Edman, J.C.; Emans, S.J.; Kish, E.C.; Pasternak, R.H.; Slap, G.B. Adolescent medicine: Workforce trends and recommendations. *Arch. Pediatr. Adolesc. Med.* **2010**, *164*, 1086–1090. [CrossRef] [PubMed]

96. The Match, National Resident Matching Program. Results and Data. 2018 Appointment Year. Available online: http://www.nrmp.org/wp-content/uploads/2018/02/Results-and-Data-SMS-2018.pdf (accessed on 2 July 2018).

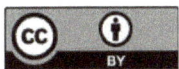

medical sciences

MDPI

Review

Sleep Disturbances in Child and Adolescent Mental Health Disorders: A Review of the Variability of Objective Sleep Markers

Suman K. R. Baddam [1,*], Craig A. Canapari [2], Stefon J. R. van Noordt [1] and Michael J. Crowley [1]

[1]   Yale Child Study Center, Yale School of Medicine, New Haven, CT 06510, USA;
     stefonv0@gmail.com (S.J.R.v.N.); Michael.Crowley@yale.edu (M.J.C.)
[2]   Division of Pulmonary Medicine, Department of Pediatrics, Yale School of Medicine,
     New Haven, CT 06510, USA; craig.canapari@yale.edu
*   Correspondence: suman.baddam@yale.edu; Tel.: +1-210-296-8283

Received: 25 March 2018; Accepted: 29 May 2018; Published: 4 June 2018

Abstract: Sleep disturbances are often observed in child and adolescent mental health disorders. Although previous research has identified consistent subjective reports of sleep disturbances, specific objective sleep markers have not yet been identified. We evaluated the current research on subjective and objective sleep markers in relation to attention deficit hyperactivity disorders, autism spectrum disorders, anxiety and depressive disorders. Subjective sleep markers are more consistent than objective markers of actigraphy, polysomnography, and circadian measures. We discuss the causes of variability in objective sleep findings and suggest future directions for research.

Keywords: sleep; mental health; electroencephalography (EEG); children; adolescents; Attention Deficit Hyperactivity Disorder (ADHD); anxiety; autism; arousal

1. Introduction

Significant neurobiological, physiological, and social changes occur during childhood and adolescence [1,2], including changes in circadian and sleep systems that regulate sleep duration and timing [3]. The duration of sleep decreases as development progresses, from about 14.5 h at 6 months of age to 8 h at age 16 years [4]. Other macrostructural changes, including changes in sleep stages, sleep architecture, and sleep efficiency, occur during childhood and adolescence [5]. Also, circadian changes, such as a shift toward later circadian chronotype and evening-type sleep patterns, emerge in adolescence [6]. These changes in sleep patterns across development, especially in the context of mental health problems, can be difficult for some youth.

Along with changes in sleep patterns, many youth develop mental health disorders in childhood and adolescence [7]. Attention Deficit Hyperactivity Disorder (ADHD) (8.6%), mood disorders (3.7%) [8], and autism spectrum disorders (0.7%) (ASD) [9] are common mental health problems in children that show an onset in early childhood [10]. In adolescents, common mental health issues include anxiety disorders (31.9%), behavior disorders (19.1%), mood disorders (14.3%), and substance use disorders (11.4%) [11]. Further, child and adolescent mental health disorders are characterized by significant comorbidity with a wide range of severity [8,11,12].

Sleep difficulties in youth with mental health problems are common, including increased sleep latency, nocturnal awakenings, nightmares, snoring, restless sleep, excessive daytime sleepiness, bedtime struggles, and fear of dark [13]. Sleep problems are known to have complex bidirectional relationships with childhood psychiatric disorders [14]. Historically, the evidence linking subjective sleep reports with reliable objective sleep markers in youth with mental health disorders has been inconsistent. Although youth with anxiety, depression, ADHD, or ASD often report subjective sleep disturbances [15–17], there is a paucity of evidence on reliable objective markers of sleep in pediatric mental health disorders [17,18]. An earlier meta-analysis of children with ADHD identified sleep onset difficulties, bedtime resistance and difficulty with waking up in morning on subjective reports, high sleep onset latency and true sleep on actigraphy, and low sleep efficiency on polysomnography [19]. However, a recent meta-analysis only identified high percentage of stage 1 sleep as the significant finding in children with ADHD [20]. In major depressive disorder (MDD), a systematic analysis identified decreased sleep onset latency and rapid eye movement (REM) abnormalities as reliable sleep findings [21]. Objective sleep markers such as REM abnormalities, prolonged sleep onset latency, sleep fragmentation, and reduced sleep efficiency were identified in some studies of pediatric mental health disorders. However, several other studies have not shown any differences in objective sleep markers between children with mental health disturbances and healthy controls [22].

Herein, we review the literature on objective markers of sleep disturbances in the context of youth mental health disorders. We focused on current research studies and literature predominantly published during the last decade which includes objective measurements of sleep (polysomnography (PSG) or actigraphy) or circadian rhythms. Specifically, we examined studies in children and adolescents with anxiety disorders, depressive disorders, ADHD, and ASD diagnosed by diagnostic and statistical manual of mental disorders (DSM) criteria. We excluded studies of children with primary sleep disorders. From the selected studies, we identified objective sleep markers and their associations with subjective reports of sleep disturbances.

2. Objective and Subjective Markers of Sleep Disturbances

Objective markers of sleep disturbances include measurements by PSG, actigraphy, and measures of circadian biology. Polysomnography, the most widely used and validated standard for the evaluation of sleep, is a multi-modal instrument which assesses a range of physiological changes in electroencephalography (EEG), respiration, and heart rate [23], with an established scoring method to identify macrostructural sleep characteristics [24,25]. Actigraphy, a wrist-based instrument that measures movement by an accelerometer, is another reliable tool for measuring sleep and wake rhythms [23,26]. Circadian rhythms are assessed using laboratory-based protocols [27], including assessment of melatonin and cortisol [28]. Arousals from sleep, defined as behavioral awakenings, an abrupt shift in the EEG frequency and desynchronization of EEG [29], have been examined in research studies as markers of sleep instability. Brief arousals from sleep, referred to as microarousals and cyclic alternating patterns, are used as markers of sleep disturbances [30,31] whereas subjective sleep patterns are assessed from several instruments including Children's Sleep Habits Questionnaire [32], Adolescent Sleep-Wake Scale, Sleep Disturbances Scale for Children, Sleep Self-report, School Sleep Habits Survey [33], and sleep diaries.

2.1. Sleep in Anxiety and Depressive Disorders

Subjectively, parents of children with generalized anxiety disorder (GAD) report resistance to bedtime, delay in sleep onset, short sleep duration, high anxiety before sleep, and daytime sleepiness [34]. Similarly, adolescents with anxiety have high bedtime worries/fears, insomnia symptoms, daytime sleepiness on self-reports and high sleep onset latency, total sleep time and wake after sleep onset duration, and low sleep efficiency on sleep diaries [35]. In depression, children and adolescents typically report insomnia and, in some cases, hypersomnia, with severe depression associated with comorbid insomnia and hypersomnia [15]. In MDD, sleep diaries indicate subjective sleep complaints such as long sleep latency, a high number of awakenings, and high wake after sleep onset, although, these subjective reports are less common than in anxious children and adolescents [36]. Gender differences emerged in depression with females showing greater numbers of sleep complaints than males [15].

Recent actigraphy studies did not reveal any differences between children with GAD and healthy controls, despite reported subjective sleep disturbances [34]. However, a recent study in adolescents with GAD showed long sleep onset latencies, but unexpectedly greater sleep duration, compared to typically developing children [35]. Few studies have examined sleep patterns of children and adolescents with depression using actigraphy. Adolescent males with depression showed a shift toward later circadian phases from weekdays to weekends [37]. Short sleep duration and lower sleep efficiency were identified in adolescents with the seasonal affective disorder, a variant of depressive disorder [38].

Polysomnography in anxiety disorders showed reduced latency to REM [39], high sleep onset latency in children [36,39], low sleep efficiency and a high number of sleep arousals compared to controls. In multiple night PSG, youth with an anxiety disorder had greater sleep onset latency on the first night compared to the second night [36]. At-home PSG, in contrast to in-lab PSG, showed children with GAD had high sleep efficiency and fewer REM periods. The authors explained that children with anxiety had high bedtime resistance at home and went to bed later, which led to high sleep efficiency (from decreased sleep onset latency and decreased wake after sleep onset) [40]. In depression, low sleep efficiency, low proportion of slow wave sleep, and a high number of arousals have been observed [41] along with decreased total sleep time [42]. Interestingly, the dissipation of slow wave activity was slower and flatter [42], suggesting differences in the homeostatic dissipation of sleep pressure in children with depression. However, in the PSG study by Forbes et al., no differences were observed in depression when compared to healthy controls [36].

Lower nighttime cortisol, a marker of circadian and arousal differences, was observed in prepubertal children with anxiety [43], but no differences were observed in adolescents [44] or MDD [43]. However, adolescents with depression show higher peri sleep onset cortisol than healthy controls [44]. Additionally, arousal assessed in anxiety disorders showed pre-sleep arousal levels correlated with objective sleep findings—with pre-sleep somatic and cognitive arousal negatively correlated with REM sleep and total sleep time, respectively [40].

Eveningness chronotype assessed by chronotype questionnaires was consistently high in children with depression [45] and adolescent males [37] and was associated with the earlier development of depression symptoms [46] and circadian phase delay [47]. Later chronotype and social jetlag were observed in adolescent females with the seasonal affective disorder [38]. Circadian period, as measured by actigraphy, was found to be high in male and low in female children and adolescents with depression, in combination with low circadian amplitude [48].

2.2. Summary of Sleep in Anxiety and Depressive Disorders

In summary, children and adolescents with anxiety disorders show reliable subjective reports of greater sleep onset latency, bedtime fears, and greater wake after sleep onset duration [34,36]. Interestingly, findings on actigraphy do not show differences in sleep in children [34] but show high sleep onset latency and high sleep duration in adolescents with anxiety when compared to healthy controls [35]. PSG results corresponded with the findings of increased sleep onset latency, low sleep efficiency, and low slow wave sleep in anxiety and depression [36,41]. However, in a comparative study, sleep findings on PSG (sleep onset latency, sleep duration, sleep efficiency) were significantly greater in anxiety than depression and healthy controls, but similar in youth with depression and healthy controls [36]. Sleep efficiency was also inconsistent when assessed by PSG conducted at home versus the laboratory [34,40]. Cortisol level separated in some studies but not in others [43,44]. Chronotype differences, such as evening chronotype, phase delay, and social jet lag were consistently present in children and adolescents with depression [37,45,46]. The sleep findings of individual anxiety and depressive disorder studies are presented in Table A1 (Appendix A).

2.2.1. Sleep in Attention Deficit Hyperactivity Disorder

In children with ADHD, subjective reports indicate a wide range of sleep problems, including difficulty with sleep onset, daytime sleepiness [49–56], anxiety prior to sleep [50,53,55,57], high severity of insomnia [50,53,55,56], high awakenings at night [50,51,53,56], difficulty waking up, less refreshing sleep [54], insufficient sleep [57], resistance to bedtime [51], and restless sleep [55]. However, a study by Mullin et al. identified no differences in subjective reports of sleep on sleep diary measures [58].

On actigraphy, children with ADHD have been identified to take longer to fall asleep [52,53,59], have lower sleep efficiency, lower sleep time [53,54], greater sleep fragmentation [59], and a high wake after sleep onset duration [59]. Greater day-to-day variability in sleep onset is present in youth with ADHD when compared to children with other psychiatric disorders and healthy controls [52]. However, sleep findings in actigraphy were not significantly different in other studies comparing children [60] and adolescents [58] with ADHD to healthy controls.

In-home PSG has shown that children with ADHD have short sleep duration, short REM sleep, a smaller percentage of REM sleep, and longer sleep onset latency [57]. However, in-lab studies of children with ADHD compared to healthy controls show greater REM duration [56,61], sleep period [61], and REM latency [49], as well as shorter total sleep time and less sleep in stage 1 and stage 3 [56]. These contrasting results are worth considering as no significant differences were present in other studies measuring overnight PSG [50,55,62] or Multiple Sleep Latency Test (MSLT—an objective assessment of sleepiness conducted with multiple naps during the day using EEG) [55]. High microarousals with increased motor activity during light and REM sleep was present in children with ADHD [63]. Cyclic alternating patterns, a marker of sleep instability and arousal, were found to be lower in children with ADHD, suggesting a state of hypoarousal in ADHD [49,64]. However, others have reported no differences in cyclic alternating patterns [62].

Cortisol levels vary across the day in children with ADHD, being lower in the morning and higher in the evening [65]. One study showed high urinary melatonin levels in children with ADHD [66], whereas another study did not show any differences in the melatonin levels in children with ADHD compared to typically developing children [67]. However, later melatonin onset at bedtime and earlier melatonin offset were present in children with ADHD [67]. Evening chronotype in children with ADHD was associated with resistance to bedtime [68] and delayed melatonin onset [69].

2.2.2. Summary of Sleep in Attention Deficit Hyperactivity Disorder

Overall, children with ADHD subjectively report sleep onset difficulties, daytime sleepiness, anxiety before sleep, and awakenings at night [50,53,55,57], corroborated on actigraphy by increased sleep onset latency, lower sleep time, and lower sleep efficiency [52,53,59]. However, at least one study did not find any differences between ADHD and typically developing children on actigraphy [58]. In PSG, longer sleep onset latency and shorter sleep duration were observed along with REM abnormalities in youth with ADHD [49,51,57]. In-lab vs. home PSG produced variable REM findings [57,61], whereas multiple studies did not identify objective sleep differences in PSG between youth with ADHD and healthy controls [50,55,62]. High melatonin and cortisol were identified [65,66], but the differences were not replicated in other studies [67]. Evening chronotype was common in ADHD and associated with resistance to bedtime [68,70]. The sleep findings of ADHD studies are presented in Table A2 (Appendix A).

2.3. Sleep in Autism Spectrum Disorders

Subjective reports of sleep in children with ASD include long mean sleep latency [71–73], short sleep duration, high nighttime awakenings, anxiety before sleep, and bedtime resistance [73]. Low functioning children with ASD are reported to have more severe sleep disturbances, including more frequent night awakenings, greater bedtime resistance, delay in sleep onset, later bedtimes and wake times, and less sleep than high functioning children with ASD [74]. However, a recent study did not find differences between typically developing children and children with ASD in subjective reports of sleep [72].

On actigraphy, preschool, school-aged children, and adolescents with ASD confirmed the subjective sleep findings, with long sleep latency, decreased sleep duration, and increased wake after sleep onset duration [73,75]. Other findings include low sleep efficiency in children [71,73,76] and adolescents [77] with ASD. Recent work also showed greater night-to-night variability in wake time, wake after sleep onset periods, and sleep efficiency in children with ASD [78], whereas greater variability in sleep onset latency has been reported in high functioning adolescents with ASD [76].

Polysomnography findings show short total sleep time, short REM latency [79], long sleep onset latency, less slow-wave sleep, low microarousals, and more sleep-wake transitions in children with ASD compared to typically developing children [72]. Low proportion of slow wave sleep and light sleep (high arousals) have been associated with high repetitive behaviors and poor social behaviors and intellectual measures [72]. Severe autism was linked to more pronounced sleep abnormalities with high sleep onset latency, high wake after sleep onset duration, low total sleep time, low slow wave sleep, and prolonged REM latency. Cyclic alternating patterns, the marker of arousal and sleep instability measured by visual inspection of sleep EEG, are greater among children with regressive autism compared to non-regressed children with autism and typically developing children [74]. Poor sleepers in autism have more affective problems, fewer social interactions, and longer sleep latency [80]. Moreover, youth with ASD also show low sleep efficiency, low sleep duration, and high variability in sleep latency from night 1 to 2 [80].

High salivary cortisol and overall blunted cortisol rhythms were identified in children with autism, with higher cortisol levels associated with severe symptoms of autism [81]. Melatonin secretion rate has been found to decrease in prepubertal children with autism [82], but not in adolescents [77]. Other studies did not identify differences in measures of cortisol or melatonin in children [83] or adolescents with autism [77].

2.4. Summary of Sleep in Autism Spectrum Disorders

Collectively, children and adolescents with autism commonly have reports of longer sleep latency, short sleep duration, and high resistance to bedtime on subjective measures [71,73]. Actigraphy validates the subjective findings of long sleep latency and short sleep time along with low sleep efficiency [71,73,77]. The PSG findings consisted of short total sleep time, short REM latency, low sleep efficiency, and low slow wave sleep [72,74,79], with severe autism associated with more severe sleep abnormalities as well as cyclic alternating patterns [72,74]. Melatonin and cortisol abnormalities were identified in children with autism but were not identified in adolescents [77,81,82]. The findings in actigraphy, PSG, and circadian measures were not consistently identified across studies. The sleep findings of autism spectrum disorder studies are presented in Table A3 (Appendix A).

3. Discussion

The goal of this review was to identify objective sleep characteristics associated with mental health disorders in children and adolescents. Collectively, the findings highlight that subjective reports of sleep problems are common in mental health disorders but do not necessarily coincide with reliable objective markers of sleep disturbances measured by actigraphy and PSG. High sleep onset latency, short sleep duration, and resistance to bedtime were commonly present in subjective measures of anxiety, ADHD, and ASD across diagnostic categories [34,35,49,57,72,73]. Although actigraphy showed high sleep onset latency [35,53,59], low sleep efficiency, and shorter sleep duration in ADHD and autism [71,73,75], these findings were not specific for a single disorder. Similarly, PSG showed long sleep onset latency, low sleep efficiency and low slow wave sleep as the common objective findings in autism [72,74,79], ADHD [56,57], anxiety, and depression [36,41], but were not specific for individual disorders and also varied across studies. However, severe autism was associated with more abnormal sleep findings [72,74,80]. The location of the study (at home vs. in-lab PSG) also produced variable findings in anxiety [34,40] and ADHD [57,61], and sleep findings also varied on multi-night PSG assessments [36,55]. Overall, specific macrostructural findings in mental health disorders were not identified. Nonspecificity of objective sleep findings in child and adolescent mental health disorders have been documented in the literature [13,14].

The overlapping objective sleep findings observed across child and adolescent mental health disorders suggest possible common sleep mechanisms. Child and adolescent mental health disorders often present with high rates of comorbidity [8,11]. When controlling for comorbid psychiatric symptoms, objective sleep markers show little differentiation in a study of sleep markers in ADHD [53]. In another study comparing diagnostic categories, child and adolescent psychiatric symptoms did not vary in sleep and cortisol measures [84], highlighting possible common pathways to objective sleep markers. However, severe mental health symptoms [72,74] and the presence of multiple comorbid mental health disorders have been associated with greater objective sleep disturbances [41]. Also, mental health symptoms, especially anxiety, present as temporary state and stable trait characteristics [85], both of which are known to affect sleep and cortisol measures [78,83] differentially. Delineating state and trait characteristics in mental health may be important for identifying sleep pathology. Considering the heterogeneity of state-trait characteristics and common sleep findings across diagnostic categories, identifying specific biobehavioral phenotypes based on biological phenotypes (such as attention, arousal, motivation) could assist with mapping reliable objective sleep markers across disorders and diagnostic categories [86,87].

Reliable macrostructural sleep findings have consistently eluded child and adolescent mental health disorders. Technical and methodological characteristics of actigraphy and PSG should be acknowledged when evaluating the findings of objective sleep markers. Actigraphy may overestimate sleep [88] during periods of inactivity. In actigraphy, greater night-to-night variability is found in ADHD [52,89] and autism [76,78], hence, an extended duration of measurement is needed to identify reliable results. Similarly, night-to-night variability is identified in PSG studies [90]. Therefore, single night PSG, commonly used in research studies [49,50,56,72,91], may be insufficient for identifying objective findings because of "first night effect". Sleep findings often are different on the first night of sleep in the lab because of novel sleeping environment. "First night effect", associated with high sleep latency, has been identified in children with ADHD [55,92] and autism [80] on multi-night studies. Given that sleep efficiency increases and wake after sleep onset decreases on the second night [93], multiple nights of PSG may be necessary to identify reliable objective differences in sleep [94]. The location of the sleep study (home vs. in-lab PSG) produces varying sleep findings in youth with anxiety [39,40] and ADHD [49,57], suggesting sleep environment moderates sleep phenotypes. The macrostructural characteristics of sleep identified with EEG have not revealed reliable differences in past studies of child and adolescent mental health disorders [13,14]. Macrostructural characteristics of sleep are assessed by visual scoring with rules that were originally established in 1968 [25]. Manual sleep scoring [24,25] can be problematic as it has low correspondence for delineating electrophysiological activity and does not take into account the temporal and spatial resolution or autonomic changes [95] during sleep. Examining the microarchitectural characteristics of sleep at greater temporal resolution using spectral methods [96] may help identify specific sleep findings in child and adolescent psychiatric disorders [97].

Arousals from sleep are an integral part of the sleep process [98] and are associated with measurable changes in the EEG [29]. Arousals associated with awakenings, microarousals (less than 3 s), and cyclic alternating patterns (CAP) that reflect sleep stage instability have been evaluated as objective markers of poor sleep [30,31]. High awakenings at night are common in anxiety [34,36], ADHD [50,55,57], and autism from subjective reports whereas arousals, microarousals and CAP are assessed by PSG and include EEG, behavioral, and autonomic components [30]. Frequent PSG arousals from sleep are identified in children with depression [41] and ADHD [63] and low microarousals in autism [72]. High cyclic alternating pattern, the marker of sleep instability and arousal [99], was reported in a regressive form of autism [74] with no differences in another study [79]. Low CAP in ADHD [49,64] is in line with evidence of a hypoarousal state in ADHD; however, other studies have failed to replicate this finding [62]. It is worth noting that microarousals and CAPs are manually scored, which likely contributes to their low reliability across studies. Computer-assisted techniques to identify EEG, respiratory and autonomic arousals during sleep in children and adolescents are likely to enhance the reliability of objective findings of sleep disruption [100].

Generalized CNS arousal, defined as optimal sensory, motor, and affective drive, is necessary for survival and interaction with the environment [101,102], and is, therefore, a critical biological process operating during sleep, wakefulness, and affective modulation. Hypothalamic-pituitary-adrenal (HPA) axis and the locus coeruleus-norepinephrine system are essential for the optimal functioning of the arousal system [103]. Dysregulation of arousal systems along with the HPA axis has been proposed in the pathophysiology of depression [104], autism [105] and ADHD [106]. Cortisol is an essential hormone of the HPA axis and was examined in several studies. High daytime cortisol has been reported in anxiety [43] and autism [81], and low daytime cortisol in ADHD [65], suggesting neuroendocrinal differences in sleep-wake systems. However, other studies have not corroborated these findings [43,44,77]. Methodological differences in measuring cortisol are present across studies which likely contributes to the inconsistent findings [107]. Heart-rate variability, a measure of autonomic arousal, has been observed to be higher in children with autism [91] and ADHD [108]. Research on arousal using reliable cortical and autonomic measures and methods in youth [109] are needed to identify more stable objective markers of sleep disturbances, particularly those that emphasize measurement reliability.

4. Future Directions

We conducted this review to identify objective sleep markers associated with mental health disorders in children and adolescents. Several subjective sleep markers were found to be more consistent and common across child mental health disorders than objective sleep markers, which were not specific and varied across studies. A gap exists in identifying the pathophysiology of sleep disturbances and their links to mental health disorders in youth. Future research should focus on these links to clarify objective markers of sleep and their association with subjective reports and mental health symptoms. Also, mental health symptoms are heterogeneous and cross existing boundaries of syndromes, hence using biobehavioral phenotypes based on pathophysiology may help identify reliable objective markers of sleep [110]. It is essential to control for circadian, homeostatic, and environmental factors (light, physical activity) [111] that impact objective findings of sleep. Multimethod assessments using actigraphy, PSG, EEG, and subjective measures are needed [88] as single measurement methods identify specific markers unique to the method. Detailed analysis of EEG using spectral analysis may also reveal subtle findings not identified by manual scoring methods. Lastly, examining dysregulation and variability of arousal patterns within biobehavioral phenotypes across sleep and mental health may identify specific treatments and help advance the mission of precision medicine [86].

Author Contributions: S.B. identified the studies for the review. S.B., C.C., S.v.N., and M.C. reviewed the studies and wrote the manuscript.

Funding: This research received no external funding.

Acknowledgments: We acknowledge no funding for this research. We would like to acknowledge Alexandra Nasser for helpful comments on the manuscript.

Conflicts of Interest: The authors declare no conflict of interest.

Appendix A

Table A1. Subjective and objective sleep patterns in anxiety and depressive disorders.

Author	Description of Study	Demographics	Measures	Significant Results	Additional Comments
Alfano et al., 2010 [16]	Cross-sectional study of children's subjective sleep patterns and arousal in anxiety disorders.	Generalized Anxiety disorder = 16 Seasonal Affective Disorder = 10 Social Phobia = 13 Age = 7–14 years	Children's Sleep Habits Questionnaire (CSHQ)	Children with GAD had higher difficulty sleeping when compared to other anxiety disorders.	Higher latino children than other ethnicities were present in the study.
			Pre-sleep Arousal Scale for Children	Pre-sleep cognitive and somatic arousal higher in children with generalized anxiety disorder.	
Alfano et al., 2015 [34]	Cross-sectional study of subjective and objective sleep patterns of children with generalized anxiety disorder (GAD).	GAD (M:F) = 19:20 Age = 8.6 ± 1.5 years Control (M:F) = 17:19 Age = 8.8 ± 1.3 years	CSHQ Sleep Self Report	High bedtime resistance, high sleep onset latency; high sleep anxiety, daytime sleepiness, parasomnias, and low sleep duration in children with GAD.	Parent reports and child reports show weak correlation. Anxiety Disorder Interview Schedule used for diagnosing anxiety disorder.
			Actigraphy for 7 days	No significant differences in any of the actigraphy measured sleep variables.	
Alfano et al., 2013 [39]	Cross-sectional study of objective sleep patterns (PSG) of children with GAD.	GAD (M:F) = 6:9 Age = 8.5 ± 1.5 years Control (M:F) = 6:9 Age = 8.9 ± 1.3 years Age range = 7–11 years	Polysomnography (PSG)	High sleep latency and low REM latency observed in GAD. Total recording time higher in Generalized Anxiety Disorder.	Anxiety Diagnostic Interview Schedule used for diagnosing anxiety disorder. Sample size was small in the study.
Patriquin et al., 2014 [41]	Cross-sectional study of objective sleep patterns of children with GAD using in-home PSG.	GAD (M:F) = 8:8 Age = 8.8 ± 1.3 years Control (M:F) = 8:8 Age = 8.4 ± 1.3 years	In-home PSG for one night	Children with GAD had higher sleep efficiency and fewer REM periods than controls. No difference in pre-sleep cognitive and somatic arousal.	
Mullin et al., 2017 [35]	Cross-sectional study of subjective and objective sleep patterns of children and adolescents with GAD.	GAD = 26 Age = 15.1 ± 1.9 years Control = 17 Age = 15.5 ± 1.5 years	Sleep Diary Children's Report of Sleep Problems	High bedtime worries, insomnia symptoms, high sleep onset latency, high wake after sleep onset duration, and low sleep efficiency in self reports of adolescents with GAD. High sleep onset latency, poor sleep quality and high waketime anxiety reported by adolescents with GAD on sleep diaries.	77% of the adolescents with GAD were taking psychiatric medications.
			Actigraphy for 7 days	High sleep onset latency and longer sleep time in adolescents with GAD.	

Table A1. *Cont.*

Author	Description of Study	Demographics	Measures	Significant Results	Additional Comments
Forbes et al., 2008 [39]	Cross-sectional study of subjective and objective findings of sleep in MDD, Anxiety Disorder and healthy controls.	MDD = 128, Age = 12.0 ± 2.3 years Anxiety Disorder = 24, Age = 12.2 ± 3.1 years Control = 101, Age = 10.9 ± 2.2 years	Sleep logs PSG for 3 nights	No significant difference in the sleep logs. For anxiety, significant high number of awakenings, long sleep latency, high stage 1 and stage 2 sleep, low sleep efficiency and high number of arousals observed in children with anxiety disorder. No differences between MDD and controls on PSG measures.	
Forbes et al., 2006 [44]	Cross-sectional study of cortisol levels in children and adolescents with affective disorders.	MDD Children = 76, Age = 10.49 ± 1.42 years Adolescents = 40, Age = 13.98 ± 1.36 years Anxiety Children = 18, Age = 10.49 ± 1.38 years Adolescents = 14, Age = 13.38 ± 1.99 years Healthy controls Children = 44, Age = 10.36 ± 1.43 years Adolescents = 32, Age = 13.44 ± 1.61 years	Plasma cortisol sampled every 20 min	Children with anxiety had higher peri sleep onset cortisol than children with depression or control children. Adolescents with depression had higher peri sleep onset cortisol than children with depression and control adolescents.	
Feder et al., 2004 [43]	Cross-sectional in-lab study of cortisol in children with anxiety and depression.	MDD = 76 Age = 9.3 ± 1.5 years Anxious = 31 Age = 8.7 ± 1.7 years Healthy controls = 17 Age = 9.2 ± 1.2 years	24 h blood cortisol sampling	Children with anxiety had lower nighttime cortisol than depression and sluggish rise in the cortisol. Depressed children did not show cortisol differences from healthy children.	
Armitage et al., 2004 [48]	Cross-sectional study of objective sleep patterns of children and adolescents with depression and healthy controls.	MDD (M:F) = 31:28 Age = 12.3 ± 2.9 years Healthy controls (M:F) = 20:21 Age = 12.4 ± 2.8 years	Actigraphy for five days	Adolescents with Major depressive disorders had lower activity levels, dampened circadian amplitude, lower light exposure and spent less time in bright light than healthy controls. Preteen girls with Major depressive disorder had low light exposure, spent less time in bright light, and had lower circadian amplitude.	More than half of the sample had comorbid psychiatric disorders.
Shahid et al., 2012 [41]	PSG study of children and adolescents in the inpatient unit.	Number (M:F) = 56:50 Age = 13.4 ± 1.7 years	Polysomnography	High levels of insomnia, low sleep efficiency, high arousals from slow wave sleep were present in all disorders. High number of diagnoses (4–7) than low number of diagnoses (1–3) were associated with low slow wave sleep, high arousals from slow wave sleep, and decreased REM sleep.	Majority of the medications were on psychotropic medications.

Table A1. *Cont.*

Author	Description of Study	Demographics	Measures	Significant Results	Additional Comments
Santangeli et al., 2017 [42]	Cross-sectional study of subjective and objective sleep patterns in adolescents with depression and healthy controls.	Depressive Disorder (M:F) = 8:0 Age = 16.9 ± 1.0 years Healthy controls (M:F) = 10:0 Age = 16.2 ± 0.7 years	Overnight polysomnography	Decreased total sleep time and slower dissipation of slow wave sleep pressure and happening later on in the night in adolescents with depression. Negative correlation of severity of depression and slow wave dissipation and depression observed in the frontal area.	
de Souza et al., 2014 [47]	Cross-sectional study of chronotype and social jet lag in children and adolescents.	N = 351 Age = 12–21 years	Munich Chronotype Questionnaire	Sleep phase delay was associated with higher levels of depression. No differences in social jetlag findings.	
Borisenkov et al., 2015 [38]	Cross-sectional study of chronotype and sleep in adolescents with depression.	Number (M:F) = 1517:1918 Age = 14.8 ± 2.6 years	Munich Chronotype Questionnaire and Seasonal Pattern Assessment Questionnaire	Later bedtimes and waketimes, longer sleep onset latency, low sleep efficiency, and more sleep inertia observed in Seasonal Affective Disorder. Circadian phase delay, and social jetlag observed in females with Seasonal affective disorder. Depressed boys were more prone to eveningness than healthy controls.	Female gender, increased age, and latitude increased likelihood of Seasonal affective disorder.
Chiu et al., 2017 [45]	Cross-sectional study of chronotype in depression.	2139 students (grades 1–7) 1708 parents	Questionnaires for subjective sleep quality, and Morningness Eveningness Questionnaire	Eveningness chronotype associated with depression after controlling for sleep quality. Eveningness chronotype associated with parental report of emotional and behavioral problems.	
Haraden et al., 2017 [46]	Longitudinal study of chronotype in adolescents with depression and healthy controls.	Male = 111, Age = 14.8 ± 2.28 years Female = 144, Age = 15.1 ± 2.33 years	Morningness Eveningness Scale	Evening chronotype associated with the earlier onset of depression symptoms.	
Merikanto et al., 2017 [37]	Cross-sectional study of chronotype and sleep in adolescents with depression and healthy controls.	Depressive Disorder (M:F) = 9:0 Age = 14.5-17.5 years Healthy controls (M:F) = 8:0 Age = 14.5-17.5 years	Horne Ostberg Morningness Eveningness Questionnaire Actigraphy for 25 days (25 to 44 days)	Evening chronotype was high in adolescent males with depression. Earlier circadian phase on school days and greater shift to later circadian phase was observed in depressed boys.	

M: Male; F: female; REM: rapid eye movement; ADHD: Attention Deficit Hyperactivity Disorder; MDD: major depressive disorder.

Table A2. Subjective and objective sleep parameters in attention deficit hyperactivity disorder.

Author	Description of Study	Demographics	Measures	Significant Results	Additional Comments
Hvolby et al., 2008 [52]	Cross-sectional evaluation of objective sleep in children with ADHD, psychiatric disorders and healthy controls.	ADHD (M:F) = 37:8 Age = 5 years 9 months–10 years 11 months Psychiatric control (M:F) = 55:9 Age = 6 years 2 months–12 years 4 months Healthy Controls, (M:F) = 61:36 Age = 6 years–11 years 1 months	Actigraphy	Long sleep onset latency, greater day to day variability in sleep onset latency in children with ADHD when compared to healthy children and psychiatric controls.	
Owens et al., 2009 [54]	Cross-sectional evaluation of subjective and objective sleep patterns of children with ADHD and healthy controls.	ADHD (M:F) = 82:25 Age 10.2 ± 2.0 years Control (M:F) = 23:23 Age = 10.3 ± 2.6 years	Electronic sleep diaries	Children with ADHD report less sleep, more difficulty waking up in the morning, and more daytime sleepiness. Parental reports suggest more reports of sleep difficulties such as difficulty getting out of bed, difficulty getting ready for bed, and difficulty falling asleep than healthy children.	
			Actigraphy	Lower sleep efficiency, shorter total sleep time in children with ADHD.	
Mullin et al., 2011 [58]	Cross-sectional study of children and adolescents with ADHD, Bipolar disorder and healthy controls.	ADHD combined (M:F) = 11:3 Age = 15.1 ± 2.1 years Bipolar Disorder (M:F) = 6:7 Age = 14.4 ± 2.1 years Healthy controls (M:F) = 11:10 Age = 14.1 ± 2.0 years	Sleep diary	Children with ADHD did not differ from the controls in any of the subjective sleep parameters.	Children with ADHD on medication.
			actigraphy	No differences in sleep between adolescents with ADHD and controls.	
Moreau et al., 2014 [53]	Cross-sectional study of subjective and objective sleep patterns in children with ADHD	ADHD (M:F) = 24:17 Age = 9.7 ± 1.6 years Healthy controls (M:F) = 24:17 Age = 9.5 ± 1.6 years	Children's Sleep Habits Questionnaire Insomnia severity index and Sleep Diary	Sleep onset delay, sleep anxiety, daytime sleepiness and high insomnia score in children with ADHD	Three fourths of the children with ADHD children were taking stimulants. Having a medication on board or comorbidity was not associated with differences in sleep disturbances in ADHD.
			Actigraphy for 5 days	Total sleep time, and sleep efficiency were lower and sleep onset latency significantly higher in children with ADHD. Mean activity was higher in children with ADHD. Higher deviation of sleep onset latency and higher deviation In mean activity in children with ADHD than controls.	
Jeong et al., 2014 [59]	Cross-sectional study of objective sleep patterns in children with ADHD and healthy controls	ADHD (M:F) = 37:0 Age = 8.7 ± 2.1 years Healthy controls (M:F) = 32:0 Age = 9.3 ± 1.9 years	Actigraphy for 3 days	Children with ADHD had longer sleep latency, wake after sleep and greater sleep fragmentation than healthy controls.	
Bergwerf et al., 2016 [60]	Cross-sectional study of objective sleep patterns in children with ADHD and healthy controls	ADHD (M:F) = 47:16 Age = 9.7 ± 1.6 years Healthy controls (M:F) = 32:29 Age = 10.1 ± 1.6 years	Actigraphy	No differences of measured sleep patterns in children with ADHD and controls. No significant night-to-night variability in children with ADHD when compared to controls.	Long duration in bed, high nocturnal activity, and high average wake bout duration in children with ADHD but did not reach significance.

Table A2. *Cont.*

Author	Description of Study	Demographics	Measures	Significant Results	Additional Comments
Gruber et al., 2009 [57]	Cross-sectional study of subjective and objective sleep patterns in children with ADHD and healthy controls.	ADHD (M:F) = 10:5 Age = 8.93± 1.39 years Healthy controls (M:F) = 13:10 Age = 8.61 ± 1.27 years	Children's Sleep Habits Questionnaire In home olysomnography one night	Parents of children with ADHD report lower sleep time, high sleep anxiety, daytime sleepiness, sleep onset difficulties and high awakenings at night. Children with ADHD had shorter sleep duration and shorter Rem sleep duration, total sleep time, and smaller percentage of REM sleep.	No medication in the past seven days. Children with ADHD scored high on the internalizing symptoms than healthy controls.
Kirov et al., 2004 [6]	Cross-sectional study of objective sleep findings in children with ADHD and healthy controls.	ADHD = 17 Age = 11.2 ± 2.0 years Control = 17 Age = 11.2 ± 2.3 years	Polysomnography	Greater REM sleep duration, high sleep period time identified in children with ADHD. High movements in light sleep stages and high movement related epochs in children with ADHD.	
Miano et al., 2006 [64]	Cross-sectional study of objective sleep patterns in children with ADHD and healthy controls.	ADHD (M:F) = 18:2, Age range = 6–13 years Healthy Controls (M:F) = 11:9, Age range = 6–13 years	Two-night polysomnography	Children with ADHD have increased sleep period, total sleep time and high sleep stage shifts. Low cyclic alternating patterns in stage 2 sleep observed in ADHD.	
Kirov et al., 2007 [65]	Cross-sectional study of objective sleep patterns in children with co-morbid ADHD and controls.	ADHD and Tic Disorder (M:F) = 18:1 Age 11.0 ± 2.2 years Control (M:F) = 17:2 Age = 11.0 ± 2.2 years	Polysomnography	High sleep period time, short REM latency and high REM sleep in children with ADHD. High microarousals, increased motor activity during light and REM sleep also observed in children with ADHD.	
Pribodova et al., 2010 [53]	Cross-sectional study of subjective and objective sleep patterns in children with ADHD and healthy controls.	ADHD (M:F) = 26:5 Age = 9.3± 1.7 years Healthy controls (M:F) = 22:4 Age = 9.2 ± 1.5 years	Pediatric sleep questionnaire Two-night polysomnography	Children with ADHD had restless sleep, difficulty with falling asleep and high leg movements. Children with ADHD had increased wakefulness, reduced sleep efficiency, and prolonged sleep onset latency on first when compared to second night. No night to night variability in control subjects. Multiple sleep latency test did not show differences.	
Choi et al., 2010 [54]	Cross-sectional study of subjective and objective sleep patterns in children with ADHD and healthy controls.	ADHD (M:F) = 24:3 Age = 9.0 ± 2.1 years Healthy controls (M:F) = 23:3 Age = 8.4 ± 1.5 years	Children's Sleep Habits Questionnaire Overnight Polysomnography	Children with ADHD have more difficulty with sleep onset, less sleep duration, more awakenings at night, more daytime sleepiness, and more parasomnias. Total sleep disturbance scores higher in children with ADHD. No significant differences in the PSG sleep characteristics of children with ADHD and controls.	High internalizing, externalizing and affective problems in children with ADHD.

Table A2. *Cont.*

Author	Description of Study	Demographics	Measures	Significant Results	Additional Comments
Gruber et al., 2012 [31]	In home study of children with ADHD using polysomnography.	ADHD (M:F) = 17:9 Age = 8.46 ± 1.5 years Healthy controls (M:F) = 30:19 Age = 8.6 ± 1.2 years	Children's Sleep Habits Questionnaire In home Polysomnography	High sleep onset latency, high sleep anxiety, daytime sleepiness, awakenings at night, resistance to bedtime and low total sleep time in children with ADHD. No significant differences on PSG measures in children with ADHD and healthy controls.	
Imeraj et al., 2012 [65]	Cross-sectional study of cortisol patterns in children with ADHD and healthy controls.	ADHD (M:F) = 9:2 Age = 8.8 ± 1.5 years ADHD + ODD (M:F) = 17:5 Age = 9.0 ± 1.5 years Healthy controls (M:F) = 26:7 Age = 8.8 ± 1.6 years	Salivary cortisol measured five times a day for five days	Cortisol lower in the morning and higher in the evening.	
Prihodova et al., 2012 [62]	Cross-sectional study of subjective and objective sleep of children with ADHD using polysomnography.	ADHD (M:F) = 12:2 Age = 9.6± 1.6 years Healthy controls (M:F) = 8:4 Age = 9.0 ± 1.6 years	Two-night polysomnography	No significant changes in macro and microstructural differences among ADHD and controls.	Recruited from the clinic by the DSM criteria. Children with ADHD had high internalizing symptoms than healthy controls.
Akinci et al., 2015 [49]	Cross-sectional study of subjective and objective sleep patterns in children with ADHD and healthy controls.	ADHD (M:F) = 20:8 Age = 8–12 years Healthy controls (M:F) = 9:6 Age = 9–13 years	Pittsburgh Sleep Quality Index (PSQI) Laboratory polysomnography	On PSQI, low sleep quality, high sleep latency and low sleep efficiency were present in children with ADHD. High REM latency and high REM sleep percentage was present in children with ADHD. Low oxygen saturation at night and awake period and increased leg movements in ADHD. Cyclical alternating patterns (CAP) were low in ADHD.	Children were free of medication use.
Virring et al., 2016 [56]	Cross-sectional study of subjective and objective sleep patterns in children with ADHD and healthy controls.	ADHD n = 76 Age = 9.6 ± 18 years, 74% male Controls = 25 Age = 9.4 ± 1.5 years 68% male.	Sleep Diary Children's Sleep Habits Survey Polysomnography	Children with ADHD differed from healthy controls in all the measures on the Children's Sleep Habits Questionnaire Scale Children with ADHD had longer sleep onset latency than the control group on sleep diaries. Sleep latency, number of sleep cycles, and REM sleep higher, and total sleep time, Stage 3 and stage 1 sleep lower in children with ADHD than controls.	Sleep measures did not differ among the different ADHD subtypes. Children diagnosed with ADHD with and without comorbidity did not differ in sleep measures.
Van der Heijden et al., 2005 [69]	Cross-sectional study of objective sleep patterns in children with ADHD and healthy controls.	ADHD with sleep onset insomnia (M:F) = 66:21, Age = 8.8 ± 1.7 years ADHD without sleep onset insomnia (M:F) = 26:7, Age = 8.2 ± 2.0 years	Actigraphy and melatonin	Children with ADHD and sleep onset insomnia had significantly longer sleep onset latency, later bedtime and waketime. Melatonin onset significantly later in children with ADHD and sleep onset insomnia.	
Buber et al., 2016 [66]	Cross-sectional study of urinary melatonin in children with ADHD and healthy controls.	ADHD (M:F) = 23:4 Age = 9.3 ± 2.6 years Healthy controls (M:F) = 21:7 Age = 10.5 ± 2.7 years	24 h urinary melatonin levels measured in the morning and evening	High urinary melatonin levels present daytime, nighttime and 24 h levels in children with ADHD.	

Table A2. *Cont.*

Author	Description of Study	Demographics	Measures	Significant Results	Additional Comments
Novakova et al., 2011 [6?]	Cross-sectional study of salivary melatonin in children with ADHD and healthy controls.	ADHD (M:F) = 30:4 Age = 6–12 years Healthy controls (M:F) = 26:17 Age = 6–12 years	24 h salivary melatonin	No differences in salivary melatonin levels between ADHD and control subjects.	Duration of the melatonin signal was shortened in 10–12 year old sub sample with ADHD.
Doi et al., 2015 [?]	Cross-sectional study of chronotype in children with behavioral problems.	Number (M:F) = 342: 312 Age = 4–6 years	Munich Chronotype Questionnaire	Chronotype was associated with inattention/hyperactivity problems.	

M: Male; F: female; REM: rapid eye movement; ADHD: Attention Deficit Hyperactivity Disorder.

Table A3. Subjective and objective sleep findings in autism spectrum disorders (ASD).

Author	Description of Study	Demographics	Measures	Significant Results	Additional Comments
Allik et al., 2006 [?]	Cross-sectional study of subjective and objectively measured sleep in ASD, high functioning autism and Healthy Controls.	ASD (M:F) = 17:2 High functioning autism (M:F) = 11:2 Control (M:F) = 28:4 Age = 8.5–12.8 years	Sleep Diary for one week	High sleep onset latency, poor sleep efficiency and low sleep quality observed in autism and high functioning autism on sleep diaries.	
			Actigraphy for one week	No differences in sleep on actigraphy between autism spectrum and healthy controls.	
Goodlin-Jones et al., 2008 [?]	Cross-sectional study of subjective and objective sleep characteristics in preschool children with autism, children with developmental delay, and healthy controls.	Autism Spectrum Disorder = 68 Age = 2.3–5.6 years Developmental Disability = 57 Age = 2.0–5.7 years Healthy Controls = 69 Age = 2.0–5.1 years	Children's Sleep Habits Questionnaire and daily sleep diary	Sleep diary and actigraphy measures were concordant with each other for start of sleep, sleep duration, sleep onset latency, number of naps, nap duration, wake after sleep duration, and 24 h sleep duration.	
			Actigraphy	Children with Autism had significantly shorter 24 h sleep duration, shorter naps, less time in bed than children with developmental disability and healthy children. Developmentally disabled children had more fragmented sleep, with high number and duration of awakenings than autism and healthy controls.	
Souders et al., 2009 [?]	Cross-sectional study of subjective and objectively measured sleep in Autism Spectrum Disorder and Healthy Controls.	Autism Spectrum (M:F) = 44:15 Control (M:F) = 26:14	Children's Sleep Habits Questionnaire	Longer sleep onset latency, high sleep anxiety, bedtime resistance, and parasomnias, and short sleep duration in Autism.	
			Actigraphy for 10 days	Longer Sleep latency, short sleep duration, increased wake after sleep onset duration, and low sleep efficiency in children with Autism.	

Table A3. Cont.

Author	Description of Study	Demographics	Measures	Significant Results	Additional Comments
Goldman et al., 2017 [77]	Cross-sectional study of subjective and objective sleep patterns of children with autism spectrum disorders and healthy controls.	Autism spectrum disorder (M:F) = 20:8; Age = 15.6 ± 2.8 years; Typically developing children = (M:F) = 6:7; Age = 15.6 ± 2.1 years	Adolescent Sleep Wake Scale; Actigraphy	More difficulty going to bed and falling asleep on self-reports of children with autism spectrum disorder. / Sleep latency was longer and sleep efficiency lower in autism spectrum disorder. Cortisol and dim light melatonin onset not significantly different between children with autism and healthy controls.	
Baker et al., 2013 [76]	Longitudinal study of subjective and objectively measured sleep in High Functioning Autism and healthy controls.	High Functioning Autism (M:F) = 22:5; Control (M:F) = 26:14; Age = 15.5 ± 1.3 years	Sleep Diary for 7 days, and modified School Sleep Habits Survey; Actigraphy	Difficulties with falling asleep and high daytime fatigue in adolescents with high functioning autism. / High sleep onset latency and low sleep efficiency that are both variable in Autism than healthy controls.	Night to night variability of sleep latency, sleep onset time, sleep offset time and sleep period higher at follow up.
Fletcher et al., 2017 [78]	Longitudinal study of subjective and objectively measured sleep in Autism and healthy controls	Autism (M:F) = 17:5; Control (M:F) = 14:15; Age = 6–13 years; At follow up 7–14 year	Children's Sleep Habits Questionnaire; Actigraphy	Higher global scores on Children's sleep habits questionnaire in children with Autism at baseline and follow up / Low sleep efficiency, highly variable sleep efficiency in Autism. High variability in wake time and wake after sleep onset in Autism.	Significant difference in IQ between children with Autism and typically developing children.
Makow et al., 2006 [80]	Cross-sectional study of subjective and objective sleep in children with ASD and healthy controls.	ASD = 21; Healthy Controls = 10; Age = 4–10 years	Children's Sleep Habits Questionnaire; Two-night polysomnography	High bedtime resistance, sleep onset delay, low sleep duration, high sleep anxiety in children with autism when compared to healthy controls. / Low sleep efficiency, high sleep latency observed in children with Autism.	
Miano et al., 2007 [79]	Cross-sectional study of subjective and objective sleep in children with ASD and healthy controls.	ASD (M:F) = 16; Age = 9.4 ± 4.5 years; Controls (M:F) = 9:9; Age = 10.2 ± 2.9 years	Sleep Questionnaires; Polysomnography	Difficulty initiating sleep and maintaining sleep, and daytime sleepiness in ASD. / Short total sleep time, short REM latency, reduced time in bed in ASD than healthy controls.	

Table A3. *Cont.*

Author	Description of Study	Demographics	Measures	Significant Results	Additional Comments
Giannotti et al., 2011 [?]	Cross-sectional study of subjective and objectively measured sleep in Autism (regressed and non-regressed) and Healthy Controls.	Autism (regressed) M:F = 16:6 Age = 5.5 ± 2.1 years; Autism (non-regressed) M:F = 14:4 Age = 5.1 ± 3.9 years; Healthy Children M:F = 9:3 Age = 5.8 ± 2.4 years	Children's Sleep Habits Questionnaire; Polysomnography for two consecutive nights	Shorter total sleep time, later bedtimes and later waketimes in the regressed and non-regressed children. High number of awakenings at night, bedtime resistance, sleep onset delay, later bedtimes and waketimes that are severe in regressed than non-regressed children with Autism. Total sleep time, sleep efficiency less in regressed and non-regressed Autism than typically developing children. Awakenings per hour, REM sleep less in regressed than non-regressed children than typically developing children. Slow wave sleep, REM percentage less in regressed autism than typically developing children. Stage 2 sleep high in regressed autism than typically developing children.	Autism children had mild mental retardation and borderline intellectual functioning.
Lambert et al., 2016 [72]	Cross-sectional study of subjective and objective measures of sleep in children with autism and healthy controls.	Autism = 11 Age = 6–13 years; Control = 13 Age = 7–12 years	Children's Sleep Habits Questionnaire; Polysomnography	No differences in subjective measures of children with Autism and healthy controls. Longer sleep latency, low slow wave sleep, low sleep spindles and K complexes in Autism. Higher stage transitions from stage 1 to wake and low microarousals per hour of sleep in Autism.	Low slow wave sleep and light sleep associated with high repetitive behaviors. The groups differed significantly in anxiety, affective and attentional problems.
Harder et al., 2016 [91]	Cross-sectional study of objective sleep patterns in ASD and Healthy Controls.	Autism Disorder (M:F) = 21:0 Age = 4–10 years; Typically Developing Children (M:F) = 18:5 Age = 4–10 years	Polysomnography; Heart rate variability	Low stage 3 sleep in children with Autism than healthy controls. Children with ASD had higher HR during N2, and REM sleep. ASD children had higher values of normalized Low Frequency (Heart rate variability) in REM and normalized lower High Frequency heart rate variability in REM. Higher Low Frequency to High Frequency ratio in REM.	

Table A3. *Cont.*

Author	Description of Study	Demographics	Measures	Significant Results	Additional Comments
Tordjman et al., 2005 [82]	Cross-sectional study of circadian measures of sleep in ASD and healthy controls.	Autism Disorder (M:F) = 33:17 Age = 11.5 ± 4.5 years Typically Developing Children (M:F) = 49:39 Age = 11.0 ± 4.4 years	Urinary melatonin	Nocturnal melatonin secretion rate lower in autism, specifically in prepubertal children, marked in males. Melatonin levels negatively correlated with impairment in verbal communication and play.	Children diagnosed by Autism Diagnostic Observation Schedule. Twenty children taking medication.
Corbett et al., 2014 [83]	Cross-sectional study of objective measures of sleep in children with autism and healthy controls.	ASD = 46 Age = 10.3 ± 1.7 years Typically developing children = 48 Age = 9.9 ± 1.6 years	Salivary cortisol	No differences in Cortisol Awakening Response between children with autism and typically developing children.	
Tordjman et al., 2014 [81]	Cross-sectional study of circadian measures of sleep in ASD and healthy controls.	Autism Disorder (M:F) = 36:19 Age = 11.3 ± 4.1 years Typically Developing Children (M:F) = 22:10 Age = 11.7 ± 4.9 years	Salivary cortisol collected five times a day	Salivary cortisol measured high in Autism and flat cortisol daytime and night slopes in children and adolescents with Autism. Higher cortisol levels in children with severe impairments in social interaction.	Children diagnosed by Autism Diagnostic Observation Schedule.

M: Male; F: female; ASD: Autism Spectrum Disorder; IQ: intelligence quotient; HR: heart rate; REM: rapid eye movement.

References

1. Sturman, D.A.; Moghaddam, B. The neurobiology of adolescence: Changes in brain architecture, functional dynamics, and behavioral tendencies. *Neurosci. Biobehav. Rev.* **2011**, *35*, 1704–1712. [CrossRef] [PubMed]
2. Cicchetti, D. Socioemotional, Personality, and biological development: Illustrations from a Multilevel Developmental Psychopathology Perspective on Child Maltreatment. *Annu. Rev. Psychol.* **2016**, *67*, 187–211. [CrossRef] [PubMed]
3. Skeldon, A.C.; Derks, G.; Dijk, D.-J. Modelling changes in sleep timing and duration across the lifespan: Changes in circadian rhythmicity or sleep homeostasis? *Sleep Med. Rev.* **2016**, *28*, 96–107. [CrossRef] [PubMed]
4. Iglowstein, I.; Jenni, O.G.; Molinari, L.; Largo, R.H. Sleep Duration from Infancy to Adolescence: Reference Values and Generational Trends. *Pediatrics* **2003**, *111*, 302–307. [CrossRef] [PubMed]
5. Ohayon, M.M.; Carskadon, M.A.; Guilleminault, C.; Vitiello, M.V. Meta-Analysis of Quantitative Sleep Parameters from Childhood to Old Age in Healthy Individuals: Developing Normative Sleep Values across the Human Lifespan. *Sleep* **2004**, *27*, 1255–1273. [CrossRef] [PubMed]
6. Crowley, S.J.; Acebo, C.; Carskadon, M.A. Sleep, circadian rhythms, and delayed phase in adolescence. *Sleep Med.* **2007**, *8*, 602–612. [CrossRef] [PubMed]
7. Polanczyk, G.V.; Salum, G.A.; Sugaya, L.S.; Caye, A.; Rohde, L.A. Annual Research Review: A meta-analysis of the worldwide prevalence of mental disorders in children and adolescents. *J. Child Psychol. Psychiatry* **2015**, *56*, 345–365. [CrossRef] [PubMed]
8. Merikangas, K.R.; He, J.-P.; Brody, D.; Fisher, P.W.; Bourdon, K.; Koretz, D.S. Prevalence and treatment of mental disorders among US children in the 2001-2004 NHANES. *Pediatrics* **2010**, *125*, 75–81. [CrossRef]
9. Baxter, A.J.; Brugha, T.S.; Erskine, H.E.; Scheurer, R.W.; Vos, T.; Scott, J.G. The epidemiology and global burden of autism spectrum disorders. *Psychol. Med.* **2015**, *45*, 601–613. [CrossRef] [PubMed]
10. Kessler, R.C.; Angermeyer, M.; Anthony, J.C.; DE Graaf, R.; Demyttenaere, K.; Gasquet, I.; DE Girolamo, G.; Gluzman, S.; Gureje, O.; Haro, J.M.; et al. Lifetime prevalence and age-of-onset distributions of mental disorders in the World Health Organization's World Mental Health Survey Initiative. *World Psychiatry Off. J. World Psychiatr. Assoc.* **2007**, *6*, 168–176.
11. Merikangas, K.R.; He, J.; Burstein, M.; Swanson, S.A.; Avenevoli, S.; Cui, L.; Benjet, C.; Georgiades, K.; Swendsen, J. Lifetime Prevalence of Mental Disorders in U.S. Adolescents: Results from the National Comorbidity Survey Replication–Adolescent Supplement (NCS-A). *J. Am. Acad. Child Adolesc. Psychiatry* **2010**, *49*, 980–989. [CrossRef]
12. Strang, J.F.; Kenworthy, L.; Daniolos, P.; Case, L.; Wills, M.C.; Martin, A.; Wallace, G.L. Depression and anxiety symptoms in children and adolescents with autism spectrum disorders without intellectual disability. *Res. Autism Spectr. Disord.* **2012**, *6*, 406–412. [CrossRef] [PubMed]
13. Ivanenko, A.; Crabtree, V.M.; Obrien, L.M.; Gozal, D. Sleep complaints and psychiatric symptoms in children evaluated at a pediatric mental health clinic. *J. Clin. Sleep Med.* **2006**, *2*, 42–48. [PubMed]
14. Alfano, C.A.; Gamble, A.L. The Role of Sleep in Childhood Psychiatric Disorders. *Child Youth Care Forum* **2009**, *38*, 327–340. [CrossRef] [PubMed]
15. Liu, X.; Buysse, D.J.; Gentzler, A.L.; Kiss, E.; Mayer, L.; Kapornai, K.; Vetró, A.; Kovacs, M. Insomnia and hypersomnia associated with depressive phenomenology and comorbidity in childhood depression. *Sleep* **2007**, *30*, 83–90. [CrossRef] [PubMed]
16. Alfano, C.A.; Pina, A.A.; Zerr, A.A.; Villalta, I.K. Pre-Sleep Arousal and Sleep Problems of Anxiety-Disordered Youth. *Child Psychiatry Hum. Dev.* **2010**, *41*, 156–167. [CrossRef] [PubMed]
17. Ramtekkar, U.; Ivanenko, A. Sleep in Children with Psychiatric Disorders. *Semin. Pediatr. Neurol.* **2015**, *22*, 148–155. [CrossRef] [PubMed]
18. Gregory, A.M.; Sadeh, A. Sleep, emotional and behavioral difficulties in children and adolescents. *Sleep Med. Rev.* **2012**, *16*, 129–136. [CrossRef] [PubMed]
19. Cortese, S.; Faraone, S.V.; Konofal, E.; Lecendreux, M. Sleep in children with attention-deficit/hyperactivity disorder: Meta-analysis of subjective and objective studies. *J. Am. Acad. Child Adolesc. Psychiatry* **2009**, *48*, 894–908. [CrossRef] [PubMed]

20. Díaz-Román, A.; Hita-Yáñez, E.; Buela-Casal, G. Sleep Characteristics in Children with Attention Deficit Hyperactivity Disorder: Systematic Review and Meta-Analyses. *J. Clin. Sleep Med.* **2016**, *12*, 747–756. [CrossRef] [PubMed]

21. Augustinavicius, J.L.S.; Zanjani, A.; Zakzanis, K.K.; Shapiro, C.M. Polysomnographic features of early-onset depression: A meta-analysis. *J. Affect. Disord.* **2014**, *158*, 11–18. [CrossRef] [PubMed]

22. Urrila, A.S.; Paunio, T.; Palomäki, E.; Marttunen, M. Sleep in adolescent depression: Physiological perspectives. *Acta Physiol.* **2015**, *213*, 758–777. [CrossRef] [PubMed]

23. Ancoli-Israel, S.; Cole, R.; Alessi, C.; Chambers, M.; Moorcroft, W.; Pollak, C.P. The role of actigraphy in the study of sleep and circadian rhythms. *Sleep* **2003**, *26*, 342–392. [CrossRef] [PubMed]

24. Berry, R.B.; Brooks, R.; Gamaldo, C.; Harding, S.M.; Lloyd, R.M.; Quan, S.F.; Troester, M.T.; Vaughn, B.V. *AASM Manual for the Scoring of Sleep and Associated Events: Rules, Terminology and Technical Specifications is the Definitive Reference for Sleep Scoring. Version 2.4.*; AASM: Darien, IL, USA, 2017.

25. Kales, A.; Rechtschaffen, A.; University of California, L.A.; Brain Information Service; National Institute of Neurological Diseases and Blindness (U.S.). *A Manual of Standardized Terminology, Techniques and Scoring System for Sleep Stages of Human Subjects*; United States Government Printing Office: Washington, DC, USA, 1968.

26. Meltzer, L.J.; Montgomery-Downs, H.E.; Insana, S.P.; Walsh, C.M. Use of actigraphy for assessment in pediatric sleep research. *Sleep Med. Rev.* **2012**, *16*, 463–475. [CrossRef] [PubMed]

27. Carskadon, M.A.; Acebo, C.; Richardson, G.S.; Tate, B.A.; Seifer, R. An Approach to Studying Circadian Rhythms of Adolescent Humans. *J. Biol. Rhythm.* **1997**, *12*, 278–289. [CrossRef] [PubMed]

28. Morris, C.J.; Aeschbach, D.; Scheer, F.A.J.L. Circadian system, sleep and endocrinology. *Mol. Cell. Endocrinol.* **2012**, *349*, 91–104. [CrossRef] [PubMed]

29. Bonnet, M.H.; Carley, D.; Carskadon, M.; Easton, P.; Guilleminault, C.; Harper, R.; Hayes, B.; Hirshkowitz, M.; Ktonas, P.; Keenan, S.; et al. EEG arousals: Scoring rules and examples. A preliminary report from the Sleep Disorders Atlas Task Force of the American Sleep Disorder Association. *Sleep* **1992**, *15*, 173–184.

30. Halász, P.; Terzano, M.; Parrino, L.; Bódizs, R. The nature of arousal in sleep. *J. Sleep Res.* **2004**, *13*, 1–23. [CrossRef] [PubMed]

31. Terzano, M.G.; Mancia, D.; Salati, M.R.; Costani, G.; Decembrino, A.; Parrino, L. The cyclic alternating pattern as a physiologic component of normal NREM sleep. *Sleep* **1985**, *8*, 137–145. [CrossRef] [PubMed]

32. Owens, J.; Spirito, A.; McGuinn, M. The Children's Sleep Habits Questionnaire (CSHQ): Psychometric properties of a survey instrument for school-aged children. *Sleep* **2000**, *23*, 1043–1051. [CrossRef] [PubMed]

33. Erwin, A.M.; Bashore, L. Subjective Sleep Measures in Children: Self-Report. *Front. Pediatr.* **2017**, *5*. [CrossRef] [PubMed]

34. Alfano, C.A.; Patriquin, M.A.; De Los Reyes, A. Subjective—Objective Sleep Comparisons and Discrepancies among Clinically-Anxious and Healthy Children. *J. Abnorm. Child Psychol.* **2015**, *43*, 1343–1353. [CrossRef] [PubMed]

35. Mullin, B.C.; Pyle, L.; Haraden, D.; Riederer, J.; Brim, N.; Kaplan, D.; Novins, D. A Preliminary Multimethod Comparison of Sleep among Adolescents with and Without Generalized Anxiety Disorder. *J. Clin. Child Adolesc. Psychol.* **2017**, *46*, 198–210. [CrossRef] [PubMed]

36. Forbes, E.E.; Bertocci, M.A.; Gregory, A.M.; Ryan, N.D.; Axelson, D.A.; Birmaher, B.; Dahl, R.E. Objective Sleep in Pediatric Anxiety Disorders and Major Depressive Disorder. *J. Am. Acad. Child Adolesc. Psychiatry* **2008**, *47*, 148–155. [CrossRef] [PubMed]

37. Merikanto, I.; Partonen, T.; Paunio, T.; Castaneda, A.E.; Marttunen, M.; Urrila, A.S. Advanced phases and reduced amplitudes are suggested to characterize the daily rest-activity cycles in depressed adolescent boys. *Chronobiol. Int.* **2017**, *34*, 967–976. [CrossRef] [PubMed]

38. Borisenkov, M.F.; Petrova, N.B.; Timonin, V.D.; Fradkova, L.I.; Kolomeichuk, S.N.; Kosova, A.L.; Kasyanova, O.N. Sleep characteristics, chronotype and winter depression in 10–20-year-olds in northern European Russia. *J. Sleep Res.* **2015**, *24*, 288–295. [CrossRef] [PubMed]

39. Alfano, C.A.; Reynolds, K.; Scott, N.; Dahl, R.E.; Mellman, T.A. Polysomnographic sleep patterns of non-depressed, non-medicated children with generalized anxiety disorder. *J. Affect. Disord.* **2013**, *147*, 379–384. [CrossRef] [PubMed]

40. Patriquin, M.A.; Mellman, T.A.; Glaze, D.G.; Alfano, C.A. Polysomnographic sleep characteristics of generally-anxious and healthy children assessed in the home environment. *J. Affect. Disord.* **2014**, *161*, 79–83. [CrossRef] [PubMed]

41. Shahid, A.; Khairandish, A.; Gladanac, B.; Shapiro, C. Peeking into the minds of troubled adolescents: The utility of polysomnography sleep studies in an inpatient psychiatric unit. *J. Affect. Disord.* **2012**, *139*, 66–74. [CrossRef] [PubMed]

42. Santangeli, O.; Porkka-Heiskanen, T.; Virkkala, J.; Castaneda, A.E.; Marttunen, M.; Paunio, T.; Urrila, A.S. Sleep and slow-wave activity in depressed adolescent boys: A preliminary study. *Sleep Med.* **2017**, *38*, 24–30. [CrossRef] [PubMed]

43. Feder, A.; Coplan, J.D.; Goetz, R.R.; Mathew, S.J.; Pine, D.S.; Dahl, R.E.; Ryan, N.D.; Greenwald, S.; Weissman, M.M. Twenty-four-hour cortisol secretion patterns in prepubertal children with anxiety or depressive disorders. *Biol. Psychiatry* **2004**, *56*, 198–204. [CrossRef] [PubMed]

44. Forbes, E.E.; Williamson, D.E.; Ryan, N.D.; Birmaher, B.; Axelson, D.A.; Dahl, R.E. Peri-Sleep-Onset Cortisol Levels in Children and Adolescents with Affective Disorders. *Biol. Psychiatry* **2006**, *59*, 24–30. [CrossRef] [PubMed]

45. Chiu, W.-H.; Yang, H.-J.; Kuo, P.-H. Chronotype preference matters for depression in youth. *Chronobiol. Int.* **2017**, *34*, 933–941. [CrossRef] [PubMed]

46. Haraden, D.A.; Mullin, B.C.; Hankin, B.L. The relationship between depression and chronotype: A longitudinal assessment during childhood and adolescence. *Depression Anxiety* **2017**, *34*, 967–976. [CrossRef] [PubMed]

47. De Souza, C.M.; Hidalgo, M.P.L. Midpoint of sleep on school days is associated with depression among adolescents. *Chronobiol. Int.* **2014**, *31*, 199–205. [CrossRef] [PubMed]

48. Armitage, R.; Hoffmann, R.; Emslie, G.; Rintelman, J.; Moore, J.; Lewis, K. Rest-activity cycles in childhood and adolescent depression. *J. Am. Acad. Child Adolesc. Psychiatry* **2004**, *43*, 761–769. [CrossRef] [PubMed]

49. Akinci, G.; Oztura, I.; Hiz, S.; Akdogan, O.; Karaarslan, D.; Ozek, H.; Akay, A. Sleep Structure in Children With Attention-Deficit/Hyperactivity Disorder. *J. Child Neurol.* **2015**, *30*, 1520–1525. [CrossRef] [PubMed]

50. Choi, J.; Yoon, I.-Y.; Kim, H.-W.; Chung, S.; Yoo, H.J. Differences between objective and subjective sleep measures in children with attention deficit hyperactivity disorder. *J. Clin. Sleep Med.* **2010**, *6*, 589–595. [PubMed]

51. Gruber, R.; Fontil, L.; Bergmame, L.; Wiebe, S.T.; Amsel, R.; Frenette, S.; Carrier, J. Contributions of circadian tendencies and behavioral problems to sleep onset problems of children with ADHD. *BMC Psychiatry* **2012**, *12*, 212. [CrossRef] [PubMed]

52. Hvolby, A.; Jørgensen, J.; Bilenberg, N. Actigraphic and Parental Reports of Sleep Difficulties in Children With Attention-Deficit/Hyperactivity Disorder. *Arch. Pediatr. Adolesc. Med.* **2008**, *162*, 323. [CrossRef] [PubMed]

53. Moreau, V.; Rouleau, N.; Morin, C.M. Sleep of Children with Attention Deficit Hyperactivity Disorder: Actigraphic and Parental Reports. *Behav. Sleep Med.* **2014**, *12*, 69–83. [CrossRef] [PubMed]

54. Owens, J.; Sangal, R.B.; Sutton, V.K.; Bakken, R.; Allen, A.J.; Kelsey, D. Subjective and objective measures of sleep in children with attention-deficit/hyperactivity disorder. *Sleep Med.* **2009**, *10*, 446–456. [CrossRef] [PubMed]

55. Prihodova, I.; Paclt, I.; Kemlink, D.; Skibova, J.; Ptacek, R.; Nevsimalova, S. Sleep disorders and daytime sleepiness in children with attention-deficit/hyperactivity disorder: A two-night polysomnographic study with a multiple sleep latency test. *Sleep Med.* **2010**, *11*, 922–928. [CrossRef] [PubMed]

56. Virring, A.; Lambek, R.; Thomsen, P.H.; Møller, L.R.; Jennum, P.J. Disturbed sleep in attention-deficit hyperactivity disorder (ADHD) is not a question of psychiatric comorbidity or ADHD presentation. *J. Sleep Res.* **2016**, *25*, 333–340. [CrossRef] [PubMed]

57. Gruber, R.; Xi, T.; Frenette, S.; Robert, M.; Vannasinh, P.; Carrier, J. Sleep disturbances in prepubertal children with attention deficit hyperactivity disorder: A home polysomnography study. *Sleep* **2009**, *32*, 343–350. [CrossRef] [PubMed]

58. Mullin, B.C.; Harvey, A.G.; Hinshaw, S.P. A preliminary study of sleep in adolescents with bipolar disorder, ADHD, and non-patient controls. *Bipolar Disord.* **2011**, *13*, 425–432. [CrossRef] [PubMed]

59. Jeong, J.-H.; Lee, H.K.; Kim, N.-Y.; Park, M.-H.; Kim, T.-W.; Seo, H.-J.; Lim, H.-K.; Hong, S.-C.; Han, J.-H. Sleep and cognitive problems in patients with attention-deficit hyperactivity disorder. *Neuropsychiatr. Dis. Treat.* **2014**, *10*, 1799. [CrossRef] [PubMed]

60. Bergwerff, C.E.; Luman, M.; Oosterlaan, J. No objectively measured sleep disturbances in children with attention-deficit/hyperactivity disorder. *J. Sleep Res.* **2016**, *25*, 534–540. [CrossRef] [PubMed]

61. Kirov, R.; Kinkelbur, J.; Heipke, S.; Kostanecka-Endress, T.; Westhoff, M.; Cohrs, S.; Ruther, E.; Hajak, G.; Banaschewski, T.; Rothenberger, A. Is there a specific polysomnographic sleep pattern in children with attention deficit/hyperactivity disorder? *J. Sleep Res.* **2004**, *13*, 87–93. [CrossRef] [PubMed]

62. Příhodová, I.; Paclt, I.; Kemlink, D.; Nevšímalová, S. Sleep microstructure is not altered in children with attention-deficit/hyperactivity disorder (ADHD). *Physiol. Res.* **2012**, *61*, 125–133. [PubMed]

63. Kirov, R.; Banaschewski, T.; Uebel, H.; Kinkelbur, J.; Rothenberger, A. REM-sleep alterations in children with co-existence of tic disorders and attention-deficit/hyperactivity disorder: Impact of hypermotor symptoms. *Eur. Child Adolesc. Psychiatry* **2007**, *16*, 45–50. [CrossRef] [PubMed]

64. Miano, S.; Donfrancesco, R.; Bruni, O.; Ferri, R.; Galiffa, S.; Pagani, J.; Montemitro, E.; Kheirandish, L.; Gozal, D.; Villa, M.P. NREM Sleep Instability is Reduced in Children With Attention-Deficit/Hyperactivity Disorder. *Sleep* **2006**, *29*, 797–803. [PubMed]

65. Imeraj, L.; Antrop, I.; Roeyers, H.; Swanson, J.; Deschepper, E.; Bal, S.; Deboutte, D. Time-of-day effects in arousal: Disrupted diurnal cortisol profiles in children with ADHD. *J. Child Psychol. Psychiatry* **2012**, *53*, 782–789. [CrossRef] [PubMed]

66. Büber, A.; Çakaloz, B.; Işıldar, Y.; Ünlü, G.; Bostancı, H.E.; Aybek, H.; Herken, H. Increased urinary 6-hydroxymelatoninsulfate levels in attention deficit hyperactivity disorder diagnosed children and adolescent. *Neurosci. Lett.* **2016**, *617*, 195–200. [CrossRef] [PubMed]

67. Nováková, M.; Paclt, I.; Ptáček, R.; Kuželová, H.; Hájek, I.; Sumová, A. Salivary Melatonin Rhythm as a Marker of the Circadian System in Healthy Children and Those With Attention-Deficit/Hyperactivity Disorder. *Chronobiol. Int.* **2011**, *28*, 630–637. [CrossRef] [PubMed]

68. Durmuş, F.B.; Arman, A.R.; Ayaz, A.B. Chronotype and its relationship with sleep disorders in children with attention deficit hyperactivity disorder. *Chronobiol. Int.* **2017**, *34*, 886–894. [CrossRef] [PubMed]

69. Van der Heijden, K.B.; Smits, M.G.; Van Someren, E.J.W.; Boudewijn Gunning, W. Idiopathic Chronic Sleep Onset Insomnia in Attention-Deficit/Hyperactivity Disorder: A Circadian Rhythm Sleep Disorder. *Chronobiol. Int.* **2005**, *22*, 559–570. [CrossRef] [PubMed]

70. Doi, Y.; Ishihara, K.; Uchiyama, M. Associations of chronotype with social jetlag and behavioral problems in preschool children. *Chronobiol. Int.* **2015**, *32*, 1101–1108. [CrossRef] [PubMed]

71. Allik, H.; Larsson, J.-O.; Smedje, H. Sleep Patterns of School-Age Children with Asperger Syndrome or High-Functioning Autism. *J. Autism Dev. Disord.* **2006**, *36*, 585–595. [CrossRef] [PubMed]

72. Lambert, A.; Tessier, S.; Rochette, A.-C.; Scherzer, P.; Mottron, L.; Godbout, R. Poor sleep affects daytime functioning in typically developing and autistic children not complaining of sleep problems: A questionnaire-based and polysomnographic study. *Res. Autism Spectr. Disord.* **2016**, *23*, 94–106. [CrossRef]

73. Souders, M.C.; Mason, T.B.A.; Valladares, O.; Bucan, M.; Levy, S.E.; Mandell, D.S.; Weaver, T.E.; Pinto-Martin, J. Sleep Behaviors and Sleep Quality in Children with Autism Spectrum Disorders. *Sleep* **2009**, *32*, 1566–1578. [CrossRef] [PubMed]

74. Giannotti, F.; Cortesi, F.; Cerquiglini, A.; Vagnoni, C.; Valente, D. Sleep in children with autism with and without autistic regression. *J. Sleep Res.* **2011**, *20*, 338–347. [CrossRef] [PubMed]

75. Goodlin-Jones, B.; Tang, K.; Liu, J.; Anders, T.F. Sleep patterns in preschool-age children with autism, developmental delay, and typical development. *J. Am. Acad. Child Adolesc. Psychiatry* **2008**, *47*, 930–938. [CrossRef] [PubMed]

76. Baker, E.; Richdale, A.; Short, M.; Gradisar, M. An investigation of sleep patterns in adolescents with high-functioning autism spectrum disorder compared with typically developing adolescents. *Dev. Neurorehabilit.* **2013**, *16*, 155–165. [CrossRef] [PubMed]

77. Goldman, S.E.; Alder, M.L.; Burgess, H.J.; Corbett, B.A.; Hundley, R.; Wofford, D.; Fawkes, D.B.; Wang, L.; Laudenslager, M.L.; Malow, B.A. Characterizing Sleep in Adolescents and Adults with Autism Spectrum Disorders. *J. Autism Dev. Disord.* **2017**, *47*, 1682–1695. [CrossRef] [PubMed]

78. Fletcher, F.E.; Foster-Owens, M.D.; Conduit, R.; Rinehart, N.J.; Riby, D.M.; Cornish, K.M. The developmental trajectory of parent-report and objective sleep profiles in autism spectrum disorder: Associations with anxiety and bedtime routines. *Autism* **2017**, *21*, 493–503. [CrossRef] [PubMed]

79. Miano, S.; Bruni, O.; Elia, M.; Trovato, A.; Smerieri, A.; Verrillo, E.; Roccella, M.; Terzano, M.G.; Ferri, R. Sleep in children with autistic spectrum disorder: A questionnaire and polysomnographic study. *Sleep Med.* **2007**, *9*, 64–70. [CrossRef] [PubMed]

80. Malow, B.A.; Marzec, M.L.; McGrew, S.G.; Wang, L.; Henderson, L.M.; Stone, W.L. Characterizing Sleep in Children with Autism Spectrum Disorders: A Multidimensional Approach. *Sleep* **2006**, *29*, 1563–1571. [CrossRef] [PubMed]

81. Tordjman, S.; Anderson, G.M.; Kermarrec, S.; Bonnot, O.; Geoffray, M.-M.; Brailly-Tabard, S.; Chaouch, A.; Colliot, I.; Trabado, S.; Bronsard, G.; et al. Altered circadian patterns of salivary cortisol in low-functioning children and adolescents with autism. *Psychoneuroendocrinology* **2014**, *50*, 227–245. [CrossRef] [PubMed]

82. Tordjman, S.; Anderson, G.M.; Pichard, N.; Charbuy, H.; Touitou, Y. Nocturnal excretion of 6-sulphatoxymelatonin in children and adolescents with autistic disorder. *Biol. Psychiatry* **2005**, *57*, 134–138. [CrossRef] [PubMed]

83. Corbett, B.A.; Schupp, C.W. The cortisol awakening response (CAR) in male children with autism spectrum disorder. *Horm. Behav.* **2014**, *65*, 345–350. [CrossRef] [PubMed]

84. Hatzinger, M.; Brand, S.; Perren, S.; von Wyl, A.; Stadelmann, S.; von Klitzing, K.; Holsboer-Trachsler, E. Pre-schoolers suffering from psychiatric disorders show increased cortisol secretion and poor sleep compared to healthy controls. *J. Psychiatr. Res.* **2012**, *46*, 590–599. [CrossRef] [PubMed]

85. Endler, N.S.; Kocovski, N.L. State and trait anxiety revisited. *J. Anxiety Disord.* **2001**, *15*, 231–245. [CrossRef]

86. Insel, T.R. The nimh research domain criteria (rdoc) project: Precision medicine for psychiatry. *Am. J. Psychiatry* **2014**, *171*, 395–397. [CrossRef] [PubMed]

87. Insel, T.R.; Cuthbert, B.; Garvey, M.; Heinssen, R.; Pine, D.S.; Quinn, K.; Sanislow, C.; Wang, P. Research Domain Criteria (RDoC): Toward a new classification framework for research on mental disorders. *Am. J. Psychiatry* **2010**, *167*, 748–751. [CrossRef] [PubMed]

88. Sadeh, A. The role and validity of actigraphy in sleep medicine: An update. *Sleep Med. Rev.* **2011**, *15*, 259–267. [CrossRef] [PubMed]

89. Gruber, R.; Sadeh, A. Sleep and Neurobehavioral Functioning in Boys with Attention-Deficit/ Hyperactivity Disorder and No Reported Breathing Problems. *Sleep* **2004**, *27*, 267–273. [CrossRef] [PubMed]

90. Kushida, C.A.; Littner, M.R.; Morgenthaler, T.; Alessi, C.A.; Bailey, D.; Coleman, J.; Friedman, L.; Hirshkowitz, M.; Kapen, S.; Kramer, M.; et al. Practice Parameters for the Indications for Polysomnography and Related Procedures: An Update for 2005. *Sleep* **2005**, *28*, 499–523. [CrossRef] [PubMed]

91. Harder, R.; Malow, B.A.; Goodpaster, R.L.; Iqbal, F.; Halbower, A.; Goldman, S.E.; Fawkes, D.B.; Wang, L.; Shi, Y.; Baudenbacher, F.; et al. Heart rate variability during sleep in children with autism spectrum disorder. *Clin. Auton. Res.* **2016**, *26*, 423–432. [CrossRef] [PubMed]

92. Kirov, R.; Uebel, H.; Albrecht, B.; Banaschewski, T.; Yordanova, J.; Rothenberger, A. Attention-deficit/hyperactivity disorder (ADHD) and adaptation night as determinants of sleep patterns in children. *Eur. Child Adolesc. Psychiatry* **2012**, *21*, 681–690. [CrossRef] [PubMed]

93. Newell, J.; Mairesse, O.; Verbanck, P.; Neu, D. Is a one-night stay in the lab really enough to conclude? First-night effect and night-to-night variability in polysomnographic recordings among different clinical population samples. *Psychiatry Res.* **2012**, *200*, 795–801. [CrossRef] [PubMed]

94. Le Bon, O.; Staner, L.; Hoffmann, G.; Dramaix, M.; San Sebastian, I.; Murphy, J.R.; Kentos, M.; Pelc, I.; Linkowski, P. The first-night effect may last more than one night. *J. Psychiatr. Res.* **2001**, *35*, 165–172. [CrossRef]

95. Himanen, S.-L.; Hasan, J. Limitations of Rechtschaffen and Kales. *Sleep Med. Rev.* **2000**, *4*, 149–167. [CrossRef] [PubMed]

96. Malinowska, U.; Durka, P.J.; Blinowska, K.J.; Szelenberger, W.; Wakarow, A. Micro- and macrostructure of sleep EEG. *IEEE Eng. Med. Biol. Mag.* **2006**, *25*, 26–31. [CrossRef] [PubMed]

97. Lofthouse, N.; Gilchrist, R.; Splaingard, M. Mood-related Sleep Problems in Children and Adolescents. *Child Adolesc. Psychiatr. Clin. N. Am.* **2009**, *18*, 893–916. [CrossRef] [PubMed]

98. Bonnet, M.H.; Arand, D.L. EEG Arousal Norms by Age. *J. Clin. Sleep Med.* **2007**, *3*, 271–274. [PubMed]

99. Parrino, L.; Grassi, A.; Milioli, G. Cyclic alternating pattern in polysomnography: What is it and what does it mean? *Curr. Opin. Pulm. Med.* **2014**, *20*, 533–541. [CrossRef] [PubMed]

100. Paruthi, S.; Chervin, R.D. Approaches to the assessment of arousals and sleep disturbance in children. *Sleep Med.* **2010**, *11*, 622–627. [CrossRef] [PubMed]

101. Calderon, D.P.; Kilinc, M.; Maritan, A.; Banavar, J.R.; Pfaff, D. Generalized CNS arousal: An elementary force within the vertebrate nervous system. *Neurosci. Biobehav. Rev.* **2016**, *68*, 167. [CrossRef] [PubMed]

102. Satpute, A.B.; Kragel, P.A.; Barrett, L.F.; Wager, T.D.; Bianciardi, M. Deconstructing arousal into wakeful, autonomic and affective varieties. *Neurosci. Lett.* **2018**. [CrossRef] [PubMed]

103. Tsigos, C.; Chrousos, G.P. Hypothalamic–pituitary–adrenal axis, neuroendocrine factors and stress. *J. Psychosom. Res.* **2002**, *53*, 865–871. [CrossRef]

104. Hegerl, U.; Sander, C.; Hensch, T. Arousal Regulation in Affective Disorders. *Syst. Neurosci. Depression* **2016**, 341–370.

105. McDonnell, A.; McCreadie, M.; Mills, R.; Deveau, R.; Anker, R.; Hayden, J. The role of physiological arousal in the management of challenging behaviours in individuals with autistic spectrum disorders. *Res. Dev. Disabil.* **2015**, *36*, 311–322. [CrossRef] [PubMed]

106. Lecendreux, M.; Konofal, E.; Bouvard, M.; Falissard, B.; Mouren-Simeoni, M.-C. Sleep and Alertness in Children with ADHD. *J. Child Psychol. Psychiatry* **2000**, *41*, 803–812. [CrossRef] [PubMed]

107. Hansen, Å.M.; Garde, A.H.; Persson, R. Sources of biological and methodological variation in salivary cortisol and their impact on measurement among healthy adults: A review. *Scand. J. Clin. Lab. Investig.* **2008**, *68*, 448–458. [CrossRef] [PubMed]

108. Imeraj, L.; Antrop, I.; Roeyers, H.; Deschepper, E.; Bal, S.; Deboutte, D. Diurnal variations in arousal: A naturalistic heart rate study in children with ADHD. *Eur. Child Adolesc. Psychiatry* **2011**, *20*, 381–392. [CrossRef] [PubMed]

109. Baumert, M.; Kohler, M.; Kabir, M.; Kennedy, D.; Pamula, Y. Cardiorespiratory response to spontaneous cortical arousals during stage 2 and rapid eye movement sleep in healthy children. *J. Sleep Res.* **2010**, *19*, 415–424. [CrossRef] [PubMed]

110. Cuthbert, B.N.; Insel, T.R. Toward the future of psychiatric diagnosis: The seven pillars of RDoC. *BMC Med.* **2013**, *11*, 126. [CrossRef] [PubMed]

111. Frank, E.; Sidor, M.M.; Gamble, K.L.; Cirelli, C.; Sharkey, K.M.; Hoyle, N.; Tikotzky, L.; Talbot, L.S.; McCarthy, M.J.; Hasler, B.P. Circadian clocks, brain function, and development. *Ann. N. Y. Acad. Sci.* **2013**, *1306*, 43–67. [CrossRef] [PubMed]

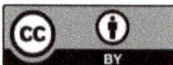

medical
sciences

MDPI

Review

Narcolepsy and Psychiatric Disorders: Comorbidities or Shared Pathophysiology?

Anne Marie Morse [1] and Kothare Sanjeev [2,*]

[1] Division of Child Neurology and Sleep Medicine, Geisinger Medical Center, Danville, PA 17820, USA; amorse@geisinger.edu

[2] Division of Pediatric Neurology, Pediatric Sleep Program (Neurology), Department of Pediatrics, Cohen Children's Medical Center, Lake Success, NY 11042, USA

* Correspondence: skothare@northwell.edu; Tel.: +1-516-465-5255; Fax: +718-347-2240

Received: 3 January 2018; Accepted: 6 February 2018; Published: 15 February 2018

Abstract: Narcolepsy and psychiatric disorders have a significant but unrecognized relationship, which is an area of evolving interest, but unfortunately, the association is poorly understood. It is not uncommon for the two to occur co-morbidly. However, narcolepsy is frequently misdiagnosed initially as a psychiatric condition, contributing to the protracted time to accurate diagnosis and treatment. Narcolepsy is a disabling neurodegenerative condition that carries a high risk for development of social and occupational dysfunction. Deterioration in function may lead to the secondary development of psychiatric symptoms. Inversely, the development of psychiatric symptoms can lead to the deterioration in function and quality of life. The overlap in pharmaceutical intervention may further enhance the difficulty to distinguish between diagnoses. Comprehensive care for patients with narcolepsy should include surveillance for psychiatric illness and appropriate treatment when necessary. Further research is necessary to better understand the underlying pathophysiology between psychiatric disease and narcolepsy.

Keywords: narcolepsy; schizophrenia; attention deficit hyperactivity disorder; depression; anxiety; psychiatric disorders

1. Introduction

Narcolepsy is a disabling neurodegenerative condition that is characterized by the pentad features of excessive daytime sleepiness (EDS), sleep fragmentation, sleep related hallucinations, sleep paralysis, and cataplexy; brief episodes of loss of tone frequently provoked by strong emotions. Instability in the transition between wakefulness and rapid eye movement (REM) sleep causes these symptoms.

Diagnosis is generally made based on the presence of EDS and findings of an average sleep latency of ≤ 8 and the presence of two or more sleep onset REM periods (SOREMPs) on sleep testing. SOREMPs are the presence of REM sleep within 15 minutes of sleep onset, as opposed to the typical cycle taking about 90–120 min. Alternatively, it may be diagnosed by evaluating cerebrospinal fluid (CSF) hypocretin (HRT), which is found to be low in narcolepsy type 1. It is estimated to affect about 1 in 2000 individuals and frequently can take as long as 8–10 year to be accurately diagnosed [1].

Narcolepsy has long been described to have a high co-morbidity for psychiatric disease [2], which is frequently quoted as the cause for delay in diagnosis. The underpinnings of the development of psychiatric symptoms, however, remain unclear. It has been suggested that psychiatric symptoms are either a result of the chronic disabling nature of the disease or it may represent a "shared pathophysiology" or a combination of both.

Improved familiarity with psychiatric illnesses that may share similar features to narcolepsy or may be comorbid (Figure 1) may improve therapeutic outcomes. Consideration of narcolepsy as a part of the differential diagnosis for psychiatric disease may reduce time to diagnosis. Additionally, regular assessment for co-occurring psychiatric disorders in narcolepsy patients may also improve quality of life and functionality.

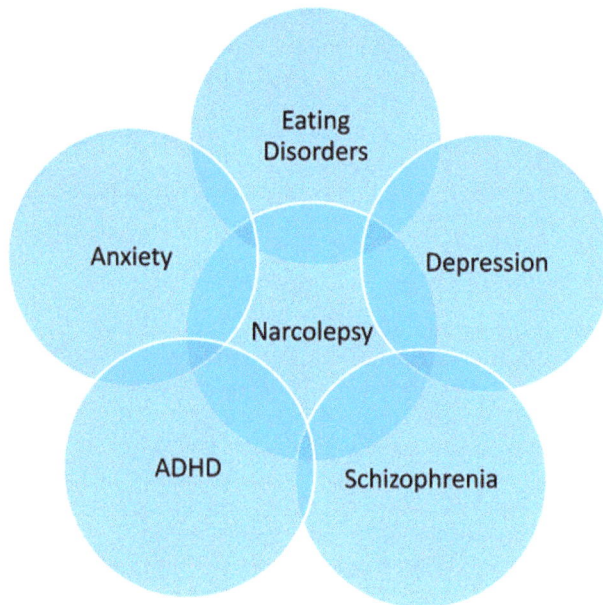

Figure 1. Venn Diagram of the overlapping relationship between highlighting the intimate relationship between psychiatric disorders and narcolepsy [3–12]. ADHD: attention deficit hyperactivity disorder.

2. Attention Deficit Hyperactivity Disorder

Attention deficit hyperactivity disorder (ADHD) is characterized by symptoms of inattention, impulsivity and hyperactivity [13]. Many clinicians perceive ADHD to be the antithesis of narcolepsy; however, there is a significant clinical similarity. Historically, there has even been the suggestion for various overlap syndromes, such as Syndrome Z and Primary Disorder of Vigilance, which were defined by a combination of narcolepsy and ADHD symptoms [14,15].

Recently, there is increasing evidence that sleep dysfunction is intimately related to the development of attention deficit hyperactivity disorder (ADHD). Restricted, dysfunctional, or fragmented sleep may precipitate ADHD features [16,17]. On the other hand, problems with sleep may represent an intrinsic component of ADHD [18]. Individuals with ADHD have an increased association with restless legs syndrome/periodic limb movements in sleep (RLS/PLMS), obstructive sleep apnea/snoring, rhythmic movement disorder (body rocking and head banging), and parasomnias [9,17,18]. The presence of ADHD symptoms in children and adolescents with narcolepsy were found to be about two-fold higher than in controls [9]. Retrospectively, adults with narcolepsy had been found to have a much greater likelihood of having a diagnosis of ADHD in childhood compared to controls [11].

Alternatively, these features may be related to or even confused with the sense of cognitive impairments such as mental fog and difficulty thinking. Cognitive features, such as mental fogginess, have been found to be among the most significant symptoms affecting the daily life of patients with narcolepsy [19]. Hyperactivity seen in ADHD may, in fact, be a compensatory response for individuals who are under-aroused or sleepy [11]. ADHD symptoms have been shown to contribute to poor quality of life and increased frequency of depressive symptoms [20] similar to narcolepsy.

Pharmaceutical interventions for ADHD has overlap (Figure 2) with treatment used in narcolepsy for excessive daytime sleepiness, potentially masking the clinical features of narcolepsy [21,22]. There has been consideration for hypocretin deficiency to be causative for the shared symptoms in narcolepsy and ADHD. However, ADHD symptoms have been found in narcolepsy type 1 and type 2, suggesting that hypocretin deficiency may be unrelated to shared symptomatology. This has been further confirmed with CSF hypocretin evaluation [9]. Therefore, symptoms of EDS, fatigue, and sleep fragmentation may be the cause for ADHD symptoms, which may also explain similar findings in other sleep wake disorders [23].

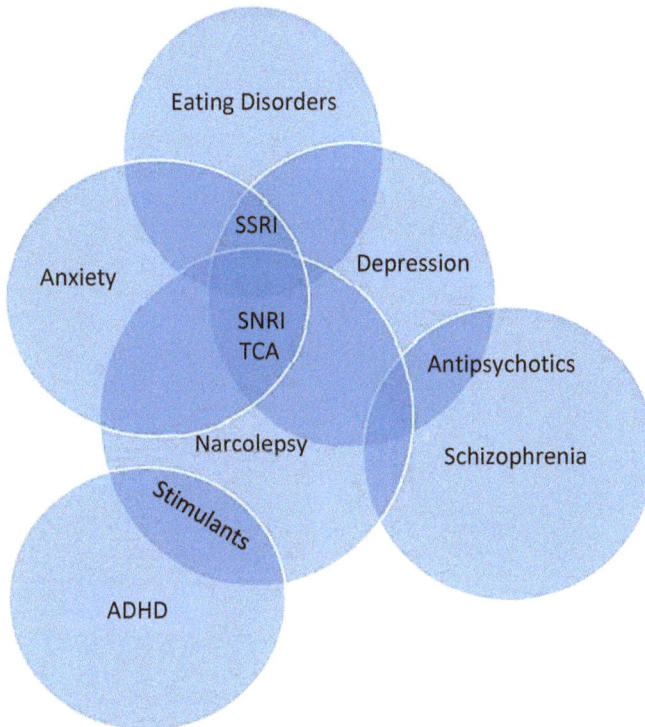

Figure 2. Venn diagram of the overlapping relationship in pharmaceutical treatment for narcolepsy and select psychiatric disorders [4–6,9–11,24,25]. Overlapping benefit of pharmaceutical treatment is found in most treatments, except antipsychotics, which can exacerbate symptoms of narcolepsy. SNRI: Serotonin norepinephrine reuptake inhibitor; TCA: tricyclic antidepressant; SSRI: selective serotonin reuptake inhibitor; ADHD: attention deficit hyperactivity disorder.

3. Depression

Depressed mood is the most commonly described psychiatric symptom in narcolepsy literature [26–28]. Studies evaluating narcoleptic patients with self-reported questionnaires have found up to 57% suffered from depression [26,27]. It is frequently suggested that this is due to the significant overlap in symptoms, such as disordered nocturnal sleep, social withdrawal, impaired attention, fatigue, and weight gain (Table 1). However, when excluding symptoms that may represent overlap, a higher level of depressive symptoms is still present in patients with narcolepsy, including features of anhedonia, pathological guilt, and crying [28]. Depressed mood and sleepiness have been found to be the main limiting factors in maintaining attention in patients with narcolepsy [29].

Additionally, depression has been found to be a major independent risk factor for impaired quality of life [30].

Table 1. Comparison of symptoms of narcolepsy and depression [6,12,28].

Narcolepsy	Depression
Severe Excessive Daytime Sleepiness	Fatigue/lack of energy
Sleep Fragmentation	Sleep Initiation/maintenance difficulties +/- psychosis
Hallucinations (Visual/multi-modal)	Psychomotor agitation/retardation
Cataplexy	Reduced Cognition/Poor school performance
Sleep Paralysis	Withdrawn from friends/family
Negative effect on school/work performance	Guilt
Negative effect on socialization	Appetite changes (weight gain/loss)
Weight gain	Suicide

The chronicity and debilitating nature of narcolepsy may provide the psychological substrate for development of depression. However, Lee et al. identified more than 50% of patients who had narcolepsy and comorbid depression had been diagnosed with depression prior to narcolepsy [10]. Therefore, a shared pathophysiology related to hypocretin deficiency should be considered. Recent research has suggested HRT deficiency impedes appropriate emotional input processing within the amygdala [31]. Further support for this concept was found in the post-mortem evaluation of CSF HRT in depressed patients who completed suicide, which also demonstrated lowered levels of HRT [32]. However, these findings have been inconsistent in other studies [33].

4. Anxiety Disorders

Anxiety disorders are receiving increasing attention as co-morbidity in narcolepsy, but references are still relatively scarce. Anxiety disorders, such as panic attacks and social phobias, have been reported in as many as 53% of patients with narcolepsy [6]. The time course of development for specific anxiety disorders has been suggested to vary by type. For instance, obsessive compulsive disorder and social phobia are more frequently present before the diagnosis of narcolepsy, while panic disorder or simple phobia occur afterward [34]. It has been suggested that these symptoms may be a result of a perceived loss of personal control, such as is experienced with a cataplectic event. Alternatively, it may be related to a fragmented perception of reality due to experienced hallucinations [7].

5. Eating Disorders

Patient with narcolepsy are frequently overweight [3]. It has been found that children with narcolepsy, regardless of pharmaceutical treatment or presence of cataplexy, have higher body mass index (BMIs) [8]. There have been suggestions that these findings are related to a combination of the reduction in basal metabolism and physical activity due to sleepiness [3].

There is additional evidence that these patients are at increased risk for various eating disorders. For example, Fortuyn et al. found narcoleptic patients to report irresistible and persistent craving for food, specifically binge eating with lack of control and restrictive actions to correct binging [25]. Eating disorders, such as anorexia/bulimia nervosa, are typically driven by a desire for specific body habitus. There has been some suggestion of fear of becoming fat endorsed by some patients, but in general, this is not the underlying motive for such behaviors in patients with narcolepsy [5,25]. These patterns of behavior require further exploration as hypocretin stimulates appetite [35]. Therefore, a deficiency would be expected to result in decreased food seeking behavior and weight loss. However, fragmented sleep can modify leptin and ghrelin secretion, thus supporting the increased appetite and weight gain, besides the low basal metabolic rate [36].

6. Schizophrenia

Schizophrenia and narcolepsy have significant overlap in symptoms including hallucinations, sleep fragmentation, and psychosis (Table 2). In general, hallucinations present in narcolepsy are visual, whereas in schizophrenia they are more so auditory [12]. However, it is not uncommon for hallucinations in narcolepsy to be complex multi-sensory phenomena, which can lead to confusion. Comorbid schizophrenia and narcolepsy has been reported, but is thought to be rare [4] (Table 3).

Table 2. Comparison of symptoms of narcolepsy and schizophrenia [4,7,37].

Narcolepsy	Schizophrenia
Excessive Daytime Sleepiness	Excessive Daytime Sleepiness/Mania
Sleep Fragmentation	Sleep initiation or maintenance difficulties
Hallucinations (Visual/multi-modal)	Hallucinations (auditory)
Cataplexy	Catatonia
Sleep Paralysis	PLMD/RLS
Nocturnal Movement Disorders (PLMs)	Reduced REM latency/increased REM density
Reduced REM Latency (SOREMPs)	Social Isolation
Negative effect on socialization	Memory loss, slowness in activity, mental confusion
Negative effect on school/work performance	

Table 3. Review of psychiatric disorders in narcolepsy.

Reference	Study Details	ADHD	Depression	Anxiety	Eating Disorders	Schizophrenia	Undassified Mental Illness	Addictive Behavior
Lecendreux, 2015 [9]	Cross Sectional Survey 108 children with NwC/NwoC </= 18 years old 67 Controls	35.3% NwC 19.7% NwoC 4.8% controls	N/A	N/A	N/A	N/A	N/A	N/A
Modestino, 2013 [11]	Retrospective (ADHD symptoms in childhood)161 adults NwC/NwoC 117 controls	37% Nw/woC	10.55% Nw/woC	N/A	N/A	N/A	N/A	N/A
Lee, 2017 [10]	Case Contro l258 Nw/woC 2580 Controls	8.8% Nw/woC 0.9% controls (*baseline)	32.7% Nw/woC 6.3% control	N/A	N/A	N/A	N/A	N/A
Black, 2017 [24]	Retrospective (medical claims data analysis) 9312 Nw/woC 46559 Controls	N/A	37.9% Nw/woC 13.8% Controls (* mood disorders)	25.1% Nw/woC 11.9% Controls	17.3% Nw/woC 8.4% Controls (*obesity)	N/A	62.3% Nw/woC 31.2% Controls	N/A
Fortuyn, 2011 [6]	Case Control 60 Nw/woC 120 Controls	N/A	13% Nw/woC 5% Controls	35% Nw/woC 3% Controls	N/A	N/A	N/A	N/A
Canellas, 2014 [4]	Case series 10 Narcolepsy Patients	N/A	N/A	N/A	N/A	100% overlap	N/A	N/A
Dahmen, 2008 [1]	Case Control 116 Nw/woC 80 Controls	N/A	N/A	N/A	13% Nw/woC 18% Controls *Eat40 Score Nw/woC 2x higher than Controls*	N/A	N/A	N/A
Chabas, 2007 [3]	Case Control 13 Nw/woC 9 Controls	N/A	N/A	N/A	*Bulimia* 46% Nw/woC 11% control	N/A	N/A	N/A
Fortuyn, 2008 [25]	Case Control 60 NwC 120 Controls	N/A	N/A	N/A	Eating Disoder NOS 15-25% NwC 0% controls	Eating Disoder NOS 15-25% NwC 0% controls	N/A	N/A
Barateau, 2016 [38]	Case Control 710 Controls 243 NwC 116 NwoC 91 IH	N/A	N/A	N/A	N/A	N/A	N/A	*Alcohol* 7.5% NwC 15.2% controls NSD in IH, control, and NwoC *Tobacco* 37.2% NwC 21.7% controls Illicit Drugs NSD in groups

NwC: narcolepsy with cataplexy, NwoC: narcolepsy without cataplexy, Nw/woC: narcolepsy with or without cataplexy, IH: Idiopathic Hypersomnia, NSD no significant differences. N/A: Not applicable.

7. Pathophysiology Overlap

There are only about 70,000 hypocretin cells (HRT-1 and HRT-2), which are concentrated in the lateral hypothalamus. The understood role of hypocretin at this time is in relation to arousal and reward circuitry. Although small in number, the axons of these cells project widely throughout the cortex in varying densities. Hypocretin and dopamine have significant overlap, particularly in the basal forebrain, thalamic paraventricular nucleus, and prefrontal cortex [39]. There are similar overlapping circuits for hypocretin and other monoamines, such as serotonin and norepinephrine. Hypocretin has been shown to have direct excitatory effects on serotonergic neurons, especially in the dorsal raphe nucleus [40]. Similarly, there is a direct excitatory effect on the noradrenergic system, with HRT-1 having five times the excitatory effect of HRT-2 [41]. The understanding of the relationship between HRT and various neurotransmitters is rapidly evolving. This intimate interconnectivity leads to the speculation for a shared pathophysiology for narcolepsy and psychiatric illness, but definitive evidence is still lacking.

8. Conclusions

The presence of psychiatric illness in narcolepsy patients is common. The timeline for development of psychiatric symptoms is poorly defined, which may represent contribution of influencing factors such as age of onset, gender, and duration of illness. There is suggestion that the behavioral phenotype of narcolepsy encompasses various traits of psychiatric disease [28]. Alternative considerations include a secondary development of psychiatric illness, such as depression and anxiety, due to the deleterious effects on reduced quality of life in narcolepsy versus a shared pathophysiology for both narcolepsy and psychiatric disease.

Narcolepsy is associated with an increased risk for poor quality of life which also results in a high socioeconomic burden. Additionally, it has been found to be associated with a 1.5-fold increase in mortality risk compared to those without narcolepsy [34]. It is unclear how the high burden of co-morbid psychiatric disease contributes to this overall. The presence of persistent depressive symptoms has been shown to be an independent risk factor for impaired quality of life [30]. Excessive daytime sleepiness has also been suggested to increase risk for suicidal ideation, which is amplified in the setting of co-morbid depression [42].

A large, systematic, US population–based analysis of medical comorbidities associated with narcolepsy confirmed the findings that there is an excessive prevalence for psychiatric illness. These findings were highlighted by significantly higher psychiatric medication use, psychiatry office visits, and mental illness–related service costs [24]. The consideration for a diagnosis of narcolepsy should be considered in atypical and refractory psychiatric illness. It is important to provide a comprehensive psychiatric evaluation in all patients with narcolepsy to improve identification of co-morbid psychiatric illness and provide appropriate treatment.

The pharmaceutical treatments used in both narcolepsy and psychiatric illness can lend to further difficulty correctly identifying narcolepsy (Figure 2). On the other hand, a paradoxical effect may occur in some cases that may provide guidance for the correct diagnosis. For instance, use of anti-psychotics in schizophrenia can worsen features of narcolepsy and stimulant therapy for narcolepsy may enhance features of psychosis.

9. Future Directions

Future studies should focus on identifying the most effective approach to treating patients with narcolepsy and co-morbid psychiatric illness. The high burden of comorbid disease is debilitating and based on current literature is not being adequately treated. Additionally, the cause for increased mortality in patients with narcolepsy remains unclear. Future studies are needed to clarify if this is a result of narcolepsy as an independent risk factor or the cumulative effect of medical and psychiatric co-morbidities present.

Hypocretin neurons have been identified as a part of the central reward circuitry. Therefore, evaluation of the relationship of HRT deficiency with development of psychiatric symptoms may provide further insight to the underlying pathophysiology. In addition, these findings may also identify unique therapeutic strategies for both narcolepsy and mental illness.

Conflicts of Interest: The authors declare no conflict of interest. No off label use of drugs or products have been discussed in the manuscript.

References

1. Thorpy, M.; Morse, A.M. Reducing the clinical and socioeconomic burden of narcolepsy by earlier diagnosis and effective treatment. *Sleep Med. Clin.* **2017**, *12*, 61–71. [CrossRef] [PubMed]
2. Lishman, W. The psychologIcal consequences of cerebral disorder. In *Organic Psychiatry*; Blackwell Science: Baskı, UK , 1998; pp. 315–323.
3. Chabas, D.; Foulon, C.; Gonzalez, J.; Nasr, M.; Lyon-Caen, O.; Willer, J.-C.; Derene, J.-P.; Arnulf, I. Eating disorder and metabolism in narcoleptic patients. *Sleep* **2007**, *30*, 1267–1273. [CrossRef] [PubMed]
4. Canellas, F.; Lin, L.; Julià, M.R.; Clemente, A.; Vives-Bauza, C.; Ollilla, H.M.; Chul Hong, S.; Arboleya, S.M.; Einen, M.A.; Faraco, J.; et al. Dual cases of type 1 narcolepsy with schizophrenia and other psychotic disorders. *J. Clin. Sleep. Med.* **2014**, *10*, 1011–1018. [CrossRef] [PubMed]
5. Dahmen, N.; Becht, J.; Engel, A.; Thommes, M.; Tonn, P. Prevalence of eating disorders and eating attacks in narcolepsy. *Neuropsychiatr. Dis. Treat.* **2008**, *4*, 257–261. [PubMed]
6. Fortuyn, H.A.D.; Lappenschaar, G.; Furer, J.W.; Hodiamont, P.P.; Rijnders, C.A.; Renier, W.O.; Buitelaar, J.K.; Overeem, S. Anxiety and mood disorders in narcolepsy. *Gen. Hosp. Psychiatr.* **2010**, *32*, 49–556. [CrossRef] [PubMed]
7. Fortuyn, H.A.D.; Lappenschaar, G.; Nienhuis, F.J.; Furer, J.W.; Hodiamont, P.P.; Rijnders, C.A.; Lammers, G.J.; Renier, W.O.; Buitelaar, J.K.; Overeem, S. Psychotic symptoms in narcolepsy: Phenomenology and a comparison with schizophrenia. *Gen. Hosp. Psychiatr.* **2009**, *31*, 146–154. [CrossRef] [PubMed]
8. Kotagal, S.; Krahn, L.E.; Slocumb, N. A putative link between childhood narcolepsy and obesity. *Sleep Med.* **2004**, *5*, 147–150. [CrossRef] [PubMed]
9. Lecendreux, M.; Lavault, S.; Lopez, R.; Inocente, C.O.; Konofal, E.; Cortese, S.; Franco, P.; Arnulf, P.; Dauvilliers, Y. Attention-deficit/hyperactivity disorder (ADHD) symptoms in pediatric narcolepsy: A cross-sectional study. *Sleep* **2015**, *38*, 1285–1295. [CrossRef] [PubMed]
10. Lee, M.J.; Lee, S.Y.; Yuan, S.S.; Yang, C.-J.; Yang, K.-C.; Lee, T.-L.; Sun, C.-C.; Shyu, Y.-C.; Wang, L.-J. Comorbidity of narcolepsy and depressive disorders: A nationwide population-based study in Taiwan. *Sleep Med.* **2017**, *39*, 95–100. [CrossRef] [PubMed]
11. Modestino, E.J.; Winchester, J. A retrospective survey of childhood ADHD symptomatology among adult narcoleptics. *J. Atten. Disord.* **2013**, *17*, 574–582. [CrossRef] [PubMed]
12. Vourdas, A.; Shneerson, J.; Gregory, C.; Smith, I.E.; King, M.A.; Morrish, E.; McKenna, P.J. Narcolepsy and psychopathology: Is there an association? *Sleep Med.* **2002**, *3*, 353–360. [CrossRef]
13. Ghanizadeh, A. Agreement between diagnostic and statistical manual of mental disorders, and the proposed DSM-V attention deficit hyperactivity disorder diagnostic criteria: An exploratory study. *Compr. Psychiat.* **2013**, *54*, 7–10. [CrossRef] [PubMed]
14. Weinberg, W.A.; Brumback, R.A. Primary disorder of vigilance: A novel explanation of inattentiveness, daydreaming, boredom, restlessness, and sleepiness. *J. Pediatr.* **1990**, *116*, 720–725. [CrossRef]
15. Sultan, S.; Bertrim, S.; Kimoff, R.; Baltzan, M. Syndrome Z: A description of a possible narcolepsy spectrum disorder. *Sleep* **1998**, *21*, 88.
16. Beebe, D.W. Neurobehavioral morbidity associated with disordered breathing during sleep in children: A comprehensive review. *Sleep* **2006**, *29*, 1115–1134. [CrossRef] [PubMed]
17. Gruber, R. Sleep characteristics of children and adolescents with attention deficit-hyperactivity disorder. *Child Adolesc. Psychiatr. Clin.* **2009**, *18*, 863–876. [CrossRef] [PubMed]
18. Hvolby, A. Associations of sleep disturbance with ADHD: Implications for treatment. *ADHD Atten. Deficit Hyperact. Disord.* **2015**, *7*, 1–18. [CrossRef] [PubMed]

19. Maski, K.; Steinhart, E.; Williams, D.; Scammell, T.; Flygare, J.; McCleary, K.; Gow, M. Listening to the patient voice in narcolepsy: Diagnostic delay, disease burden, and treatment efficacy. *J. Clin. Sleep Med.* **2017**, *13*, 419–425. [CrossRef] [PubMed]

20. Craig, S.G.; Weiss, M.D.; Hudec, K.L.; Gibbins, C. The functional impact of sleep disorders in children with ADHD. *J. Atten. Disord.* **2017**, 1087054716685840. [CrossRef] [PubMed]

21. Alberto, K.; García-García, F. Current and emerging options for the drug treatment of narcolepsy. *Drugs* **2013**, *73*, 1771–1781.

22. Cortese, S.; Holtmann, M.; Banaschewski, T.; Buitelaar, J.; Coghill, D.; Danckaerts, M.; Dittman, R.W.; Graham, J.; Taylor, E.; Sergeant, J. Practitioner review: Current best practice in the management of adverse events during treatment with ADHD medications in children and adolescents. *J. Child Psychol. Psychiatr.* **2013**, *54*, 227–246. [CrossRef] [PubMed]

23. Hysing, M.; Sørensen, L.; Plessen, K.; Adolfsdottir, S.; Lundervold, A. Review: Recommendations for the assessment and management of sleep disorders in ADHD. *Evid. Based Ment. Health* **2014**, *17*, 22. [PubMed]

24. Black, J.; Reaven, N.; Funk, S.; McGaughey, K.; Ohayon, M.M.; Guilleminault, C.; Ruoff, C. Medical comorbidity in narcolepsy: Findings from the burden of narcolepsy disease (BOND) study. *Sleep Med.* **2017**, *33*, 13–18. [CrossRef] [PubMed]

25. Fortuyn, H.A.D.; Swinkels, S.; Buitelaar, J.; Renier, W.O.; Furer, J.W.; Rijnders, C.A.; Hodiamont, P.P.; Overeem, S. High prevalence of eating disorders in narcolepsy with cataplexy: A case-control study. *Sleep* **2008**, *31*, 335–341. [CrossRef] [PubMed]

26. Daniels, E.; King, M.A.; Smith, I.E.; Shneerson, J.M. Health-related quality of life in narcolepsy. *J. Sleep Res.* **2001**, *10*, 75–81. [CrossRef] [PubMed]

27. Dauvilliers, Y.; Paquereau, J.; Bastuji, H.; Drouot, X.; Weil, J.S.; Viot-Blanc, V. Psychological health in central hypersomnias: The french harmony study. *J. Neurol. Neurosurg. Psychiatr.* **2009**, *80*, 636–641. [CrossRef] [PubMed]

28. Fortuyn, H.A.D.; Mulders, P.; Renier, W.; Buitelaar, J.; Overeem, S. Narcolepsy and psychiatry: An evolving association of increasing interest. *Sleep Med.* **2011**, *12*, 714–719. [CrossRef] [PubMed]

29. Zamarian, L.; Högl, B.; Delazer, M.; Hingerl, K.; Gabelia, D.; Mitterling, T.; Brandauer, E.; Frauscher, B. Subjective deficits of attention, cognition and depression in patients with narcolepsy. *Sleep Med.* **2015**, *16*, 45–51. [CrossRef] [PubMed]

30. Vignatelli, L.; Plazzi, G.; Peschechera, F.; Delaj, L.; D'Alessandro, R. A 5-year prospective cohort study on health-related quality of life in patients with narcolepsy. *Sleep Med.* **2011**, *12*, 1–23. [CrossRef] [PubMed]

31. Schwartz, S.; Ponz, A.; Poryazova, R.; Werth, E.; Boesiger, P.; Khatami, R.; Bassetti, C.L. Abnormal activity in hypothalamus and amygdala during humour processing in human narcolepsy with cataplexy. *Brain* **2007**, *131*, 514–522. [CrossRef] [PubMed]

32. Brundin, L.; Björkqvist, M.; Petersén, Å.; Träskman-Bendz, L. Reduced orexin levels in the cerebrospinal fluid of suicidal patients with major depressive disorder. *Eur. Neuropsychopharmacol.* **2007**, *17*, 573–579. [CrossRef] [PubMed]

33. Schmidt, F.M.; Arendt, E.; Steinmetzer, A.; Bruegel, M.; Kratzsch, J.; Strauss, M.; Baum, P.; Hegerl, U.; Schönknecht, P. CSF-hypocretin-1 levels in patients with major depressive disorder compared to healthy controls. *Psychiatr. Res.* **2011**, *190*, 240–243. [CrossRef] [PubMed]

34. Ohayon, M.M.; Black, J.; Lai, C.; Eller, M.; Guinta, D.; Bhattacharyya, A. Increased mortality in narcolepsy. *Sleep* **2014**, *37*, 439–444. [CrossRef] [PubMed]

35. Baumann, C.R.; Bassetti, C.L. Hypocretins (orexins): Clinical impact of the discovery of a neurotransmitter. *Sleep Med. Rev.* **2005**, *9*, 253–268. [CrossRef] [PubMed]

36. Garcia-Garcia, F.; Juárez-Aguilar, E.; Santiago-García, J.; Cardinali, D.P. Ghrelin and its interactions with growth hormone, leptin and orexins: Implications for the sleep–wake cycle and metabolism. *Sleep Med. Rev.* **2014**, *18*, 89–97. [CrossRef] [PubMed]

37. Taylor, S.F.; Tandon, R.; Shipley, J.E.; Eiser, A.S.; Goodson, J. Sleep onset REM periods in schizophrenic patients. *Biol. Psychiatr.* **1991**, *30*, 205–209. [CrossRef]

38. Barateau, L.; Jaussent, I.; Lopez, R.; Boutrel, B.; Leu-Semenescu, S.; Arnulf, I.; Dauvilliers, Y. Smoking, alcohol, drug use, abuse and dependence in narcolepsy and idiopathic hypersomnia: A case-control study. *Sleep.* **2016**, *39*, 573–580. [CrossRef] [PubMed]

39. Deutch, A.Y.; Bubser, M. The orexins/hypocretins and schizophrenia. *Schizophr. Bull.* **2007**, *33*, 1277–1283. [CrossRef] [PubMed]
40. Liu, R.J.; van den Pol, A.N.; Aghajanian, G.K. Hypocretins (orexins) regulate serotonin neurons in the dorsal raphe nucleus by excitatory direct and inhibitory indirect actions. *J. Neurosci.* **2002**, *22*, 9453–9464. [PubMed]
41. Mieda, M.; Tsujino, N.; Sakurai, T. Differential roles of orexin receptors in the regulation of sleep/wakefulness. *Front. Endocrinol.* **2013**, *4*, 57. [CrossRef] [PubMed]
42. Chellappa, S.L.; Araújo, J.F. Excessive daytime sleepiness in patients with depressive disorder. *Rev. Bras. Psiquiatr.* **2006**, *28*, 126–129. [CrossRef] [PubMed]

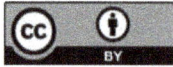

medical sciences

MDPI

Review

Traumatic Brain Injury, Sleep Disorders, and Psychiatric Disorders: An Underrecognized Relationship

Anne M. Morse [1],* and David R. Garner [2]

[1] Janet Weis Children's Hospital, Department of Pediatric Neurology and Sleep Medicine, Geisinger Medical Center, MC 14-12, 100 N Academy Blvd, Danville, PA 17822, USA

[2] Department of Pediatrics, Geisinger Medical Center, Danville, PA 17822, USA; Drgarner@geisinger.edu

* Correspondence: amorse@geisinger.edu

Received: 28 December 2017; Accepted: 5 February 2018; Published: 15 February 2018

Abstract: Traumatic brain injury (TBI) is commonplace among pediatric patients and has a complex, but intimate relationship with psychiatric disease and disordered sleep. Understanding the factors that influence the risk for the development of TBI in pediatrics is a critical component of beginning to address the consequences of TBI. Features that may increase risk for experiencing TBI sometimes overlap with factors that influence the development of post-concussive syndrome (PCS) and recovery course. Post-concussive syndrome includes physical, psychological, cognitive and sleep–wake dysfunction. The comorbid presence of sleep–wake dysfunction and psychiatric symptoms can lead to a more protracted recovery and deleterious outcomes. Therefore, a multidisciplinary evaluation following TBI is necessary. Treatment is generally symptom specific and mainly based on adult studies. Further research is necessary to enhance diagnostic and therapeutic approaches, as well as improve the understanding of contributing pathophysiology for the shared development of psychiatric disease and sleep–wake dysfunction following TBI.

Keywords: traumatic brain injury; anxiety; depression; post-traumatic stress; attention deficit disorder; sleep–wake disorders

---

1. Introduction

Traumatic brain injuries (TBI) are common in the pediatric population and can have neurocognitive consequences. Understanding the factors that influence risk for a child or adolescent to experience a TBI is an important first step in exploring the consequences of TBI. Several studies have reported specific risk factors, including pre-existing psychiatric and behavioral problems to increase the likelihood to sustain a traumatic brain injury in the pediatric population (Table 1). For instance, recent studies have shown that attention deficit hyperactivity disorder (ADHD), aggression, psychiatric prescription medication use, and use of mental health services increase the risk of TBI [1,2]. These factors have been ascertained by both prospective and retrospective analysis. The results of these findings highlight some overlap, but also identify some discrepancy in risk factors, leading one to question the influence of recall bias, influence of etiology of TBI or other contributing factors to these differences (Table 2) [1–7].

Table 1. Factors associated with increased risk for youth to experience traumatic brain injuries (TBI) [8,9].

TBI Risk Factors
Low Socioeconomic Status
Overcrowded households
Disadvantaged neighborhoods
High incidence of adverse life events
Young maternal age
Older siblings with few younger siblings
Previous TBI

Table 2. Comparison of risk factors for TBI and the development of post-concussive syndrome (PCS) based on retrospective and prospective studies [1–7].

Retrospective	Prospective	Overlap	Discrepancy
Male gender	Male gender		
Lower socioeconomic status (SES)	Behavioral problems		
Behavioral problems	Adverse family events		SES status
Attention deficit hyperactivity	during childhood	Male Gender	Maternal features
disorder (ADHD)	Punitive parenting practices	Behavioral Problems	Cognitive baseline
Cognitive problems	Maternal depression		Sports Participation
Contact Sports Participation	Maternal age		
Competitive Sports Participation	Maternal education		

Post-concussive syndrome (PCS) is defined by symptoms occurring after a head injury including, but not limited to, somatic, sleep, cognitive and/or emotional/behavioral difficulties (Table 3) [10–14]. It was previously thought that approximately 15% of those who suffer a single mild TBI (mTBI) will develop chronic PCS; however, McInnes found that this number is likely significantly higher [15]. In fact, a large proportion will continue to have a measurable impairment more than a year out from the injury [15]. In 2012, an estimated 329,290 children, younger than 20, were treated in United States emergency departments for TBI [16]. Among this demographic, the rate of emergency department visits for sports and recreation-related injuries with TBI more than doubled between 2001 and 2012 [16]. In fact, approximately 20% of 8–12th grade students were identified as having had at least one concussion, with 5.5% sustaining recurrent injuries [3]. It is important to identify associated risk factors for TBI within this group, as well as contributors to successful recovery to improve incidence and reduce morbidity.

Table 3. Post-concussive symptoms and prevalence [10–14,17–23].

	Post-Concussive Symptoms	Prevalence
	Headache	25–47%
	Nausea	7–12%
Physical	Dizziness	30%
	Fatigue	16–40%
	Problems with Balance and Gait	24–34%
	Light and Sound Sensitivity	1–4%
Emotional	Emotional Lability	1–40%
	Increased Anxiety	8–17%
Cognitive	Cognitive Deficits	7–22%
	Language Impairment	1–68%
	Disorientation and Amnesia	21–30%
Sleep	Sleep–Wake Disturbance	13–67%

The clinical course following TBI is influenced by multiple factors. Pre-injury behavior and functioning are strong predictors for the long-term development of behavioral problems and worsening of symptoms of psychiatric disorders [24–26]. For instance, children experiencing a significant life stressor prior to injury have been found to be at greater risk of persistent post-concussive symptoms after TBI [13,27]. Children with behavioral problems are commonly endorsed as being at greater risk for experiencing a TBI; however, these specific behavioral disorders are not commonly well defined [4,13].

In addition to baseline behavioral and psychiatric features, sleep–wake dysfunction is also associated with TBI (Figure 1). Sleep difficulties can affect cognition (particularly attention, memory, and executive functions), behavior, and emotional problems (Table 4) [28]. Pre-existing sleep conditions enhance the likelihood of experiencing post-concussive symptoms [29]. In addition, the presence of a comorbid sleep disorder contributes to psychologic instability, resulting in increased emotional lability and behavioral problems with worsened daily executive function [28,30]. In general, symptoms from a mild TBI should disappear by 3 months, and functional status improves over the first six to twelve months without obvious regression over the first 30 months [31]. However, in patients with history of psychiatric disease and/or sleep dysfunction, recovery may be more protracted (Table 5) [10].

Table 4. TBI comorbidities and associated symptoms [4,32–40].

	Diagnoses	Signs and Symptoms
Sleep–Wake	Insomnia	Difficulty falling/staying asleep, unrefreshing sleep, insufficient number of hours of sleep despite adequate opportunity
	Sleep Apnea	Snoring, restlessness, apnea, enuresis, diaphoresis, open-mouth breathing, bruxism, sleep fragmentation
	Idiopathic Hypersomnia	Excessive daytime sleepiness, ± excessive number of hours asleep
	Narcolepsy	Excessive daytime sleepiness, cataplexy, sleep paralysis, sleep related hallucinations, sleep fragmentation
	PLMD/RLS *	PLMs >5/h on PSG; Restlessness, discomfort in arms or legs that interferes with sleep onset or maintenance, improves with movement
	CRD	Sleep difficulties that conflict with age typical circadian rhythm; When given opportunity sleeps appropriate number of hours for age
	Parasomnia	Sleep walking, sleep talking, confusional arousals, night terrors, REM behavior disorder/dream enactment behavior
Psychiatric	Anxiety	Avoidance, phobias, obsessive compulsive symptoms, generalized anxious feelings
	Depression	Fatigue, irritability, sadness, difficulty concentrating, difficulty with recall, suicidality
	ADHD	Impaired attention, hyperactivity, impaired working memory, impaired working speed
	PTSD	Headaches, decreased psychosocial recovery, sleep disturbance/nightmares, pain, flashbacks, amnesia, irritability/aggression, concentration difficulty

PLMD: periodic limb movement disorder; RLS: restless leg syndrome; CRD: circadian rhythm disorder; ADHD: attention deficit hyperactive disorder; PTSD: post-traumatic stress disorder; PLM: periodic limb movements; PSG: polysomnography; * Note: RLS is a clinical diagnosis and PLMD is a polysomnographic diagnosis.

Table 5. Risks factors associated with prolonged recovery following TBI [2,3,41–43].

Risk Factors of Protracted Recovery
Pre-injury psychiatry history
Injury Severity
Family dysfunction
Sleep–Wake Dysfunction
Re-injury
Female gender
Referral to Rehabilitation Facility
Prescription for acute headache rescue therapy
Chronic headache treatment
Presenting SCAT2 * score <80
Participation in a non-helmeted sport

* SCAT2—Sport concussion assessment tool.

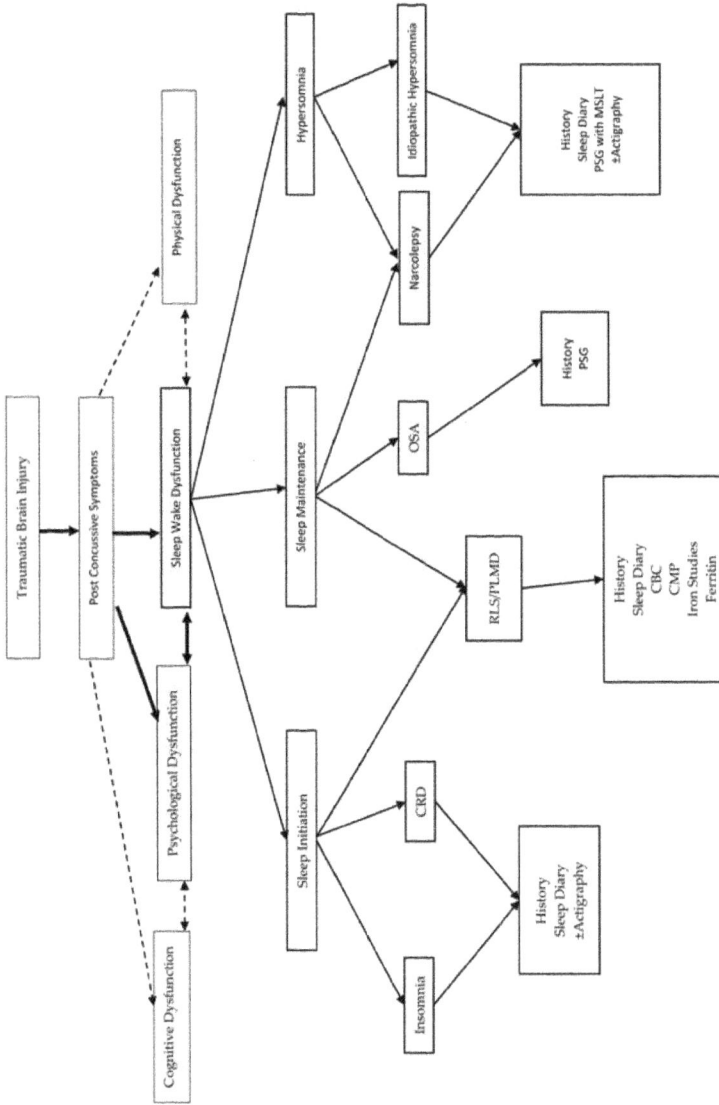

Figure 1. Traumatic brain injury and the development of post-concussive syndrome, highlighting the development of sleep wake dysfunction and its relationship to co-morbid PCS symptoms. CRD: Circadian Rhythm Disorder; CBC: Complete Blood Count; CMP: Complete Metabolic Panel; OSA: Obstructive Sleep Apnea; PSG: Polysomnography; MSLT: Multiple Sleep Latency Test; RLS: Restless Leg Syndrome; PLMD: Periodic Limb Movement Disorder.

The complexity in care of TBI patients is reflective of the multi-disciplinary needs of these patients. TBI-related morbidity may be improved with enhanced understanding of factors that not only contribute to risk for experiencing TBI, but also improved understanding and assessment of the post-concussive factors that influence the course of recovery. This manuscript will focus on the relationship of sleep and psychiatric features. It will explore the clinical relationship, examine the possible crossover in pathophysiology of TBI, sleep, and psychiatric disorders, and discuss the approaches to consider for diagnosis and treatment, highlighting the need for a comprehensive multidisciplinary evaluation to improve recovery times and outcomes [44].

2. Anxiety

Children with TBI are at a significantly higher risk than those with orthopedic injuries to present with new-onset mood and/or anxiety disorders [45]. Anxiety can be defined as the brain's response to danger causing avoidance type behavior [46]. Age at time of injury may influence the development of symptoms. Children who are younger than 10 years old are at higher risk of developing post-concussive anxiety disorders [23,47]. There is also a relation to sleep–wake dysfunction.

In general, youth with anxiety are found to have an increased rate of sleep problems with 88% of those with anxiety reporting at least one sleep problem, and 55% reporting three or more sleep problems [48]. One study also showed that sleep disturbance may vary with age, with younger children being more prone to nighttime wakings and sleep anxiety, and adolescents being more likely to experience excessive daytime sleepiness [49]. After TBI, individuals with continued symptoms of insomnia and fatigue, up to 2 years after the injury, have been found to have higher rates of depression and anxiety [50]. In fact, sleep disturbance, even in the acute post-TBI period, predicted the development of anxiety and depression in the chronic period for all severities of TBI.

3. Major Depressive Disorder

Depressive disorders occur in 10–25% of children post TBI [39,51,52]. Children greater than 12 years of age are five times more likely to experience post-traumatic depressive symptoms [51]. In general, depressed patients may have problematic sleep, as well cognitive difficulties and energy loss. Insomnia or hypersomnia is frequently one of the defining characteristics for depression. The development of depressive symptoms has been suggested to be due to either the injury itself, or as a result of other post-concussive comorbidities, such as anxiety, aggression, and sleep disturbance [53,54].

Due to their intimate relationship, the symptoms of depression and sleep–wake dysfunction influence the development and prognosis of one another. Patients identified to have a sleep disturbance ten days post TBI were 6 times more likely to have depression [54]. Sleep deprivation, defined as 6 h of sleep or less a night, in adolescents at baseline, had a 25–38% increased risk of developing depressive symptoms at follow up exams [55]. On the other hand, major depression and depressive symptoms increase the risk for the development of insomnia [56]. There is a suggestion that early onset depression may be related to the direct injury, whereas late onset depression may be due to a psychological reaction to the injury [57]. However, when including sleep symptoms as part of the evaluation, the pattern of development is less clear.

4. ADHD

ADHD has not only been shown to increase the likelihood to experience TBI, but a preexisting diagnosis of ADHD may also lead to worse outcomes after TBI [58–60]. ADHD that develops as a result of head injury is referred to as secondary ADHD or S-ADHD [61]. S-ADHD has been shown to develop in about 10–20% of patients post TBI. In one study, 15% of S-ADHD cases developed after one year and 21% after two years [9]. Increased TBI severity also increases the incidence of S-ADHD from 7–46% going from mild to severe TBI respectively [51]. Children with TBI, less than 2 years old, have double the risk for the development of S-ADHD as compared to the general population [62], thus raising the questing as to whether S-ADHD is a direct result of injury versus a biased population of children with poor self-regulation who may be more likely to participate in risk-taking behaviors resulting in injury [62].

The relationship between sleep and ADHD has a significant bidirectional effect, which is exaggerated in children following TBI [63]. Children with TBI and ADHD have a poorer sleep quality and quality of life than children with primary ADHD without TBI [64]. Evaluation of comorbid sleep dysfunction in secondary ADHD is lacking, but likely has a similar deleterious effect.

5. Post-Traumatic Stress Syndrome

Post-traumatic stress disorder (PTSD), as a part of PCS, has been well described in adults with TBI [65]. Data is lacking, however, to demonstrate the same relationship in children. Specific symptoms of PTSD present after TBI have been poorly defined in pediatric studies. There is a suggestion that children with orthopedic injuries more frequently display PTS symptoms than those with mTBI and met more symptom criteria at 12 months [40]. On the other hand, there is also a report of children with severe TBI exhibiting higher levels of PCS symptoms than those with moderate TBI or orthopedic injury [66]. Furthermore, another study demonstrated that childhood PTSD after traffic injuries was associated more with increasing age and parental PTSD, and no relationship to severity of injury [67]. The evolving anatomy and age-specific biomechanical properties of the developing child increase risk for distinct types of injuries that rarely occur in adults [68]. This may contribute to the differences observed in the development of PTS symptoms between adults and children.

Another ill-defined parameter in the literature is what symptoms of PTSD are present post TBI [69]. Persistent attention deficits at 3 months post injury have been identified as a risk factor for continued PTS symptoms at 6 months [70]. On the other hand, working memory and verbal learning deficits were found to be protective [70]. This may suggest that patients with impaired working memory and verbal learning, have impaired ability to recall the event, lending to reduced PTS symptoms [65]. Many comorbid conditions often present with TBI and can lead to shorter life expectancy, poor academic performance, and neurocognitive deficits [71]. It has been suggested in adults that sleeping difficulties may be an earlier indicator for risk of PTS disorder [72]. Another study with veterans notes that nightmares are commonly comorbid with TBI [73]. Those with insomnia and PTSD post TBI were found to have a subjective increase in sleepiness as compared to those with just PTSD and insomnia [73]. Literature evaluating sleep-specific risks associated with PTSD in pediatrics is lacking for comparison.

6. Crossover Pathophysiology of TBI, Sleep, and Psychiatric Disorders

TBI can be the result of diffuse or focal injury and frequently can be a combination of both. Diffuse injury occurs when the mechanism causes non-specific global damage, as in diffuse axonal injury or concussion. Focal injury occurs when the mechanism causes a specific targeted area of damage, such as with hematoma or contusion. These injuries may be a result of direct linear force (coup), acceleration deceleration forces (contra-coup) or a combination of both, causing shearing injuries and axonal damage [68]. In addition, there are secondary brain injuries that develop over hours to days that may result from perfusion abnormalities, neuroinflammation, excitotoxicity and dysregulated cell signaling [74,75].

The frontal–striatal circuits, which can affect executive function and wakefulness are particularly vulnerable [76]. Damage to this system is found in 18–38% of children who have suffered a TBI between the ages of 5–15 and may be related to the impaired executive function identified in the first year after injury [77]. Emotional dysregulation can also be common after TBI; this combined with executive dysfunction and hormonal imbalance can make adolescents who experience TBI more susceptible to impulsive decisions and poor choices in social situations [78]. This also may indicate why performance on neuropsychological testing may be normal; however, patients still experience significant functional impairment in real-world situations [78].

Sleep–wake dysfunction following TBI is common, affecting up to 70% of patients. The sleep–wake cycle is tightly controlled via cooperation between circadian rhythms, sleep–wake homeostasis, and external environmental factors such as medication, diet, stress, and surroundings [37]. The main sleep-promoting pathways are found in the ventrolateral (VLPO) and median preoptic nuclei (MnPO), which inhibit ascending arousal pathways in the brainstem and hypothalamus [79]. The arousal areas include histaminergic tuberomammillary nucleus, orexinergic lateral hypothalamus, noradrenergic locus coeruleus, serotonergic dorsal raphe, and the cholinergic laterodorsal tegmental and pedunculopontine tegmental nuclei [80].

Post-mortem evaluations of the brains of patients with and without TBI demonstrated a significant reduction in hypocretin neurons [81,82]. Impaired hypocretin (orexin) signaling causes excessive daytime sleepiness [37,83,84]. It has been shown that reduced cerebrospinal fluid (CSF) orexin levels are associated with a worse clinical outcome with greater likelihood for depression and sleep–wake dysfunction [85,86].

Impaired melatonin production has also been suggested to be contributory [81]. Melatonin directs this circadian regulation of sleep and wakefulness, but also has been found to have anti-inflammatory properties [37]. Melatonin may repress TBI-induced inflammation by activating mitophagy and removing damaged mitochondria [87], although it secretes directly into the third ventricle and levels can be much higher in the CSF than in the peripheral blood [88]. Peripheral sampling does provide an accurate surrogate. Melatonin production can be impacted by TBI. CSF melatonin may vary depending on time from TBI. Acutely, there is evidence of increased melatonin with decreased levels as time progresses [81,89]. These findings, however, have been inconsistent. The acute increase is suggested to be related to the anti-inflammatory properties, which may contribute to neural recovery [89,90]. Additionally, this variation may be related to the spectrum of post-traumatic sleep disorders seen (i.e., hypersomnolence to delayed sleep phase disorder) [81,91].

Circadian rhythm is associated with mood regulation, and disturbances can be linked to the development of psychiatric symptoms [37,92]. There has been the suggestion that this may be related to clock genes, which regulate circadian entrainment. Certain clock genes have been implicated in altering the homeostasis of individuals leading to psychiatric disorders such as autism, ADHD, anxiety, major depressive disorder, bipolar disorder, and schizophrenia [93]. This may represent an increased genetic susceptibility for the development of comorbid post-traumatic sleep dysfunction and mental illness.

7. Evaluation and Treatment Options

A multi-disciplinary approach should be taken in the clinical evaluation of patients following TBI. The consideration of specialties to be involved include neurology, psychiatry, sleep medicine, rehab services, social work and sports medicine, depending on the mechanism of injury. There should be a standardized intake, such as the acute concussion evaluation [10], to ensure a comprehensive evaluation of symptoms. Establishing a pre-morbid baseline may be helpful in stratifying risk for the development of PCS. In addition, it is important to identify patient-perceived impact of head injury and goals for recovery.

Treatment of sleep or psychiatric disorders post TBI is mainly based on adult studies, with limited information on treatment in pediatrics. Frequently, the treatment applied is based on recommendations that have been successful in the relevant psychiatric and sleep disorder in the non-traumatic brain injury population [94]. The approach to treatment in patients with comorbid sleep and psychiatric dysfunction should address symptoms of both processes.

In general, psychiatric medications in pediatrics are started with the lowest dosing and titrated slowly, as pediatric patients may be more susceptible to side effects of these medications [94–97]. The selection of medication is based on the psychiatric symptoms present (Table 6). Selective serotonin reuptake inhibitors are considered first-line treatment for anxiety and depression [94]. S-ADHD treatment with stimulant medication has been shown to likely be beneficial; however, there seems to be a more attenuated response for S-ADHD than that of primary ADHD [2,98,99]. Of note, those treated with psychostimulant medication prior to TBI, have been noted to have a lower risk of TBI [100]. In fact, retrospectively it was identified that most ADHD patients who sustained TBI were not pharmacologically treated prior to the injury [61,101].

PTS disorder patients with nightmares have been shown to have improvements with prazosin and/or image-rehearsal therapy with or without cognitive behavioral therapy (CBT) for insomnia [102]. CBT, for those with insomnia, has also been shown to decrease total wake time and improve sleep efficiency [103].

Table 6. Psychiatric disorders and treatments [104–110].

Psychiatric Disorder	Treatment Options
Depression	
Mild	CBT ± Exercise
Severe	CBT + SSRI ± Exercise
Suicidality	CBT + SSRI ± Hospitalization ± Exercise
With psychotic features	CBT + Antidepressant + Antipsychotic ± Exercise
Refractory	CBT + Antidepressant + Antipsychotic ± Exercise ± ECT
Anxiety	First Line: CBT ± SSRI, SNRI Second Line: CBT + SSRI, ± SNRI Third Line: CBT + SSRI + different SSRI or SNRI with Benzodiazepines used as a bridge until SSRI becomes effective.
ADHD	Stimulants [111,112] (methylphenidate, amphetamine), ± CBT, non-stimulants (atomoxetine, guanfacine, clonidine)
PTSD	CBT, Ensure Safety, Treat Comorbidities, ± Antiadrenergic medications (clonidine, guanfacine, or prazosin *)

* Prazosin is preferred in patients with PTSD nightmare disorder. CBT: cognitive behavioral therapy; ECT: electroconvulsive therapy; SSRI: selective serotonin reuptake inhibitor; SNRI selective serotonin norepinephrine reuptake inhibitor.

The approach to treating sleep–wake dysfunction is dependent on the specific sleep disorder present (Figures 1 and 2). Melatonin has also been studied for sleep disorders post TBI and although no statistical difference was found with daytime alertness, patients subjectively reported improved daytime alertness compared to baseline [113]. Amitriptyline has also been subjectively reported by patients to help with sleep disorders by increasing their sleep duration, despite any statistical difference being shown [113]. Other adult studies have shown that modafinil and armodafinil significantly improve sleep latency for those with excessive daytime sleepiness (EDS) due to mild or moderate TBI [114,115].

Studies evaluating non-pharmacological treatment are also limited. CBT has been shown to improve children's behavior post TBI [116]. Similarly, adolescents who participated in an online counselor-assisted problem solving therapy during their post-TBI hospitalization, showed less impaired functioning after [117]. In adults, blue light exposure, as a form of chronotherapy, was shown to reduce fatigue and daytime sleepiness following TBI [118]. Alternative therapies, such as acupuncture, have even demonstrated subjectively improved sleep quality, cognitive function, and the ability to taper sleep medication use [119]. Earlier recommendations include the importance of transition support including alerting school of injury and potential consequences, monitoring students for any increased needs, and offering assistance or adjusting requirements for a couple of weeks post injury [11].

A negative approach to problem solving and depression symptoms has been associated with elevated PTS symptoms and suggests that targeting negative aspects may help mitigate PTS symptoms [120]. This becomes important because adult and childhood survivors of TBI are already at elevated risk of suicidal behavior [121–123]. Symptom checklists are not adequate screening tools for all potential psychiatric outcomes, which highlights the importance of the physician's role in screening for psychiatric disorders and suicidal ideation post injury [26].

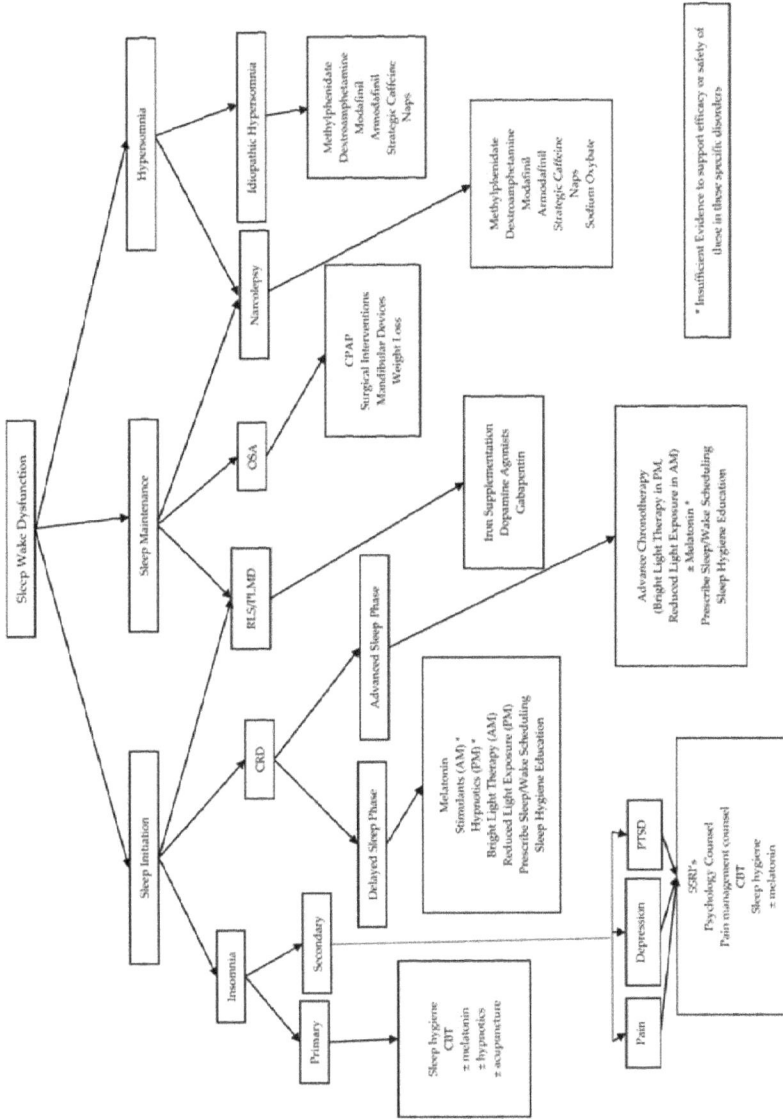

Figure 2. A disease-specific approach to treatment of sleep–wake dysfunction. CRD: Circadian Rhythm Disorder; OSA: Obstructive Sleep Apnea; RLS: Restless Leg Syndrome; PLMD: Periodic Limb Movement Disorder; CBT: Cognitive Behavioral Therapy; SSRI: Selective Serotonin Reuptake Inhibitor

8. Discussion and Future Direction

Traumatic brain injury is a significant pediatric public health concern. It is helpful to view TBI as a disease process, rather than an isolated event [38] due to the cumulative damage that can incur over time. This is evidenced by the features of post-concussive syndrome that can include evolving symptoms of physical, psychological, cognitive, and sleep–wake dysfunction. Increased comorbidity, such as co-occurrence of sleep–wake dysfunction and psychiatric illness, leads to more deleterious outcomes and a more protracted recovery. A multi-disciplinary approach is necessary to provide the comprehensive care necessary in these patients to optimize recovery.

Perception of an injury and expectations for recovery can dramatically influence patient outcomes [17]. Early incorporation of psychological support should be evaluated as a potential tool for improving outcomes in pediatrics. Adult studies have demonstrated benefit of both pharmacological treatments and non-pharmacological treatments; however, there is still a significant gap in knowledge when it comes to pediatric treatments. A targeted evaluation of these recommendations in patients by age and severity of TBI is necessary to determine whether adult treatments are appropriate and effective.

Well-defined TBI severity criteria are needed in the pediatric population. In addition, the effect of pre-morbid functioning needs to be better elucidated. Clinical studies that partner with school systems that implement baseline cognitive assessments may help in filling this data void. In order to improve understanding of how sleep and psychiatric symptoms influence recovery, longitudinal studies are needed. These studies should include well defined age at injury to better assess the effects of TBI on normal development and sleep ontogeny.

Conflicts of Interest: The authors declare no conflicts of interest.

References

1. Eme, R. ADHD: An integration with pediatric traumatic brain injury. *Expert Rev. Neurother.* **2012**, *12*, 475–483. [CrossRef] [PubMed]
2. Schachar, R.J.; Park, L.S.; Dennis, M. Mental Health Implications of Traumatic Brain Injury (TBI) in Children and Youth. *J. Can. Acad. Child Adolesc. Psychiatry* **2015**, *24*, 100–108. [PubMed]
3. Veliz, P.; McCabe, S.E.; Eckner, J.T.; Schulenberg, J.E. Prevalence of concussion among us adolescents and correlated factors. *JAMA* **2017**, *318*, 1180–1182. [CrossRef] [PubMed]
4. Li, L.; Liu, J. The effect of pediatric traumatic brain injury on behavioral outcomes: A systematic review. *Dev. Med. Child Neurol.* **2013**, *55*, 37–45. [CrossRef] [PubMed]
5. Davidson, L.L.; Hughes, S.J.; O'Connor, P.A. Preschool behavior problems and subsequent risk of injury. *Pediatrics* **1988**, *82*, 644–651. [PubMed]
6. Bijur, P.E.; Haslum, M.; Golding, J. Cognitive and behavioral sequelae of mild head injury in children. *Pediatrics* **1990**, *86*, 337–344. [PubMed]
7. McKinlay, A.; Kyonka, E.G.; Grace, R.C.; Horwood, L.J.; Fergusson, D.M.; MacFarlane, M.R. An investigation of the pre-injury risk factors associated with children who experience traumatic brain injury. *Inj. Prev.* **2010**, *16*, 31–35. [CrossRef] [PubMed]
8. Bijur, P.; Golding, J.; Haslum, M.; Kurzon, M. Behavioral predictors of injury in school-age children. *Am. J. Dis. Child.* **1988**, *142*, 1307–1312. [CrossRef] [PubMed]
9. Max, J.E.; Schachar, R.J.; Levin, H.S.; Ewing-Cobbs, L.; Chapman, S.B.; Dennis, M.; Saunders, A.; Landis, J. Predictors of attention-deficit/hyperactivity disorder within 6 months after pediatric traumatic brain injury. *J. Can. Acad. Child Adolesc. Psychiatry* **2005**, *44*, 1032–1040. [CrossRef] [PubMed]
10. Gioia, G.; Micky, C. Acute Concussion Evaluation (ACE): Physicial/Clincian Office Version. 27 April 2006. 2016. Available online: https://www.cdc.gov/headsup/pdfs/providers/ace-a.pdf (accessed on 19 September 2017).
11. Kirkwood, M.W.; Yeates, K.O.; Taylor, H.G.; Randolph, C.; McCrea, M.; Anderson, V.A. Management of pediatric mild traumatic brain injury: A neuropsychological review from injury through recovery. *Clin. Neuropsychol.* **2008**, *22*, 769–800. [CrossRef] [PubMed]

12. Mittenberg, W.; Wittner, M.S.; Miller, L.J. Postconcussion syndrome occurs in children. *Neuropsychology* **1997**, *11*, 447–452. [CrossRef] [PubMed]

13. Ponsford, J.; Willmott, C.; Rothwell, A.; Cameron, P.; Ayton, G.; Nelms, R.; Curran, C.; Ng, K.T. Cognitive and behavioral outcome following mild traumatic head injury in children. *J. Head Trauma Rehabil.* **1999**, *14*, 360–372. [CrossRef] [PubMed]

14. Yeates, K.O.; Luria, J.; Bartkowski, H.; Rusin, J.; Martin, L.; Bigler, E.D. Postconcussive symptoms in children with mild closed head injuries. *J. Head Trauma Rehabil.* **1999**, *14*, 337–350. [CrossRef] [PubMed]

15. McInnes, K.; Friesen, C.L.; MacKenzie, D.E.; Westwood, D.A.; Boe, S.G. Mild Traumatic Brain Injury (mTBI) and chronic cognitive impairment: A scoping review. *PLoS ONE* **2017**, *12*, e0174847. [CrossRef] [PubMed]

16. Coronado, V.G.; Haileyesus, T.; Cheng, T.A.; Bell, J.M.; Haarbauer-Krupa, J.; Lionbarger, M.R.; Flores-Herrera, J.; McGuire, L.C.; Gilchrist, J. Trends in Sports- and Recreation-Related Traumatic Brain Injuries Treated in US Emergency Departments: The National Electronic Injury Surveillance System-All Injury Program (NEISS-AIP) 2001–2012. *J. Head Trauma Rehabil.* **2015**, *30*, 185–197. [CrossRef] [PubMed]

17. Kenzie, E.S.; Parks, E.L.; Bigler, E.D.; Lim, M.M.; Chesnutt, J.C.; Wakeland, W. Concussion As a Multi-Scale Complex System: An Interdisciplinary Synthesis of Current Knowledge. *Front. Neurol.* **2017**, *8*, 513. [CrossRef] [PubMed]

18. Nakase-Richardson, R.; Sherer, M.; Barnett, S.D.; Yablon, S.A.; Evans, C.C.; Kretzmer, T.; Schwartz, D.J.; Modarres, M. Prospective evaluation of the nature, course, and impact of acute sleep abnormality after traumatic brain injury. *Arch. Phys. Med. Rehabil.* **2013**, *94*, 875–882. [CrossRef] [PubMed]

19. Chaput, G.; Giguere, J.F.; Chauny, J.M.; Denis, R.; Lavigne, G. Relationship among subjective sleep complaints, headaches, and mood alterations following a mild traumatic brain injury. *Sleep Med.* **2009**, *10*, 713–716. [CrossRef] [PubMed]

20. Hillier, S.L.; Sharpe, M.H.; Metzer, J. Outcomes 5 years post-traumatic brain injury (with further reference to neurophysical impairment and disability). *Brain Inj.* **1997**, *11*, 661–675. [PubMed]

21. Huang, C.T.; Lin, W.C.; Ho, C.H.; Tung, L.C.; Chu, C.C.; Chou, W.; Wang, C.H. Incidence of severe dysphagia after brain surgery in pediatric traumatic brain injury: A nationwide population-based retrospective study. *J. Head Trauma Rehabil.* **2014**, *29*, E31–E36. [CrossRef] [PubMed]

22. Morgan, A.; Ward, E.; Murdoch, B.; Kennedy, B.; Murison, R. Incidence, characteristics, and predictive factors for dysphagia after pediatric traumatic brain injury. *J. Head Trauma Rehabil.* **2003**, *18*, 239–251. [CrossRef] [PubMed]

23. Max, J.E.; Keatley, E.; Wilde, E.A.; Bigler, E.D.; Levin, H.S.; Schachar, R.J.; Saunders, A.; Ewing-Cobbs, L.; Chapman, S.B.; Dennis, M.; et al. Anxiety disorders in children and adolescents in the first six months after traumatic brain injury. *J. Neuropsychiatry Clin. Neurosci.* **2011**, *23*, 29–39. [CrossRef] [PubMed]

24. Schwartz, L.; Taylor, H.G.; Drotar, D.; Yeates, K.O.; Wade, S.L.; Stancin, T. Long-term behavior problems following pediatric traumatic brain injury: Prevalence, predictors, and correlates. *J. Pediatr. Psychol.* **2003**, *28*, 251–263. [CrossRef] [PubMed]

25. Catroppa, C.; Anderson, V.A.; Morse, S.A.; Haritou, F.; Rosenfeld, J.V. Outcome and predictors of functional recovery 5 years following pediatric traumatic brain injury (TBI). *J. Pediatr. Psychol.* **2008**, *33*, 707–718. [CrossRef] [PubMed]

26. Ellis, M.J.; Ritchie, L.J.; Koltek, M.; Hosain, S.; Cordingley, D.; Chu, S.; Selci, E.; Leiter, J.; Russell, K. Psychiatric outcomes after pediatric sports-related concussion. *J. Neurosurg. Pediatr.* **2015**, *16*, 709–718. [CrossRef] [PubMed]

27. Smyth, K.; Sandhu, S.S.; Crawford, S.; Dewey, D.; Parboosingh, J.; Barlow, K.M. The role of serotonin receptor alleles and environmental stressors in the development of post-concussive symptoms after pediatric mild traumatic brain injury. *Dev. Med. Child Neurol.* **2014**, *56*, 73–77. [CrossRef] [PubMed]

28. Shay, N.; Yeates, K.O.; Walz, N.C.; Stancin, T.; Taylor, H.G.; Beebe, D.W.; Caldwell, C.T.; Krivitzky, L.; Cassedy, A.; Wade, S.L. Sleep problems and their relationship to cognitive and behavioral outcomes in young children with traumatic brain injury. *J. Neurotrauma* **2014**, *31*, 1305–1312. [CrossRef] [PubMed]

29. Kostyun, R.O.; Milewski, M.D.; Hafeez, I. Sleep disturbance and neurocognitive function during the recovery from a sport-related concussion in adolescents. *Am. J. Sports Med.* **2015**, *43*, 633–640. [CrossRef] [PubMed]

30. Hooper, S.R.; Alexander, J.; Moore, D.; Sasser, H.C.; Laurent, S.; King, J.; Bartel, S.; Callahan, B. Caregiver reports of common symptoms in children following a traumatic brain injury. *NeuroRehabilitation* **2004**, *19*, 175–189. [PubMed]

31. Keightley, M.L.; Cote, P.; Rumney, P.; Hung, R.; Carroll, L.J.; Cancelliere, C.; Cassidy, J.D. Psychosocial consequences of mild traumatic brain injury in children: Results of a systematic review by the International Collaboration on Mild Traumatic Brain Injury Prognosis. *Arch. Phys. Med. Rehabil.* **2014**, *95*, S192–S200. [CrossRef] [PubMed]

32. Ornstein, T.J.; Sagar, S.; Schachar, R.J.; Ewing-Cobbs, L.; Chapman, S.B.; Dennis, M.; Saunders, A.E.; Yang, T.T.; Levin, H.S.; Max, J.E. Neuropsychological performance of youth with secondary attention-deficit/hyperactivity disorder 6- and 12-months after traumatic brain injury. *J. Int. Neuropsychol. Soc.* **2014**, *20*, 971–981. [CrossRef] [PubMed]

33. Brown, E.A.; Kenardy, J.A.; Dow, B.L. PTSD perpetuates pain in children with traumatic brain injury. *J. Pediatr. Psychol.* **2014**, *39*, 512–520. [CrossRef] [PubMed]

34. Kovachy, B.; O'Hara, R.; Hawkins, N.; Gershon, A.; Primeau, M.M.; Madej, J.; Carrion, V. Sleep disturbance in pediatric PTSD: Current findings and future directions. *J. Clin. Sleep Med.* **2013**, *9*, 501–510. [CrossRef] [PubMed]

35. Ruff, R.L.; Blake, K. Pathophysiological links between traumatic brain injury and post-traumatic headaches. *F1000Research* **2016**, *5*. [CrossRef] [PubMed]

36. Kenardy, J.; Le Brocque, R.; Hendrikz, J.; Iselin, G.; Anderson, V.; McKinlay, L. Impact of posttraumatic stress disorder and injury severity on recovery in children with traumatic brain injury. *J. Clin. Child Adolesc. Psychol.* **2012**, *41*, 5–14. [CrossRef] [PubMed]

37. Singh, K.; Morse, A.M.; Tkachenko, N.; Kothare, S.V. Sleep Disorders Associated With Traumatic Brain Injury-A Review. *Pediatr. Neurol.* **2016**, *60*, 30–36. [CrossRef] [PubMed]

38. Masel, B.E.; DeWitt, D.S. Traumatic brain injury: A disease process, not an event. *J. Neurotrauma* **2010**, *27*, 1529–1540. [CrossRef] [PubMed]

39. Bloom, D.R.; Levin, H.S.; Ewing-Cobbs, L.; Saunders, A.E.; Song, J.; Fletcher, J.M.; Kowatch, R.A. Lifetime and novel psychiatric disorders after pediatric traumatic brain injury. *J. Can. Acad. Child Adolesc. Psychiatry* **2001**, *40*, 572–579. [CrossRef] [PubMed]

40. Hajek, C.A.; Yeates, K.O.; Gerry Taylor, H.; Bangert, B.; Dietrich, A.; Nuss, K.E.; Rusin, J.; Wright, M. Relationships among post-concussive symptoms and symptoms of PTSD in children following mild traumatic brain injury. *Brain Inj.* **2010**, *24*, 100–109. [CrossRef] [PubMed]

41. Bock, S.; Grim, R.; Barron, T.F.; Wagenheim, A.; Hu, Y.E.; Hendell, M.; Deitch, J.; Deibert, E. Factors associated with delayed recovery in athletes with concussion treated at a pediatric neurology concussion clinic. *Childs Nerv. Syst.* **2015**, *31*, 2111–2116. [CrossRef] [PubMed]

42. Miller, J.H.; Gill, C.; Kuhn, E.N.; Rocque, B.G.; Menendez, J.Y.; O'Neill, J.A.; Agee, B.S.; Brown, S.T.; Crowther, M.; Davis, R.D.; et al. Predictors of delayed recovery following pediatric sports-related concussion: A case-control study. *J. Neurosurg. Pediatr.* **2016**, *17*, 491–496. [CrossRef] [PubMed]

43. Gilbert, K.S.; Kark, S.M.; Gehrman, P.; Bogdanova, Y. Sleep disturbances, TBI and PTSD: Implications for treatment and recovery. *Clin. Psychol. Rev.* **2015**, *40*, 195–212. [CrossRef] [PubMed]

44. Zhang, J.; Xu, Z.; Zhao, K.; Chen, T.; Ye, X.; Shen, Z.; Wu, Z.; Shen, X.; Li, S. Sleep Habits, Sleep Problems, Sleep Hygiene, and Their Associations With Mental Health Problems Among Adolescents. *J. Am. Psychiatr. Nurses Assoc.* **2017**. [CrossRef] [PubMed]

45. Luis, C.A.; Mittenberg, W. Mood and anxiety disorders following pediatric traumatic brain injury: A prospective study. *J. Clin. Exp. Neuropsychol.* **2002**, *24*, 270–279. [CrossRef] [PubMed]

46. Beesdo, K.; Knappe, S.; Pine, D.S. Anxiety and anxiety disorders in children and adolescents: Developmental issues and implications for DSM-V. *Psychiatr. Clin. N. Am.* **2009**, *32*, 483–524. [CrossRef] [PubMed]

47. Vasa, R.A.; Gerring, J.P.; Grados, M.; Slomine, B.; Christensen, J.R.; Rising, W.; Denckla, M.B.; Riddle, M.A. Anxiety after severe pediatric closed head injury. *J. Can. Acad. Child Adolesc. Psychiatry* **2002**, *41*, 148–156. [CrossRef] [PubMed]

48. Alfano, C.A.; Ginsburg, G.S.; Kingery, J.N. Sleep-related problems among children and adolescents with anxiety disorders. *J. Can. Acad. Child Adolesc. Psychiatry* **2007**, *46*, 224–232. [CrossRef] [PubMed]

49. Weiner, C.L.; Meredith Elkins, R.; Pincus, D.; Comer, J. Anxiety sensitivity and sleep-related problems in anxious youth. *J. Anxiety Disord.* **2015**, *32*, 66–72. [CrossRef] [PubMed]

50. Cantor, J.B.; Bushnik, T.; Cicerone, K.; Dijkers, M.P.; Gordon, W.; Hammond, F.M.; Kolakowsky-Hayner, S.A.; Lequerica, A.; Nguyen, M.; Spielman, L.A. Insomnia, fatigue, and sleepiness in the first 2 years after traumatic brain injury: An NIDRR TBI model system module study. *J. Head Trauma Rehabil.* **2012**, *27*, E1-14. [CrossRef] [PubMed]

51. Max, J.E.; Keatley, E.; Wilde, E.A.; Bigler, E.D.; Schachar, R.J.; Saunders, A.E.; Ewing-Cobbs, L.; Chapman, S.B.; Dennis, M.; Yang, T.T.; et al. Depression in children and adolescents in the first 6 months after traumatic brain injury. *Int. J. Dev. Neurosci.* **2012**, *30*, 239–245. [CrossRef] [PubMed]

52. Max, J.E.; Koele, S.L.; Smith, W.L., Jr.; Sato, Y.; Lindgren, S.D.; Robin, D.A.; Arndt, S. Psychiatric disorders in children and adolescents after severe traumatic brain injury: A controlled study. *J. Can. Acad. Child Adolesc. Psychiatry* **1998**, *37*, 832–840. [CrossRef] [PubMed]

53. Jorge, R.E.; Robinson, R.G.; Moser, D.; Tateno, A.; Crespo-Facorro, B.; Arndt, S. Major depression following traumatic brain injury. *Arch. Gen. Psychiatry* **2004**, *61*, 42–50. [CrossRef] [PubMed]

54. Rao, V.; McCann, U.; Han, D.; Bergey, A.; Smith, M.T. Does acute TBI-related sleep disturbance predict subsequent neuropsychiatric disturbances? *Brain Inj.* **2014**, *28*, 20–26. [CrossRef] [PubMed]

55. Roberts, R.E.; Duong, H.T. The prospective association between sleep deprivation and depression among adolescents. *Sleep* **2014**, *37*, 239–244. [CrossRef] [PubMed]

56. Roberts, R.E.; Duong, H.T. Depression and insomnia among adolescents: A prospective perspective. *J. Affect. Disord.* **2013**, *148*, 66–71. [CrossRef] [PubMed]

57. Jorge, R.E.; Robinson, R.G.; Arndt, S.V.; Forrester, A.W.; Geisler, F.; Starkstein, S.E. Comparison between acute- and delayed-onset depression following traumatic brain injury. *J. Neuropsychiatry Clin. Neurosci.* **1993**, *5*, 43–49. [CrossRef] [PubMed]

58. DiScala, C.; Lescohier, I.; Barthel, M.; Li, G. Injuries to children with attention deficit hyperactivity disorder. *Pediatrics* **1998**, *102*, 1415–1421. [CrossRef] [PubMed]

59. Hoare, P.; Beattie, T. Children with attention deficit hyperactivity disorder and attendance at hospital. *Eur. J. Emerg. Med.* **2003**, *10*, 98–100. [CrossRef] [PubMed]

60. Bonfield, C.M.; Lam, S.; Lin, Y.; Greene, S. The impact of attention deficit hyperactivity disorder on recovery from mild traumatic brain injury. *J. Neurosurg. Pediatr.* **2013**, *12*, 97–102. [CrossRef] [PubMed]

61. Gerring, J.P.; Brady, K.D.; Chen, A.; Vasa, R.; Grados, M.; Bandeen-Roche, K.J.; Bryan, R.N.; Denckla, M.B. Premorbid prevalence of ADHD and development of secondary ADHD after closed head injury. *J. Can. Acad. Child Adolesc. Psychiatry* **1998**, *37*, 647–654. [CrossRef] [PubMed]

62. Keenan, H.T.; Hall, G.C.; Marshall, S.W. Early head injury and attention deficit hyperactivity disorder: Retrospective cohort study. *BMJ* **2008**, *337*, a1984. [CrossRef] [PubMed]

63. Owens, J.A. The ADHD and sleep conundrum: A review. *J. Dev. Behav. Pediatr.* **2005**, *26*, 312–322. [CrossRef] [PubMed]

64. Ekinci, O.; Okuyaz, C.; Gunes, S.; Ekinci, N.; Orekeci, G.; Teke, H.; Cobanogullari Direk, M. Sleep and quality of life in children with traumatic brain injury and ADHD. *Int. J. Psychiatry Med.* **2017**, *52*, 72–87. [CrossRef] [PubMed]

65. Bryant, R.A.; Harvey, A.G. Postconcussive symptoms and posttraumatic stress disorder after mild traumatic brain injury. *J. Nerv. Ment. Dis.* **1999**, *187*, 302–305. [CrossRef] [PubMed]

66. Levi, R.B.; Drotar, D.; Yeates, K.O.; Taylor, H.G. Posttraumatic stress symptoms in children following orthopedic or traumatic brain injury. *J. Clin. Child Psychol.* **1999**, *28*, 232–243. [CrossRef] [PubMed]

67. de Vries, A.P.; Kassam-Adams, N.; Cnaan, A.; Sherman-Slate, E.; Gallagher, P.R.; Winston, F.K. Looking beyond the physical injury: Posttraumatic stress disorder in children and parents after pediatric traffic injury. *Pediatrics* **1999**, *104*, 1293–1299. [CrossRef] [PubMed]

68. Pinto, P.S.; Meoded, A.; Poretti, A.; Tekes, A.; Huisman, T.A. The unique features of traumatic brain injury in children. review of the characteristics of the pediatric skull and brain, mechanisms of trauma, patterns of injury, complications, and their imaging findings—Part 2. *J. Neuroimaging* **2012**, *22*, e18-41. [CrossRef] [PubMed]

69. Bryant, R. Post-traumatic stress disorder vs traumatic brain injury. *Dialogues Clin. Neurosci.* **2011**, *13*, 251–262. [PubMed]

70. Guo, X.; Edmed, S.L.; Anderson, V.; Kenardy, J. Neurocognitive predictors of posttraumatic stress disorder symptoms in children 6 months after traumatic brain injury: A prospective study. *Neuropsychology* **2017**, *31*, 84–92. [CrossRef] [PubMed]

71. Ventura, T.; Harrison-Felix, C.; Carlson, N.; Diguiseppi, C.; Gabella, B.; Brown, A.; Devivo, M.; Whiteneck, G. Mortality after discharge from acute care hospitalization with traumatic brain injury: A population-based study. *Arch. Phys. Med. Rehabil.* **2010**, *91*, 20–29. [CrossRef] [PubMed]

72. Macera, C.A.; Aralis, H.J.; Rauh, M.J.; MacGregor, A.J. Do sleep problems mediate the relationship between traumatic brain injury and development of mental health symptoms after deployment? *Sleep* **2013**, *36*, 83–90. [CrossRef] [PubMed]

73. Viola-Saltzman, M.; Watson, N.F. Traumatic brain injury and sleep disorders. *Neurol. Clin.* **2012**, *30*, 1299–1312. [CrossRef] [PubMed]

74. Robertson, C.L.; Scafidi, S.; McKenna, M.C.; Fiskum, G. Mitochondrial mechanisms of cell death and neuroprotection in pediatric ischemic and traumatic brain injury. *Exp. Neurol.* **2009**, *218*, 371–380. [CrossRef] [PubMed]

75. Kochanek, P.M.; Clark, R.S.; Ruppel, R.A.; Adelson, P.D.; Bell, M.J.; Whalen, M.J.; Robertson, C.L.; Satchell, M.A.; Seidberg, N.A.; Marion, D.W.; et al. Biochemical, cellular, and molecular mechanisms in the evolution of secondary damage after severe traumatic brain injury in infants and children: Lessons learned from the bedside. *Pediatr. Crit. Care Med.* **2000**, *1*, 4–19. [CrossRef] [PubMed]

76. Dennis, M.; Guger, S.; Roncadin, C.; Barnes, M.; Schachar, R. Attentional-inhibitory control and social-behavioral regulation after childhood closed head injury: Do biological, developmental, and recovery variables predict outcome? *J. Int. Neuropsychol. Soc.* **2001**, *7*, 683–692. [CrossRef] [PubMed]

77. Sesma, H.W.; Slomine, B.S.; Ding, R.; McCarthy, M.L. Executive functioning in the first year after pediatric traumatic brain injury. *Pediatrics* **2008**, *121*, e1686–e1695. [CrossRef] [PubMed]

78. Tlustos, S.J.; Peter Chiu, C.Y.; Walz, N.C.; Wade, S.L. Neural substrates of inhibitory and emotional processing in adolescents with traumatic brain injury. *J. Pediatr. Rehabil. Med.* **2015**, *8*, 321–333. [CrossRef] [PubMed]

79. Saper, C.B.; Fuller, P.M.; Pedersen, N.P.; Lu, J.; Scammell, T.E. Sleep state switching. *Neuron* **2010**, *68*, 1023–1042. [CrossRef] [PubMed]

80. Sukumaran, T.U. Pediatric sleep project. *Indian Pediatr.* **2011**, *48*, 843–844. [CrossRef] [PubMed]

81. Shekleton, J.A.; Parcell, D.L.; Redman, J.R.; Phipps-Nelson, J.; Ponsford, J.L.; Rajaratnam, S.M. Sleep disturbance and melatonin levels following traumatic brain injury. *Neurology* **2010**, *74*, 1732–1738. [CrossRef] [PubMed]

82. Nardone, R.; Bergmann, J.; Kunz, A.; Caleri, F.; Seidl, M.; Tezzon, F.; Gerstenbrand, F.; Trinka, E.; Golaszewski, S. Cortical excitability changes in patients with sleep-wake disturbances after traumatic brain injury. *J. Neurotrauma* **2011**, *28*, 1165–1171. [CrossRef] [PubMed]

83. Baumann, C.R.; Stocker, R.; Imhof, H.G.; Trentz, O.; Hersberger, M.; Mignot, E.; Bassetti, C.L. Hypocretin-1 (orexin A) deficiency in acute traumatic brain injury. *Neurology* **2005**, *65*, 147–149. [CrossRef] [PubMed]

84. Nishino, S.; Ripley, B.; Overeem, S.; Lammers, G.J.; Mignot, E. Hypocretin (orexin) deficiency in human narcolepsy. *Lancet* **2000**, *355*, 39–40. [CrossRef]

85. Brundin, L.; Bjorkqvist, M.; Petersen, A.; Traskman-Bendz, L. Reduced orexin levels in the cerebrospinal fluid of suicidal patients with major depressive disorder. *Eur. Neuropsychopharmacol.* **2007**, *17*, 573–579. [CrossRef] [PubMed]

86. Schwartz, S.; Ponz, A.; Poryazova, R.; Werth, E.; Boesiger, P.; Khatami, R.; Bassetti, C.L. Abnormal activity in hypothalamus and amygdala during humour processing in human narcolepsy with cataplexy. *Brain* **2008**, *131*, 514–522. [CrossRef] [PubMed]

87. Lin, C.; Chao, H.; Li, Z.; Xu, X.; Liu, Y.; Hou, L.; Liu, N.; Ji, J. Melatonin attenuates traumatic brain injury-induced inflammation: A possible role for mitophagy. *J. Pineal Res.* **2016**, *61*, 177–186. [CrossRef] [PubMed]

88. Reiter, R.J.; Tan, D.X.; Kim, S.J.; Cruz, M.H. Delivery of pineal melatonin to the brain and SCN: Role of canaliculi, cerebrospinal fluid, tanycytes and Virchow-Robin perivascular spaces. *Brain Struct. Funct.* **2014**, *219*, 1873–1887. [CrossRef] [PubMed]

89. Seifman, M.A.; Adamides, A.A.; Nguyen, P.N.; Vallance, S.A.; Cooper, D.J.; Kossmann, T.; Rosenfeld, J.V.; Morganti-Kossmann, M.C. Endogenous melatonin increases in cerebrospinal fluid of patients after severe traumatic brain injury and correlates with oxidative stress and metabolic disarray. *J. Cereb. Blood Flow Metab.* **2008**, *28*, 684–696. [CrossRef] [PubMed]

90. Parcell, D.L.; Ponsford, J.L.; Redman, J.R.; Rajaratnam, S.M. Poor sleep quality and changes in objectively recorded sleep after traumatic brain injury: A preliminary study. *Arch. Phys. Med. Rehabil.* **2008**, *89*, 843–850. [CrossRef] [PubMed]

91. Cajochen, C.; Krauchi, K.; Mori, D.; Graw, P.; Wirz-Justice, A. Melatonin and S-20098 increase REM sleep and wake-up propensity without modifying NREM sleep homeostasis. *Am. J. Physiol.* **1997**, *272*, R1189–R1196. [CrossRef] [PubMed]

92. Liberman, A.R.; Kwon, S.B.; Vu, H.T.; Filipowicz, A.; Ay, A.; Ingram, K.K. Circadian Clock Model Supports Molecular Link Between PER3 and Human Anxiety. *Sci. Rep.* **2017**, *7*, 9893. [CrossRef] [PubMed]

93. Charrier, A.; Olliac, B.; Roubertoux, P.; Tordjman, S. Clock Genes and Altered Sleep-Wake Rhythms: Their Role in the Development of Psychiatric Disorders. *Int. J. Mol. Sci.* **2017**, *18*, 938. [CrossRef] [PubMed]

94. Silver, J.M.; McAllister, T.W.; Arciniegas, D.B. Depression and cognitive complaints following mild traumatic brain injury. *Am. J. Psychiatry* **2009**, *166*, 653–661. [CrossRef] [PubMed]

95. Alderfer, B.S.; Arciniegas, D.B.; Silver, J.M. Treatment of depression following traumatic brain injury. *J. Head Trauma Rehabil.* **2005**, *20*, 544–562. [CrossRef] [PubMed]

96. Arciniegas, D.B.; Anderson, C.A.; Topkoff, J.; McAllister, T.W. Mild traumatic brain injury: A neuropsychiatric approach to diagnosis, evaluation, and treatment. *Neuropsychiatr. Dis. Treat.* **2005**, *1*, 311–327. [PubMed]

97. Arciniegas, D.B.; Silver, J.M. Pharmacotherapy of posttraumatic cognitive impairments. *Behav. Neurol.* **2006**, *17*, 25–42. [CrossRef] [PubMed]

98. Levin, H.; Hanten, G.; Max, J.; Li, X.; Swank, P.; Ewing-Cobbs, L.; Dennis, M.; Menefee, D.S.; Schachar, R. Symptoms of attention-deficit/hyperactivity disorder following traumatic brain injury in children. *J. Dev. Behav. Pediatr.* **2007**, *28*, 108–118. [CrossRef] [PubMed]

99. Willmott, C.; Ponsford, J. Efficacy of methylphenidate in the rehabilitation of attention following traumatic brain injury: A randomised, crossover, double blind, placebo controlled inpatient trial. *J. Neurol. Neurosurg. Psychiatry* **2009**, *80*, 552–557. [CrossRef] [PubMed]

100. Fann, J.R.; Leonetti, A.; Jaffe, K.; Katon, W.J.; Cummings, P.; Thompson, R.S. Psychiatric illness and subsequent traumatic brain injury: A case control study. *J. Neurol. Neurosurg. Psychiatry* **2002**, *72*, 615–620. [CrossRef] [PubMed]

101. Max, J.E.; Lansing, A.E.; Koele, S.L.; Castillo, C.S.; Bokura, H.; Schachar, R.; Collings, N.; Williams, K.E. Attention deficit hyperactivity disorder in children and adolescents following traumatic brain injury. *Dev. Neuropsychol.* **2004**, *25*, 159–177. [CrossRef] [PubMed]

102. Seda, G.; Sanchez-Ortuno, M.M.; Welsh, C.H.; Halbower, A.C.; Edinger, J.D. Comparative meta-analysis of prazosin and imagery rehearsal therapy for nightmare frequency, sleep quality, and posttraumatic stress. *J. Clin. Sleep Med.* **2015**, *11*, 11–22. [CrossRef] [PubMed]

103. Ouellet, M.C.; Morin, C.M. Efficacy of cognitive-behavioral therapy for insomnia associated with traumatic brain injury: A single-case experimental design. *Arch. Phys. Med. Rehabil.* **2007**, *88*, 1581–1592. [CrossRef] [PubMed]

104. Birmaher, B.; Brent, D.; Bernet, W.; Bukstein, O.; Walter, H.; Benson, R.S.; Chrisman, A.; Farchione, T.; Greenhill, L.; Hamilton, J.; et al. Practice parameter for the assessment and treatment of children and adolescents with depressive disorders. *J. Can. Acad. Child Adolesc. Psychiatry* **2007**, *46*, 1503–1526. [CrossRef] [PubMed]

105. Ginsburg, G.S.; Becker, E.M.; Keeton, C.P.; Sakolsky, D.; Piacentini, J.; Albano, A.M.; Compton, S.N.; Iyengar, S.; Sullivan, K.; Caporino, N.; et al. Naturalistic follow-up of youths treated for pediatric anxiety disorders. *JAMA Psychiatry* **2014**, *71*, 310–318. [CrossRef] [PubMed]

106. Ginsburg, G.S.; Kendall, P.C.; Sakolsky, D.; Compton, S.N.; Piacentini, J.; Albano, A.M.; Walkup, J.T.; Sherrill, J.; Coffey, K.A.; Rynn, M.A.; et al. Remission after acute treatment in children and adolescents with anxiety disorders: Findings from the CAMS. *J. Consult. Clin. Psychol.* **2011**, *79*, 806–813. [CrossRef] [PubMed]

107. Wolraich, M.; Brown, L.; Brown, R.T.; DuPaul, G.; Earls, M.; Feldman, H.M.; Ganiats, T.G.; Kaplanek, B.; Meyer, B.; Perrin, J.; et al. ADHD: Clinical practice guideline for the diagnosis, evaluation, and treatment of attention-deficit/hyperactivity disorder in children and adolescents. *Pediatrics* **2011**, *128*, 1007–1022. [PubMed]

108. Pliszka, S. Practice parameter for the assessment and treatment of children and adolescents with attention-deficit/hyperactivity disorder. *J. Can. Acad. Child Adolesc. Psychiatry* **2007**, *46*, 894–921. [CrossRef] [PubMed]

109. Pliszka, S.R.; Crismon, M.L.; Hughes, C.W.; Corners, C.K.; Emslie, G.J.; Jensen, P.S.; McCracken, J.T.; Swanson, J.M.; Lopez, M. The Texas Children's Medication Algorithm Project: Revision of the algorithm for pharmacotherapy of attention-deficit/hyperactivity disorder. *J. Can. Acad. Child Adolesc. Psychiatry* **2006**, *45*, 642–657. [CrossRef] [PubMed]

110. Akinsanya, A.; Marwaha, R.; Tampi, R.R. Prazosin in Children and Adolescents With Posttraumatic Stress Disorder Who Have Nightmares: A Systematic Review. *J. Clin. Psychopharmacol.* **2017**, *37*, 84–88. [CrossRef] [PubMed]

111. Cohen, J.A.; Mannarino, A.P.; Murray, L.K. Trauma-focused CBT for youth who experience ongoing traumas. *Child Abuse Negl.* **2011**, *35*, 637–646. [CrossRef] [PubMed]

112. Connor, D.F.; Grasso, D.J.; Slivinsky, M.D.; Pearson, G.S.; Banga, A. An open-label study of guanfacine extended release for traumatic stress related symptoms in children and adolescents. *J. Child Adolesc. Psychopharmacol.* **2013**, *23*, 244–251. [CrossRef] [PubMed]

113. Kemp, S.; Biswas, R.; Neumann, V.; Coughlan, A. The value of melatonin for sleep disorders occurring post-head injury: A pilot RCT. *Brain Inj.* **2004**, *18*, 911–919. [CrossRef] [PubMed]

114. Menn, S.J.; Yang, R.; Lankford, A. Armodafinil for the treatment of excessive sleepiness associated with mild or moderate closed traumatic brain injury: A 12-week, randomized, double-blind study followed by a 12-month open-label extension. *J. Clin. Sleep Med.* **2014**, *10*, 1181–1191. [CrossRef] [PubMed]

115. Kaiser, P.R.; Valko, P.O.; Werth, E.; Thomann, J.; Meier, J.; Stocker, R.; Bassetti, C.L.; Baumann, C.R. Modafinil ameliorates excessive daytime sleepiness after traumatic brain injury. *Neurology* **2010**, *75*, 1780–1785. [CrossRef] [PubMed]

116. Pastore, V.; Colombo, K.; Liscio, M.; Galbiati, S.; Adduci, A.; Villa, F.; Strazzer, S. Efficacy of cognitive behavioural therapy for children and adolescents with traumatic brain injury. *Disabil. Rehabil.* **2011**, *33*, 675–683. [CrossRef] [PubMed]

117. Wade, S.L.; Kurowski, B.G.; Kirkwood, M.W.; Zhang, N.; Cassedy, A.; Brown, T.M.; Nielsen, B.; Stancin, T.; Taylor, H.G. Online problem-solving therapy after traumatic brain injury: A randomized controlled trial. *Pediatrics* **2015**, *135*, e487–e495. [CrossRef] [PubMed]

118. Sinclair, K.L.; Ponsford, J.L.; Taffe, J.; Lockley, S.W.; Rajaratnam, S.M. Randomized controlled trial of light therapy for fatigue following traumatic brain injury. *Neurorehabil. Neural Repair* **2014**, *28*, 303–313. [CrossRef] [PubMed]

119. Zollman, F.S.; Larson, E.B.; Wasek-Throm, L.K.; Cyborski, C.M.; Bode, R.K. Acupuncture for treatment of insomnia in patients with traumatic brain injury: A pilot intervention study. *J. Head Trauma Rehabil.* **2012**, *27*, 135–142. [CrossRef] [PubMed]

120. Rhine, T.; Cassedy, A.; Yeates, K.O.; Taylor, H.G.; Kirkwood, M.W.; Wade, S.L. Investigating the Connection Between Traumatic Brain Injury and Posttraumatic Stress Symptoms in Adolescents. *J. Head Trauma Rehabil.* **2017**. [CrossRef] [PubMed]

121. Harris, E.C.; Barraclough, B. Suicide as an outcome for mental disorders. A meta-analysis. *Br. J. Psychiatry* **1997**, *170*, 205–228. [CrossRef] [PubMed]

122. Lewinsohn, P.M.; Rohde, P.; Seeley, J.R. Psychosocial characteristics of adolescents with a history of suicide attempt. *J. Can. Acad. Child Adolesc. Psychiatry* **1993**, *32*, 60–68. [CrossRef] [PubMed]

123. Teasdale, T.W.; Engberg, A.W. Suicide after traumatic brain injury: A population study. *J. Neurol. Neurosurg. Psychiatry* **2001**, *71*, 436–440. [CrossRef] [PubMed]

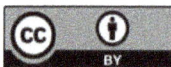

medical sciences

Review

Exploring Interventions for Sleep Disorders in Adolescent Cannabis Users

Tzvi Furer *, Komal Nayak and Jess P. Shatkin

Department of Child and Adolescent Psychiatry, Child Study Center at Hassenfeld Children's Hospital of New York at NYU Langone, One Park Avenue, 7th Floor, New York, NY 10016, USA;
Komal.Nayak@nyumc.org (K.N.); Jess.Shatkin@nyumc.org (J.P.S.)
* Correspondence: tzvi.furer@nyumc.org

Received: 8 January 2018; Accepted: 5 February 2018; Published: 8 February 2018

Abstract: This review summarizes the available literature on the intersection of adolescent cannabis use and sleep disturbances, along with interventions for adolescent cannabis users who suffer sleep impairments. Adolescents are susceptible to various sleep disorders, which are often exacerbated by the use of substances such as cannabis. The relationship between cannabis and sleep is bidirectional. Interventions to improve sleep impairments among adolescent cannabis users to date have demonstrated limited efficacy, although few studies indicating the benefits of behavioral interventions—such as Cognitive Behavior Therapy for Insomnia or Mindfulness Based Stress Reduction—appear promising in the treatment of sleep disorders, which are present for users of cannabis. Further research is necessary to elucidate the precise mechanisms by which cannabis use coexists with sleep impairments, along with effective interventions for those users who suffer sleep difficulties.

Keywords: adolescent; cannabis; sleep; interventions

1. Introduction

Adolescents undergo tumultuous changes in sleep. By early puberty, the majority of adolescents begin to show preference for later sleep and wake times [1,2], with evident symptoms of sleepiness during the daytime [3]. Several studies have demonstrated that a substantial proportion of adolescents are sleep deprived [3], which often leads to irregular sleep schedules between weekdays and weekends [1,4]. For example, 17 percent of adolescents report trouble falling asleep before 2 a.m. at least three times per week [5]. This pattern of disrupted sleep often results in circadian misalignment, with roughly one to seven percent of adolescents meeting diagnostic criteria for delayed sleep phase disorder, or DSPD [6–8]. DSPD itself typically leads to a series of negative outcomes, such as academic difficulties, irritability, and depressed mood. Delaying the middle school and, especially, high school start times is a proven intervention to not only reduce sleepiness, fatigue, and negative mood, but also improve academic performance and even reduce automobile accidents among those teens who drive [2]. The U.S. Centers for Disease Control (CDC) has, in fact, recommended that high schools not start before 8:30 a.m.; however, only 20 percent of schools in the U.S. adhere to this recommendation [2].

Adolescence is also a time of increased risk-taking behavior, including experimentation with alcohol, cannabis, and tobacco [9]. According to studies, cannabis is the most prevalent psychoactive substance used by adolescents in the United States [10]. Not surprisingly, irregular sleep schedules, daytime sleepiness, and frequency of substance use have been found to correlate with one another [11]. Multiple studies [12–14] demonstrate that sleep problems precede, and are often predictive of, future adolescent substance use. Consequently, the extant literature on substance use and sleep indicates that the effect is bidirectional, with both a lack of sleep and continued use of substances each leading to potentially more difficulties with the other [15].

Cannabis is the most common substance found in drug screens following adolescent arrests, emergency room admissions, and autopsies [16]. As of September 2017, 28 states and the District of Columbia have legalized cannabis for medical purposes within the United States, and 7 states and the District of Columbia have legalized cannabis for recreational use; in addition, several other states have proposed bills to legalize cannabis within the next few years [17]. Surveys done in states where cannabis has been legalized indicate no significant trends in increased marijuana use post-legalization, with noted decreases in cannabis use within the past 30 days for both 10th grade students in Washington as well as overall youth use in Colorado [18]. In Alaska, the percentage of all high school students using cannabis use has remained stable, even post-legalization of marijuana [18]. As of 2015, 81% of 12th grade students across the United States cited being able to access marijuana easily if they desired, while 64% of 10th grade students and 35% of 8th grade students also reported "easy" access [9].

The annual prevalence of marijuana use has largely declined from 2013 to 2016, showing a drop from 12.7% in 2013 to 9.4% in 2016 for 8th grade students while use in 10th grade students dropped from 29.8% in 2013 to 23.9% in 2016 [9]. For 12th grade students, however, the annual prevalence has held mostly steady, with annual prevalence noted as 36.4% in 2013 while documented as 35.6% in 2016. General attitudes of students have trended towards greater acceptance of marijuana use, with the perceived risk of regular cannabis use noted in 2016 as 57.5, 44, and 31% for 8th, 10th, and 12th graders, respectively. Meanwhile, perceived risk of regular cannabis use was previously greater in 2013, noted as 61, 46.5, and 39.5% for 8th, 10th, and 12th graders, respectively [9].

In this paper, we review the current literature on sleep disorders in adolescents who use cannabis, the bidirectional effects of cannabis and sleep disorders, and behavioral interventions for adolescents who use cannabis and have comorbid sleep disorders.

2. Cannabis and Sleep

It is reported that the cannabis plant has over 100 cannabinoids, of which are the active components of marijuana that work primarily on the endocannabinoid system. Delta-9-tetrahydrocannabinol (THC) and cannabidiol (CBD) are two of the most researched cannabinoids, and are classified as phytocannabinoids [17]. The stability of the circadian rhythm is impaired after administration of THC [19]. In response to chronic administration of THC, the body adapts to a state of reduced slow wave sleep [20]. THC is psychoactive via activation of specific CB1 (cannabinoid) receptors that regulate mood, appetite, and memory [21]. Activation of CB1 receptors creates the 'high' feeling reported by cannabis users, and is noted to have a biphasic effect corresponding to either high or low doses of THC. Animal model studies have defined this 'biphasic' difference based on the quantity of THC: specifically that low doses of THC produce an anxiolytic effect, while higher doses of THC can induce panic symptoms [22–24]. Use of THC overall can potentially produce either cognitive impairment or acute psychosis. CBD differs from THC in that it does not activate the CB1 cannabinoid receptors, and is therefore not 'psychoactive' [25]. CBD does not display the same intoxicating effects as THC, and is currently being researched as an adjunctive treatment for symptoms of psychosis [25]. On a molecular level, the endocannabinoid system is presumed to be involved in the regulation of the circadian sleep–wake cycle [26] and the maintenance and promotion of sleep [20]. Overall, chronic cannabis use has been found to be associated with poorer sleep quality and disruptions in sleep [27]. It is generally accepted, however, that a bidirectional effect exists between regular cannabis use and sleep impairments, although the scientific literature is limited.

It has been shown that acute exposure to cannabis can reduce sleep latency, overall time in rapid eye movement (REM) phase, and decreased REM density [28], while administration of CBD and/or THC also has profound effects on sleep. The relationship of cannabidiol with sleep has had different noted outcomes; low-dose CBD has been found to create a stimulating effect, while high dose CBD has shown to have a sedating effect [17]. Other studies of CBD have been mixed; one study demonstrated that cannabidiol blocked anxiety-induced REM sleep suppression without an effect on NREM sleep [29], while other research found that CBD injections caused an increase in the total percentage of sleep in rats [30]. Meanwhile, administration of THC may promote sleep onset and decrease total REM sleep time. Both CBD and THC have a profound effect on sleep architecture in consistent cannabis users. CBD has been found to decrease stage 3 (N3) sleep (commonly known as slow-wave sleep) when used in conjunction with THC, while THC and synthetic THC preparations have been associated with decreased sleep latency [31]. Stage 3 (N3) sleep has been shown to be important in the consolidation of hippocampus-dependent declarative memories [32], whereas previously it was theorized that REM sleep played a major role in memory consolidation [33]. This finding explains previous reports indicating the adverse effects of cannabis on working memory and the ability to maintain information [34]. Thus, the noted effects on sleep architecture play a significant role in cannabis' known effects on memory, especially in adolescents. Disturbed sleep is reported in 67–73% of adults and 33–43% of adolescents during a quit attempt [35–37] and can be seen up to 45 days post-cessation [38]. Prolonged use of cannabis followed by rapid cessation is known to result in sleep disruption and a significant REM rebound, characterized by an increase in dreaming [35,38–40].

Most available data on the effects of cannabis on sleep describes the adult population; however, emerging evidence suggests that adolescents experience these same changes in sleep [41]. Numerous studies have found a correlation between sleep duration [42], self-reported sleep problems [43], and insomnia [13] among those adolescents who use cannabis. Sleep-timing characteristics are associated with substance use [44], with demonstrated differences between individual chronotypes. Chronotypes are specific behaviors indicative of an individual's circadian rhythm, with morning chronotypes found to have earlier sleep onset and wake-up times, while evening chronotypes show later sleep onset patterns and more significant substance use behaviors [45].

Sleep also appears to have an important role in both cessation from cannabis and relapse [36]. Up to 65% of cannabis users, in fact, have identified poor sleep as the primary reason for relapse during a prior attempt at cessation. Paradoxically, cannabis has been described by users as having both a soporific and a sleep disrupting quality [46]. This observation may be due to the cyclical nature of substance use. Individuals may begin using cannabis to aid in sleep initiation, but once tolerance is established, they may require higher doses to yield the same effect. This pattern of use then leads to increased sleep disturbances during abstinence from cannabis, resulting in further relapses [37]. It is important to note that little data is available regarding regular users in natural settings, who are not seeking treatment for cannabis addiction or sleep disorders [47].

Cannabis has also been used in the medical treatment of various sleep-related disorders, including obstructive sleep apnea (OSA) and REM behavior disorder [17]. Among patients suffering from OSA, the endocannabinoid oleamide and exogenous cannabinoid THC have been found to reduce apneic events by alleviating serotonin-mediated OSA symptoms [48]. One case series has observed that cannabidiol reduced symptoms of REM behavior disorder among four adults with Parkinson's disease [49]. Finally, limited research on excessive daytime sleepiness has noted that patients who tested positive for THC (indicating recent cannabis use) were more likely to meet criteria for narcolepsy [50].

3. Interventions

Overall, there is limited data describing useful interventions for adolescents who use cannabis and suffer from sleep problems. Pharmacological interventions do not typically target the cannabis abuse itself, and most of the current treatment literature focuses on addressing symptoms of withdrawal, among which are the various sleep disturbances. Most of these studies have focused on adult patients, and little has been demonstrated in a naturalized clinical setting. Not surprisingly, both zolpidem and benzodiazepines in general have been found useful in treating sleep disturbances associated with cannabis withdrawal. Gabapentin, N-acetylcysteine (NAC), and naltrexone have each been shown to induce some reductions in the use of cannabis and in the prevention of relapse in small samples [51]. Of greater utility and relevance for most practitioners, however, are the benefits of behavioral interventions for the treatment of sleep problems relating to cannabis use. Over the past decade, numerous behavioral strategies have emerged for the treatment of insomnia and related sleep difficulties in both adults and adolescents. Often grouped under the rubric of "cognitive behavioral therapy for insomnia (CBT-I)", these various tools are, in fact, unique and variable in efficacy. Studies of CBT-I have shown improvement in sleep quality in both adults and adolescents with sleep disturbances [52–55].

Important behavioral interventions highlighted in this review include stimulus control therapy (SCT), sleep restriction therapy (SRT), bright light therapy, sleep hygiene education, cognitive therapy, behavioral relaxation, and mindfulness based stress reduction. These tools are part of an array of options available to address sleep problems, and provide unique benefits and applications. The goal of SCT is to enhance the association between the bed/bedroom and sleep. This objective is accomplished largely by reducing the amount of time spent awake in bed, in addition to removing all potentially alerting stimuli from the room (e.g., cell phone, lighted clocks, etc.) [56–58]. SCT is effective both for acute and chronic insomnia [59]. Sleep restriction therapy is commonly employed alongside SCT. In this case, the goal of treatment is to strengthen the homeostatic sleep drive by restricting the amount of time spent in bed to only that during which the individual is actually sleeping. This process involves a thorough and regular logging of sleep hours, and therefore can be a bit more labor intensive, but ultimately improves sleep efficiency markedly.

Another effective treatment for insomnia is bright light therapy, also known as heliotherapy or phototherapy. Bright light exposure works by resetting circadian rhythms, specifically in individuals with sleep-phase delays [4], with greater efficacy when applied during the morning hours [60]. Sleep hygiene education delivers basic information about sleep, providing practical advice on managing circadian rhythm, body temperature, napping, exercise, diet, caffeine, alcohol, tobacco, and drugs in an effort to improve sleep quality [61,62]. Cognitive therapy for insomnia treats sleep disturbances by restructuring maladaptive thoughts, beliefs, and attitudes. This method addresses faulty beliefs, unrealistic sleep expectations, and diminished perceptions about control of sleep [63]. Finally, behavioral relaxation/arousal reduction utilizes skills akin to those taught in mindfulness-based stress reduction (MSBR). These procedures focus on mindfulness-based exercises to reduce the physical and psychological tension associated with sleep difficulty. Procedures include practices such as meditation, deep breathing, progressive muscle relaxation, and biofeedback. Numerous studies have identified sleep improvements from these practices [64–66]. One study looked at a combination of the above behavioral interventions, structured as a six-session multicomponent treatment model to improve sleep and decrease the risk of relapse in an adolescent population of substance users [67]. Significant improvement was found in sleep efficiency, sleep onset latency, and total sleep time. Additionally, there was a decrease in substance problems found 12 months after the conclusion of the study.

4. Conclusions

Cannabis use and sleep impairments go hand-in-hand and share a bidirectional relationship with each strongly influencing the other. Although good behavioral and pharmacological strategies independently exist for the treatment of sleep disorders, targeted interventions for sleep impairments among those who regularly use cannabis are needed. Future studies should examine behavioral and psychopharmacological treatment models for sleep disturbances among adolescent marijuana users, who remain a difficult population to study. Sleep patterns are also undoubtedly affected by growth and development during adolescence, and the biological effects of cannabis may also vary throughout development. Since cannabis use typically begins in adolescence, identifying interventions that are effective, practical, and accepted by youth is essential to decrease the risk of long-term sleep disorders and other co-morbidities. In the meantime, practitioners are advised to rely primarily upon behavioral methods to improve the sleep of adolescents who use cannabis.

Conflicts of Interest: The authors declare no conflict of interest.

References

1. Wolfson, A.R.; Carskadon, M.A. Sleep schedules and daytime functioning in adolescents. *Child Dev.* **1998**, *69*, 875–887. [CrossRef] [PubMed]
2. Owens, J.A.; Belon, K.; Moss, P. Impact of Delaying School Start Time on Adolescent Sleep, Mood, and Behavior. *Arch. Pediatr. Adolesc. Med.* **2010**, *164*, 608–614. [CrossRef] [PubMed]
3. Carskadon, M.A. Patterns of sleep and sleepiness in adolescents. *Pediatrician* **1990**, *18*, 5–12.
4. Lack, L.; Bootzin, R.R. Circadian rhythm factors in insomnia and their treatment. In *Treating Sleep Disorders: Principles and Practice of Behavioural Sleep Medicine*; Perlin, M.L., Lichstein, K.L., Eds.; John Wiley & Sons: Hoboken, NJ, USA, 2003.
5. Saxvig, I.W.; Pallesen, S.; Wilhelmsen-Langeland, A.; Molde, H.; Bjorvatn, B. Prevalence and correlates of delayed sleep phase in high school students. *Sleep Med.* **2012**, *13*, 193–199. [CrossRef] [PubMed]
6. Johnson, E.; Roth, T.; Schultz, L.; Breslau, N. Epidemiology of DSM-IV insomnia in adolescence: Lifetime prevalence, chronicity, and an emergent gender difference. *Pediatrics* **2006**, *117*, 247–256. [CrossRef] [PubMed]
7. Ohayon, M.M.; Roberts, R.E.; Zulley, J.; Smirne, S.; Priest, R.G. Prevalence and patterns of problematic sleep among older adolescents. *J. Am. Acad. Child Adolesc. Psychiatry* **2000**, *39*, 1549–1556. [CrossRef] [PubMed]
8. Pelayo, R.P.; Thorpy, M.J.; Glovinsky, P. Prevalence of delayed sleep phase syndrome among adolescents. *J. Sleep Res.* **1988**, *17*, 392.
9. Johnston, L.D.; O'Malley, P.M.; Miech, R.A.; Bachman, J.G.; Schulenberg, J.E. *Monitoring the Future National Survey Results on Drug Use, 2016 Overview, Key Findings on Adolescent Drug Use*; Institute for Social Research, The University of Michigan: Ann Arbor, MI, USA, 2017.
10. Office of Applied Studies. *Year-End 1998 Emergency Department Data from the Drug Abuse Warning Network*; DHHS Publication No. SMA 00-3376, Drug Abuse Warning Network Series D-11; Substance Abuse and Mental Health Services Administration: Rockville, MD, USA, 2000.
11. Tynjala, J.; Kannas, L.; Levlahti, E. Perceived tiredness among adolescents and its association with sleep habits and use of psychoactive substances. *J. Sleep Res.* **1997**, *6*, 189–198. [CrossRef] [PubMed]
12. Mike, T.B.; Shaw, D.S.; Forbes, E.E.; Sitnick, S.L.; Hasler, B.P. The hazards of bad sleep- Sleep duration and quality as predictors of adolescent alcohol and cannabis use. *Drug Alcohol Depend.* **2016**, *168*, 335–339. [CrossRef] [PubMed]
13. Roane, B.M.; Taylor, D.J. Adolescent insomnia as a risk factor for early adult depression and substance abuse. *Sleep* **2008**, *31*, 1351–1356. [PubMed]
14. Wong, M.M.; Robertson, G.C.; Dyson, R.B. Prospective relationship between poor sleep and substance-related problems in a sample of adolescents. *Alcohol. Clin. Exp. Res.* **2015**, *39*, 355–362. [CrossRef] [PubMed]
15. Gillin, J.; Drummond, S.; Clark, C.; Moore, P. Medication and substance abuse. In *Principles and Practices of Sleep Medicine*, 4th ed.; Kryger, M., Roth, T., Dement, W., Eds.; Saunders: Philadelphia, PA, USA, 2005; pp. 1345–1358.
16. Dennis, M.; Titus, J.C.; Diamond, G.; Donaldson, J.; Godley, S.H.; Tims, F.M.; Webb, C.; Kaminer, Y.; Babor, T.; Roebuck, M.C.; et al. The Cannabis Youth Treatment (CYT) experiment: Rationale, study design and analysis plans. *Addiction* **2002**, *97* (Suppl. 1), 16–34. [CrossRef] [PubMed]
17. Babson, K.A.; Sottile, J.; Morabito, D. Cannabis, Cannabinoids, and Sleep: A Review of the Literature. *Curr. Psychiatry Rep.* **2017**, *19*, 23. [CrossRef] [PubMed]
18. Drug Policy Alliance. *So Far, So Good: What We Know about Marijuana Legalization in Colorado, Washington, Alaska, Oregon, and Washington, D.C.*; Drug Policy Alliance: New York, NY, USA, 2016.
19. Perron, R.R.; Tyson, R.L.; Sutherland, G.R. Delta9-tetrahydrocannabinol increases brain temperature and inverts circadian rhythms. *Neuroreport* **2001**, *12*, 3791–3794. [CrossRef] [PubMed]
20. Vaughn, L.K.; Denning, G.; Stuhr, K.L.; de Wit, H.; Hill, M.N.; Hillard, C.J. Endocannabinoid signaling: Has it got rhythm? *Br. J. Pharmacol.* **2010**, *160*, 530–543. [CrossRef] [PubMed]
21. Aizpurua-Olaizola, O.; Elezgarai, I.; Rico-Barrio, I.; Zarandona, I.; Etxebarria, N.; Usobiaga, A. Targeting the endocannabinoid system: Future therapeutic strategies. *Drug Discov. Today* **2017**, *22*, 105–110. [CrossRef] [PubMed]
22. Onaivi, E.S.; Green, M.R.; Martin, B.R. Pharmacological characterization of cannabinoids in the elevated plus maze. *J. Pharmacol. Exp. Ther.* **1990**, *253*, 1002–1009. [PubMed]

23. Berrendero, F.; Maldonado, R. Involvement of the opioid system in the anxiolytic-like effects induced by delta9-tetrahydrocannabinol. *Psychopharmacology* **2002**, *163*, 111–117. [CrossRef] [PubMed]

24. Valjent, E.; Mitchell, J.M.; Besson, M.J.; Caboche, J.; Maldonado, R. Behavioural and biochemical evidence for interactions between delta 9-tetrahydrocannabinol and nicotine. *Br. J. Pharmacol.* **2002**, *135*, 564–578. [CrossRef] [PubMed]

25. Iseger, T.A.; Bossong, M.G. A systematic review of the antipsychotic properties of cannabidiol in humans. *Schizophr. Res.* **2015**, *162*, 153–161. [CrossRef] [PubMed]

26. Marijuana (Cannabis). Marijuana (Cannabis): SAMHSA. Available online: www.samhsa.gov/atod/marijuana (accessed on 7 December 2017).

27. Maple, K.E.; McDaniel, K.A.; Shollenbarger, S.G.; Lisdahl, K.M. Dose-dependent cannabis use, depressive symptoms, and FAAH genotype predict sleep quality in emerging adults: A pilot study. *Am. J. Drug Alcohol. Abuse* **2016**, *42*, 431–440. [CrossRef] [PubMed]

28. Feinberg, I.; Jones, R.; Walker, J.; Cavness, C.; Floyd, T. Effects of marijuana extract and tetrahydrocannabinol on electroencephalographic sleep patterns. *Clin. Pharmacol. Ther.* **1976**, *19*, 782–794. [CrossRef] [PubMed]

29. Hsiao, Y.T.; Yi, P.L.; Li, C.L.; Chang, F.C. Effect of cannabidiol on sleep disruption induced by the repeated combination tests consisting of open field and elevated plus-maze in rats. *Neuropharmacology* **2012**, *62*, 373–384. [CrossRef] [PubMed]

30. Chagas, M.H.; Crippa, J.A.; Zuardi, A.W.; Hallak, J.E.; Machado-de-Sousa, J.P.; Hirotsu, C.; Maia, L.; Tufik, S.; Andersen, M.L. Effects of acute systemic administration of cannabidiol on sleep-wake cycle in rats. *J. Psychopharmacol.* **2013**, *27*, 312–316. [CrossRef] [PubMed]

31. Nicholson, A.N.; Turner, C.; Stone, B.M.; Robson, P.J. Effect of Delta-9-tetrahydrocannabinol and cannabidiol on nocturnal sleep and early-morning behavior in young adults. *J. Clin. Psychopharmacol.* **2004**, *24*, 305–313. [CrossRef] [PubMed]

32. Born, J. Slow-wave sleep and the consolidation of long-term memory. *World J. Biol. Psychiatry* **2010**, *11* (Suppl. 1), 16–21. [CrossRef] [PubMed]

33. Siegel, J.M. The REM sleep-memory consolidation hypothesis. *Science* **2001**, *294*, 1058–1063. [CrossRef] [PubMed]

34. Tervo-Clemmens, B.; Simmonds, D.; Calabro, F.J.; Day, N.L.; Richardson, G.A.; Luna, B. Adolescent cannabis use and brain systems supporting adult working memory encoding, maintenance and retrieval. *Neuroimage* **2017**, *169*, 496–509. [CrossRef] [PubMed]

35. Vandrey, R.; Smith, M.T.; McCann, U.D.; Budney, A.J.; Curran, E.M. Sleep disturbance and effects of extended-release zolpidem during cannabis withdrawal. *Drug Alcohol Depend.* **2011**, *117*, 38–44. [CrossRef] [PubMed]

36. Budney, A.J.; Vandrey, R.G.; Hughes, J.R.; Thostenson, J.D.; Bursac, Z. Comparison of cannabis and tobacco withdrawal: Severity and contribution to relapse. *J. Subs. Abuse Treat.* **2008**, *35*, 362–368. [CrossRef] [PubMed]

37. Bonn-Miller, M.O.; Babson, K.A.; Vandrey, R. Using cannabis to help you sleep: Heightened frequency of medical cannabis use among those with PTSD. *Drug Alcohol Depend.* **2014**, *136*, 162–165. [CrossRef] [PubMed]

38. Vandrey, R.; Budney, A.J.; Kamon, J.L.; Stanger, C. Cannabis withdrawal in adolescent treatment seekers. *Drug Alcohol Depend.* **2005**, *78*, 205–210. [CrossRef] [PubMed]

39. Allsop, D.J.; Lintzeris, N.; Copeland, J.; Dunlop, A.; McGregor, I.S. Cannabinoid replacement therapy (CRT): Nabiximols (Sativex) as a novel treatment for cannabis withdrawal. *Clin. Pharmacol. Ther.* **2015**, *97*, 571–574. [CrossRef] [PubMed]

40. Bolla, K.I.; Lesage, S.R.; Gamaldo, C.E.; Neubauer, D.N.; Funderburk, F.R.; Cadet, J.L.; David, P.M.; Verdejo-Garcia, A.; Benbrook, A.R. Sleep disturbance in heavy marijuana users. *Sleep* **2008**, *31*, 901–908. [CrossRef] [PubMed]

41. Cohen-Zion, M.; Drummond, S.P.; Padula, C.B.; Winward, J.; Kanady, J.; Medina, K.L.; Tapert, S.F. Sleep architecture in adolescent marijuana and alcohol users during acute and extended abstinence. *Addict. Behav.* **2009**, *34*, 976–979. [CrossRef] [PubMed]

42. McKnight-Eily, L.R.; Eaton, D.K.; Lowry, R.; Croft, J.B.; Presley-Cantrell, L.; Perry, G.S. Relationships between hours of sleep and health-risk behaviors in US adolescent students. *Prev. Med.* **2011**, *43*, 271–273. [CrossRef] [PubMed]

43. Johnson, E.O.; Breslau, N. Sleep problems and substance use in adolescence. *Drug Alcohol Depend.* **2001**, *64*, 1–7. [CrossRef]

44. Pasch, K.E.; Latimer, L.A.; Cance, J.D.; Moe, S.G.; Lytle, L.A. Longitudinal Bi-directional Relationships Between Sleep and Youth Substance Use. *J. Youth Adolesc.* **2012**, *41*, 1184–1196. [CrossRef] [PubMed]
45. Nguyen-Louie, T.T.; Brumback, T.; Worley, M.J.; Colrain, I.M.; Matt, G.E.; Squeglia, L.M.; Tapert, S.F. Effects of sleep on substance use in adolescents: A longitudinal perspective. *Addict. Biol.* **2017**. [CrossRef] [PubMed]
46. Ogeil, R.P.; Phillips, J.G.; Rajaratnam, S.M.; Broadbear, J.H. Risky drug use and effects on sleep quality and daytime sleepiness. *Hum. Psychopharmacol.* **2015**, *30*, 356–363. [CrossRef] [PubMed]
47. Pacek, L.R.; Herrmann, E.S.; Smith, M.T.; Vandrey, R. Sleep continuity, architecture and quality among treatment-seeking cannabis users: AN in-home, unattended polysomnographic study. *Exp. Clin. Psychopharmacol.* **2017**, *25*, 295–302. [CrossRef] [PubMed]
48. Carley, D.W.; Pavlovic, S.; Janelidze, M.; Radulovacki, M. Functional role for cannabinoids in respiratory stability during sleep. *Sleep* **2012**, *25*, 391–398. [CrossRef]
49. Chagas, M.H.; Eckeli, A.L.; Zuardi, A.W.; Pena-Pereira, M.A.; Sobreira-Neto, M.A.; Sobreira, E.T.; Camilo, M.R.; Bergamaschi, M.M.; Scenck, C.H.; Hallak, J.E.; et al. Cannabidiol can improve complex sleep-related behaviours associated with rapid eye movement sleep behavior disorder in Parkinson's disease patients: A case series. *J. Clin. Pharm. Ther.* **2014**, *39*, 564–566. [CrossRef] [PubMed]
50. Dzodzomenyo, S.; Stolfi, A.; Splaingard, D.; Early, E.; Onadeko, O.; Splaingard, M. Urine toxicology screen in multiple sleep latency test: The correlation of positive tetrahydrocannabinol, drug negative patients, and narcolepsy. *J. Clin. Sleep Med.* **2015**, *11*, 93–99. [CrossRef] [PubMed]
51. Brezing, C.A.; Levin, F.R. The current state of pharmacological treatments for cannabis use disorder and withdrawal. *Neuropsychopharmacology* **2018**, *43*, 173–194. [CrossRef] [PubMed]
52. De Bambotti, M.; Goldstone, A.; Colrain, I.M.; Baker, F.C. Insomnia disorder in adolescence: Diagnosis, impact, and treatment. *Sleep Med. Rev.* **2017**, 1–13. [CrossRef] [PubMed]
53. De Bruin, E.J.; Bogels, S.M.; Oort, F.J.; Meijer, A.M. Improvements of adolescent psychopathology after insomnia treatment: Results from a randomized controlled trial over 1 year. *J. Child Psychol. Psychiatry* **2017**. [CrossRef] [PubMed]
54. Mitchell, M.D.; Gehrman, P.; Perlis, M.L.; Umscheid, C.A. Comparative effectiveness of cognitive behavioral therapy for insomnia: A systematic review. *BMC Fam. Pract.* **2012**, *13*, 40. [CrossRef] [PubMed]
55. Wu, J.Q.; Appleman, E.R.; Salazar, R.D.; Ong, J.C. Cognitive behavioral therapy for insomnia comorbid with psychiatric and medical conditions: A meta-analysis. *JAMA Intern. Med.* **2015**, *175*, 1461–1472. [CrossRef] [PubMed]
56. Morin, C.M.; Culbert, J.P.; Schwartz, S.M. Nonpharmacological interventions for insomnia: A meta-analysis of treatment efficacy. *Am. J. Psychiatry* **1994**, *151*, 1172–1180. [PubMed]
57. Morin, C.M.; Colecchi, C.; Stone, J.; Sood, R.; Brink, D. Behavioral and pharmacological therapies for late-life insomnia: A randomized controlled trial. *JAMA* **1999**, *281*, 991–999. [CrossRef] [PubMed]
58. Murtagh, D.R.; Greenwood, K.M. Identifying Effective Psychological Treatments for Insomnia: A Meta-Analysis. *J. Consult. Clin. Psychol.* **1995**, *63*, 79–89. [CrossRef] [PubMed]
59. Bootzin, R.R.; Perlis, M.L. Chapter 2—Stimulus Control Therapy. In *Behavioral Treatments for Sleep Disorders*; Elsevier: Amsterdam, The Netherlands, 2011; pp. 21–30.
60. Guilleminault, C.; Clerk, A.; Black, J.; Labanowski, M.; Pelayo, R.; Claman, D. Nondrug treatment trials in psychophysiologic insomnia. *Arch Intern. Med.* **1995**, *155*, 838–844. [CrossRef] [PubMed]
61. Stepanski, E.J.; Wyatt, J.K. Use of sleep hygiene in the treatment of insomnia. *Sleep Med. Rev.* **2003**, *7*, 215–225. [CrossRef] [PubMed]
62. Manber, R.; Bootzin, R.R.; Acebo, C.; Carskadon, M.A. The effects of regularizing sleep-wake schedules on daytime sleepiness. *Sleep* **1996**, *19*, 432–441. [CrossRef] [PubMed]
63. Morin, C.M.; Kowatch, R.A.; Barry, T.; Walton, E. Cognitive-behavior therapy for late-life insomnia. *J. Consult. Clin. Psychol.* **1993**, *61*, 137–146. [CrossRef] [PubMed]
64. Kaplan, K.H.; Goldenberg, D.L.; Galvin-Nadeau, M. The impact of a meditation-based stress reduction program on fibromyalgia. *Gen. Hosp. Psychiatry* **1993**, *15*, 284–289. [CrossRef]
65. Carlson, L.E.; Speca, M.; Patel, K.D.; Goodney, E. Mindfulness-based stress reduction in relation to quality of life, mood, symptoms of stress, and immune parameters in breast and prostate cancer outpatients. *Psychosom. Med.* **2003**, *65*, 571–581. [CrossRef] [PubMed]

66. Cohen, L.; Warneke, C.; Fouladi, R.T.; Rodriguez, M.A.; Chaoul-Reich, A. Psychological adjustment and sleep quality in a randomized trial of the effects of a Tibetan yoga intervention in patients with lymphoma. *Cancer* **2004**, *100*, 2253–2260. [CrossRef] [PubMed]

67. Bootzin, R.R.; Stevens, S.J. Adolescents, substance abuse, and the treatment of insomnia and daytime sleepiness. *Clin. Psychol. Rev.* **2005**, *25*, 629–644. [CrossRef] [PubMed]

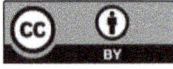

medical sciences

MDPI

Review

Cognitive and Behavioral Consequences of Sleep Disordered Breathing in Children

Irina Trosman [1,*] and Samuel J. Trosman [2]

[1] Sleep Medicine Center, Ann and Robert H. Lurie Children's Hospital of Chicago, Chicago, IL 60611, USA
[2] Head and Neck Institute, Cleveland Clinic Foundation, Cleveland, OH 44195, USA; samuel.trosman@gmail.com
* Correspondence: itrosman@luriechildrens.org; Tel.: +1-(312)-227-6740

Received: 18 September 2017; Accepted: 24 November 2017; Published: 1 December 2017

Abstract: There is now a plethora of evidence that children with sleep disordered breathing (SDB) show deficits in neurocognitive performance, behavioral impairments, and school performance. The following review will focus on the neurobehavioral impacts of SDB, pediatric sleep investigation challenges, potential mechanisms of behavioral and cognitive deficits in children with SDB, and the impact of SDB treatment.

Keywords: sleep disordered breathing; obstructive sleep apnea; children; attention; learning; behavior

1. Brief Overview of Pediatric Sleep Disordered Breathing

Sleep disordered breathing (SDB) is a term used to describe a spectrum of breathing disorders during sleep. It includes, but is not limited to, habitual snoring, obstructive sleep apnea, and sleep-related hypoventilation [1]. This review will mostly focus on primary snoring and pediatric obstructive sleep apnea.

Common nighttime symptoms of SDB include snoring, mouth breathing, apneas, gasping, labored or paradoxical breathing, excessive sweating, restless sleep, leg kicking, and hyperextension of the neck. Daytime symptoms may include inattentiveness, difficulty focusing, behavioral and mood problems, morning headaches, fatigue, excessive daytime sleepiness (EDS), and, in severe cases, failure to thrive. Persistent mouth breathing during sleep may be associated with dry mouth and complaints of thirst upon awakening.

Primary snoring (PS) is defined as snoring without associated apneas, hypopneas, hypoxemia, hypercapnia, or sleep fragmentation [2]. There is no universally accepted, clear definition of snoring. Thus, the prevalence of the condition may differ based on varying perceptions of the word's meaning across cultures. The overall prevalence of parent-reported snoring in one meta-analysis was 7.45% [3].

Obstructive Sleep Apnea (OSA) is characterized by recurrent episodes of upper airway obstruction during sleep that causes arousals, intermittent hypoxemia, and disruption of normal ventilation. According to International Classification of Sleep Disorder (ICSD)-3 criteria, OSA diagnosis requires the presence of at least one symptom (snoring, labored/obstructed breathing, or daytime consequences, such as sleepiness, hyperactivity) to be present, along with the sleep study findings [4,5].

Children with SDB may experience partial or complete obstruction of the upper airway during sleep. Recurrent episodes of airway narrowing or airway obstruction, associated with arousals or awakenings, disrupt sleep continuity. Sleep fragmentation and disrupted sleep architecture may result in nonrestorative sleep. Polysomnographic findings may include an elevated arousal index, decreased sleep efficiency, elevation of light sleep (stage N1), and reduction in overall amount of deep or Rapid eye movement (REM) sleep (stages N3 and REM) [6].

Up to 4% of typically developing children have obstructive sleep apnea, based on polysomnography (PSG) and approximately 11% have habitual snoring, based on parental report [3].

However, it is important to emphasize that the reported prevalence of SDB varies widely depending on the SDB definition and diagnostic methods deployed by investigators. For instance, the prevalence of SDB in some studies was estimated based on parental reports. However, parental reporting of snoring may not be reliable. Reporting depends on the frequency of child's co-sleeping with the parents, and co-sleeping prevalence clearly differs across cultures [7]. Other studies collected data from diagnostic testing, such as nocturnal sleep laboratory based PSG [3]. Most studies consistently report a SDB peak between 2 and 8 years of age [6,8–12].

The current gold standard for the diagnosis of OSA, as recommended by the American Academy of Pediatrics (AAP), is a PSG study [9]. The cost of the procedure and lack of accessibility may preclude patients from having an overnight sleep study. An unfamiliar environment and PSG monitoring equipment could cause sleep disruption, making sleep study interpretation a challenge.

OSA severity is determined by the frequency of obstructive apneas and hypopneas recorded on PSG. The apnea hypopnea index, or AHI, represents the average number of obstructive or partially obstructive events per hour of sleep. However, gas exchange abnormalities, such as hypoxia and hypercapnia, are frequently used as additional indicators of OSA severity.

Polysomnographic diagnostic criteria for OSA among adults and children are typically the product of expert consensus [13]. The AHI diagnostic criteria in children, when compared to adults, suffers from less available data and perhaps more heterogeneity across studies [3]. Part of the problem is that few studies have been performed to link specific levels of pediatric OSA with adverse outcomes. At present, an AHI of 1 to 5 events per hour of sleep, 5–10 per hour of sleep, and more than 10 events per hour of sleep is most often used to categorize mild, moderate, and severe OSA, respectively. However, various AHI definitions have been used in pediatric studies in the past.

Although PSG provides an objective measure of sleep disturbance, measures derived from sleep studies are often not predictive of OSA-associated morbidities [14].

2. Challenges of Pediatric Sleep Investigations Focusing on Neurobehavioral Outcomes of Sleep Disordered Breathing

Various sleep disorders may result in sleep deprivation, sleep fragmentation, EDS, and symptoms related to increases in excessive sleep pressure. These disorders may have similar impacts on mood, attention, cognition, and behavior; however, SDB has been most extensively studied in this regard.

Sleep fragmentation (resulting from respiratory related repeated arousals or brief awakenings) has been speculated to be one of the main causes of the neurobehavioral effects associated with SDB. However, changes in sleep architecture detected during PSG may be related to other co-morbid conditions, for instance "first night effect". This latest phenomenon is attributed to the use of numerous electrodes and wires during PSG studies and an unfamiliar sleep environment. The first night effect frequently distorts sleep on the first night of recording. To mitigate this, sleep centers ideally should resort to using two or three nights of PSG recordings and discard the data from the first night. However, this is frequently not feasible [15].

The most definitive demonstration of treatment consequences in severe SDB would involve a double-blind, placebo-controlled, randomized trial. This study design is very difficult for several reasons. It is impossible to withhold treatment for severe cases of SDB for ethical reasons. In addition, families and clinicians cannot be blinded to surgical intervention (i.e., adenotonsillectomy) or sham surgery.

As mentioned above, the description of SDB prevalence is fraught with difficulty due to a variety of methodological issues. Some other challenges are listed below.

- Heterogeneity in OSA severity diagnostic criteria and lack of universally accepted specific pediatric polysomnographic parameters to distinguish primary snoring from OSA [3].
- The American Academy of Sleep Medicine (AASM) in 2012 modified the obstructive hypopnea definition, making it somewhat difficult to compare results from relatively recent studies with previously published papers [16].

- SDB is most prevalent in the preschool years (3–5 years of age); however, most pediatric studies focused on school-aged children [17,18]. Sleep fragmentation, disrupted sleep architecture, hypoxia, and hypercapnia are the presumed causative mechanisms for poor functional outcomes in SDB. They may be particularly important in younger children who are most susceptible to SDB related sequelae, due to particularly rapid cerebral and functional development [19,20].
- The patient population in studies may range from general community populations to children at tertiary care institutions (TCI) or subspecialty care with variable SDB severity. This may potentially create a referral bias.
- There are difficulties in evaluating behavioral problems in children of various ages by uniform tests. Younger children may not be able to verbalize excessive daytime sleepiness or fatigue. Their manifestation of disruptive sleep or excessive daytime sleep pressure may manifest as hyperactivity, impulsivity, increased aggression or oppositional behaviors. On the contrary, excessive sleep pressure in older children may be more similar to adults and present as excessive napping, yawning, rubbing eyes, complaints of fatigue or sleepiness, irritability, etc.
- Pediatric studies frequently rely on caregiver and teacher reporting of children's behavior, attention, and hyperactivity levels as well as their estimated amount of sleep and sleep quality. These reports can be biased and affected by the caregivers' cultural preferences, educational levels, expectations, and socio-economic backgrounds.
- A variety of potentially confounding factors increases the risk of cognitive dysfunction in children with any severity of OSA, such as premature birth, lower socioeconomic status, asthma, obesity, short sleep duration, and African-American ethnicity.
- Other factors may also have a significant impact on child sleep quality, alertness level, behavior, and development, such as other sleep disorders (i.e., circadian sleep disorders, restless leg syndrome, behaviorally induced insufficiency and/or disrupted sleep, parasomnias), various medical conditions (allergies, asthma, eczema, obesity, recurrent pharyngitis, etc.), medication use (i.e., use of nasal or inhaled steroids or anti-histamines, stimulant medications), genetics, and environmental factors (such as parental smoking).

Sorting through all of these issues is a tremendously difficult task. These challenges create substantial difficulties in interpreting research results and drawing meaningful conclusions.

3. Neurobehavioral Morbidity and Sleep Disordered Breathing

One of the earliest studies to shed light on the potential causative link between OSA and its detrimental consequences on academic performance was published in 1998 [21]. A remarkable increase in the prevalence of OSA was found in first-graders whose school performance was in the lowest tenth percentile of their class. Furthermore, the children who were treated for OSA showed significant academic improvements in their school grades in subsequent years, as opposed to untreated children. Another study reported that children who snored during early childhood were at greater risk for poor academic performance in later years, long after snoring had resolved [22].

Since then, there have been numerous mostly cross-sectional studies reporting the association between OSA and neurocognitive and behavioral morbidity. Many, albeit not all, studies have shown improvements in some of these functions after OSA treatment [23–30].

Sleep Disordered Breathingand Excessive Daytime Sleepiness

The exact prevalence of excessive daytime sleepiness (EDS) in pediatric OSA is unclear. In contrast to adults, EDS does not tend to be a prominent complaint in children with SDB. EDS estimation in younger children is challenging and frequently relies on caretakers' perceptions. Adults are frequently used as surrogate reporters because children are unlikely to verbalize their symptoms. It is also important to note that behavioral sleepiness may manifest differently in children than it does in adults.

For example, children exhibit hyperactivity, inattentiveness, irritability, and/or oppositional behavior, rather than taking naps or having unintentional sleep episodes [31,32].

Several studies have examined the association between SDB and sleepiness in children by analyzing parental subjective reports. As opposed to adults with OSA, children were surprisingly relatively "protected" from OSA-induced hypersomnolence [33]. Some studies used objective measurements of EDS, such as the Multiple Sleep Latency Test (MSLT). The MSLT involves a series of brief daytime 'nap' opportunities in a comfortable sleep-conducive environment. The degree of sleepiness or "sleep pressure" is estimated by the child's ability to fall asleep during naps. The shorter the latency to sleep onset during these nap opportunities, the higher the degree of sleepiness [34]. Unfortunately, MSLT assessments are expensive and difficult to conduct in children. In addition, MSLT has not been validated for younger children and there is a limited relationship between the sleepiness derived from a MSLT and the sleepiness based on subjective reporting [35,36].

Due to lack of objective measurements of sleepiness in younger children, it is not surprising that there is a paucity of pediatric studies objectively measuring EDS in children. Based on the available limited MSLT results, it appears that EDS in children with OSA is relatively infrequent and tends to be more noticeable among those with more severe OSA and/or obese patients [35–37].

Sleep Disordered Breathing and Cognitive Function, Learning, and School Performance

Cognitive function is a mental act or process of knowledge acquisition. This process includes awareness, perception, intuition, and reasoning. Executive function encompasses the mental processes that enable children to plan, focus, remember instructions, and juggle multiple tasks successfully. Executive function is a domain that has been shown to be sensitive to intermittent hypoxemia, related to the obstructive sleep apnea syndrome. Thus, pediatric researchers focus on executive function to evaluate OSA related cognitive sequelae.

Executive function and self-regulation skills depend on working memory, mental flexibility, and self-control.

The term working memory is often used interchangeable with short-term memory. However, short-term memory is just one component of working memory. Working memory requires temporary storage of information as well as the ability to accurately manipulate this information—for instance, baking a cake by memorizing ingredients and steps without making the unfortunate mistake of addition the same ingredient twice. Working memory has been found to correlate with intellectual function better than short-term memory [38–41]. Adult research has demonstrated a link between OSA and deficits of executive function [42]. Pediatric researchers also frequently use working memory performance and executive function assessment to evaluate neurocognitive deficits inflicted by OSA.

Impairments in executive functioning have been reported in multiple studies, including the Tucson Children's Assessment of Sleep Apnea (TuCASA). The TuCASA study identified a negative correlation between AHI and immediate recall, Full Scale intelligence quotience (IQ), Performance IQ, and math achievement, while nocturnal hypoxemia adversely affected nonverbal skills [43,44].

Objective measurements of specific neuropsychological performance deficits related to sleep problems in children have been limited; however, pediatric studies have begun to identify significant differences in cognitive function between children with SDB and healthy controls.

Verbal working memory impairments associated with OSA may compromise a child's learning potential and neurocognitive development. For example, one study found significantly lower performance on measures of memory, executive function, and general intelligence in 5-year-old children with symptoms of SDB when compared to asymptomatic children [45]. Another study demonstrated decreased general intelligence, language, and visual-spatial skills in habitually snoring children [46]. The degree of neuropsychological deficits in children correlated with OSA severity [47]. In another study [48], working memory and basic attention tasks were evaluated in OSA children aged 8–12 years and compared to well-matched healthy controls. Sleep study findings and working memory functions were compared between the two groups. Compared to controls, children with OSA had poorer performance on both tasks of basic storage and central executive components in the verbal domain of working memory; however, no significant differences were detected in the visuospatial domain. The findings also suggested that AHI and oxygen saturation (SpO$_2$) nadir were associated with verbal working memory performance.

There is no consistency regarding the relationship between OSA severity and memory performance in children. While some studies revealed memory performance on standardized psychometric tests in children with OSA was significantly impaired, compared to healthy controls [49], with higher respiratory disturbance indices, correlating with greater memory deficits [50], other studies found no evidence of any differences in memory performance in children with varying degrees of OSA severity, when compared to control children [46,47,51].

School problems have been reported in multiple case-series of children with OSA [21,22,32], and such findings may underscore more extensive behavioral disturbances, such as restlessness, aggressive behavior, excessive daytime sleepiness, and poor test performances.

Sleep Disordered Breathing and Aggressive Behavior, Hyperactivity and Attention Deficit Hyperactivity Disorder

Multiple pediatric studies, based on parent or teacher surveys have found an association between childhood sleep-disordered breathing (SDB) and aggressive behavior, impulsivity, hyperactivity, and decreased attention [52–58].

For instance, one study demonstrated that in children with objectively confirmed SDB, aggressive behaviors are more frequent than in children without SDB, even when the SDB is mild [59,60]. Behavioral problems associated with sleep disordered breathing in school-aged children were also reported in the Tuscon study [60]. Another study focused on parental reporting of aggressive behavior among elementary school children. It demonstrated that aggressive children were twice as likely to have SDB symptoms compared to non-aggressive peers [61]

Multiple studies support the relationship between SBD and hyperactive behavior and inattentiveness [62]. SDB-related sleep fragmentation is speculated to be the cause of excessive daytime sleepiness, which may in turn interfere with sustained attention. Children with PS suffer from more sleepiness, inattention, and hyperactivity than healthy controls [63,64]. Despite the relative abundance of research in this area, there remain many unanswered questions regarding the relationship between sleep disturbances and attention deficit hyperactivity disorder (ADHD), and between OSA and ADHD-like symptoms in particular. The variations in diagnostic criteria for ADHD over the years (i.e., using different versions of Diagnostic and Statistical Manual of Mental Disorders criteria), the source of informant (e.g., parent, teacher, or clinical), and the reliability of rating scales used to diagnose ADHD, make the ADHD diagnosis difficult in some instances.

Interestingly, although children with ADHD appear to exhibit more sleep disturbances and symptoms of SDB than normal children [65,66] according to parental reports, only 20% of children with ADHD actually exhibited objective sleep disturbances when assessed by polysomnographic criteria [22,67]. In this study, it was also concluded that OSA is not more likely to occur among children with true ADHD when the ADHD diagnosis was established using the stringent criteria recommended by the Academy of Pediatrics and the Academy of Psychiatry.

Most studies demonstrate that parental questionnaire answers and ratings are sensitive to the behavioral aspects of SDB. Most parental ratings show that children with SDB are more symptomatic than control groups [23,68].

It is currently unclear whether sleep disturbances are intrinsic to ADHD, whether they are secondary to a co-morbid sleep disorder, or whether sleep disorders cause ADHD-like symptoms and thus result in a misdiagnosis.

In addition, some studies have shown that both children and adults with ADHD may exhibit symptoms of other sleep disorders, such as periodic limb movements of sleep, restless leg syndrome, delayed sleep phase syndrome, and initiation and maintenance insomnia [69–73].

A meta-analysis, analyzing eighteen studies published prior to 2012, was conducted to assess (1) the relationship between SDB and ADHD symptoms and (2) the extent of change in ADHD symptoms before and after adenotonsillectomy. The findings of this meta-analysis suggested that ADHD symptoms were related to SDB and improved after adenotonsillectomy [74]. However, the recent Childhood Adenotonsillectomy Trial (CHAT) study revealed no significant improvement in attention or executive function in children with non-severe OSA after adenotonsillectomy, as measured by neuropsychological testing [23].

Sleep Disordered Breathing and Depressive Symptoms

Childhood depression is a significant problem that may lead to psychosocial problems and physical disabilities. Adolescents with depression have an increased risk of suicide and substance abuse [75].

Some studies have reported a high rate of depressive and anxiety symptoms (24%) among adults with OSA [76]. However, the relationship between depressive symptoms and OSA was no longer significant after controlling for age, body mass index (BMI), and hypertension [77]. Similarly, inconsistencies regarding the relationship between depression and OSA can be found in the pediatric literature. This may be attributed to methodological differences in OSA diagnostic criteria and evaluation of depressive symptoms. OSA related sleep disturbances and impairments in daily functioning may interfere with a child's relationships with family, school, and peers [78].

A meta-analysis, designed to assess the relationship between depressive symptoms and OSA, and the efficacy of adenotonsillectomy for decreasing depressive symptoms reported a higher incidence of depressive symptoms among children with OSA, especially in males. OSA treatment with adenotonsillectomy was associated with decreased depressive symptoms when compared to pre-surgery levels. Thus, OSA screening in children and adolescents with depressive symptoms was suggested [79].

4. Are Cognitive Outcomes of Pediatric Sleep Disordered Breathing Reversed by Treatment?

Improvements in behavior, following treatment for OSA in children, were reported earlier [21,53] and suggested that at least some of the deficits may be reversible.

SDB therapeutic options include surgical interventions, with extraction of hypertrophic adenoids and tonsils being the most commonly performed procedures, as well as nonsurgical alternatives, such as watchful waiting, anti-inflammatory agents, orthodontic interventions, and positive airway pressure therapy (continuous positive airway pressure, also known as CPAP, or bi-level positive airway pressure, also known as Bi-LEVEL or Bi-PAP).

Adenotonsillectomy is considered to be the first-line treatment in children [2,80]; however, not all patients are surgical candidates and some patients will continue to have symptoms after surgery [81,82]. Other surgical interventions, such as tongue-base suspension, uvulopharyngopalatoplasty, craniofacial surgery, bariatric surgery, and in most severe cases, tracheostomy, are used in selective pediatric populations [79].

Effects of Adenotonsillectomy

Cognitive and behavioral abnormalities have been shown to be reduced after adenotonsillectomy (AT) in some [22,46,66,82–84], but not all [85], non-randomized studies, with inconsistencies in the reported effects after treatment. Previous studies have been limited by small samples, lack of randomization or appropriate controls, heterogeneous study groups, and frequent reliance on parent questionnaires, rather than on neuropsychological testing [66,84,86].

CHAT was the first large randomized controlled trial conducted to evaluate the efficacy of early adenotonsillectomy (eAT) versus watchful waiting with supportive care (WWSC) in children with OSA, with respect to cognitive, behavioral, quality-of-life, and sleep factors [23]. The primary outcome was a neurobehavioral measure of attention and executive function. Children 5 to 9 years of age with

OSA without significant gas exchange abnormalities were randomly assigned to either an eAT group or a strategy of WWSC. They were evaluated at baseline and 7 months later. The primary outcome was evaluated by Developmental Neuropsychological Assessment (NEPSY), a test that has well-established psychometric properties [87].

Secondary outcomes included caregiver and teacher ratings of behavior, symptoms of the obstructive sleep apnea syndrome, sleepiness, global quality of life, and disease-specific quality of life.

The results revealed no correlation between the severity of the obstructive sleep apnea syndrome and treatment, with respect to the primary outcomes (attention and executive-function). However, eAT was found to reduce OSA symptoms and improve secondary outcomes (behavior, quality of life, and polysomnographic findings) [23]. In addition, the study secondary analysis revealed improvement in a time measure of selective attention and visual scanning in eAT group [88]. Interestingly, PSG of almost half of WWSC children had normalized by seven months. This finding suggested that non-severe OSA in school-age children may recover over time, without surgical intervention [89].

Positive Airway Pressure Therapy

There are few published studies examining functional outcomes, such as neurocognitive outcomes, of children treated with positive airway pressure (PAP). An early study found that children with OSA who used PAP for 6 months had less daytime sleepiness, but no significant improvements in behavior, temperament or school performance. This study did not specifically assess attention, nor did it differentiate participants who were adherent to treatment from those who were not. It also used a school performance measure that was of unproven sensitivity to OSA. These methodological factors may have obscured changes in functioning for those individuals who were more adherent to PAP [90]. Another small outcomes analysis looked at self-reported academic grades, self- and parent-reported academic quality of life, and objectively-measured attention scores. These were assessed before and after PAP treatment in 13 obese adolescents with OSA as well as 15 untreated obese controls without OSA. The study demonstrated that non-adherent participants showed worsening functioning over time, while PAP users showed stable or improved functioning, similar to controls [91].

However, adherence with PAP therapy in adolescents with OSA is often a concern. Adolescents are notorious for diminished adherence to medical regimens and those who were prescribed PAP for OSA tended to follow this pattern as well [92].

In a study evaluating the effect of positive airway pressure therapy on neurobehavioral characteristics in a heterogeneous group of 52 children and adolescents, at baseline and after 3 months of treatment, PAP usage was associated with significant changes in neurobehavioral parameters, even in a heterogeneous group of children with OSA that included very young children and children with developmental delays [93].

Although it is difficult to get children to wear the PAP apparatus, it is important to encourage at least partial adherence to PAP therapy as those children who are even partially compliant with PAP therapy can display improved attention and academic functioning.

5. Potential Mechanisms of Neurobehavioral and Cognitive Dysfunction in Pediatric Sleep Disordered Breathing

The exact mechanisms by which OSA elicits neural deficits remain relatively unknown. Most likely, both the sleep fragmentation and episodic hypoxia associated with SDB lead directly to systemic inflammatory vascular changes in the brain [66,94,95]. Levels of inflammatory markers, such as C-reactive protein (CRP), interferon (IFN)-γ, tumor necrosis factor (TNF)-α and cytokine interleukin (IL)-6 have been shown to be elevated in children with SDB [96–99].

The findings linking vascular function and cognitive outcomes have been confirmed in several studies, such that the presence of endothelial dysfunction in OSA may serve as a surrogate reporter of altered cognitive functioning [100,101].

The frontal and hippocampal regions of the brain, which are implicated in the regulation of behavior and memory, respectively, appear to be most vulnerable to the effects of OSA. In children, gains in executive function skills occur during developmental periods, corresponding to the neuronal myelination and maturation of the prefrontal cortex [102,103]. Executive function is considered critical for school-age children, to develop complex problem solving [104] and to be able to perform other volitional tasks in response to new situations with demands on working memory [105]. If left untreated, OSA causes neuropsychological or executive dysfunction in developing children. If these skills are permanently impaired before maturation of the prefrontal cortex, this could severely alter a child's cognitive potential, ultimately impacting both the child's health and his or her functioning level in society.

In one study, researchers wanted to investigate the brains of children with OSA to see if there was any evidence of changes in the brain and if these changes were associated with any learning problems. They studied 31 children (19 with OSA and 12 healthy controls, aged 6–16 years). Participants underwent PSG and neuropsychological assessments, such as IQ tests and tests of their ability to perform tasks involving decision-making. Some of the children also had specialized scans of their brains (known as proton magnetic resonance spectroscopic imaging, or MRS) to measure the levels of certain metabolites produced as a result of brain activity. The researchers then compared the neuropsychological test scores with the levels of the metabolites. They found that relative to controls, children with severe OSA had lower IQs and a decreased ability to perform tasks involving decision-making. Children with OSA also had changes in metabolites in the brain, similar to those seen in diseases in which there is damage to brain cells. Compared to controls, children with OSA scored significantly lower on tests of overall intelligence and some aspects of higher-level thinking called "executive functions," but the groups did not differ on tests involving sustained attention, motor skills, or visuospatial skills. Tests of memory did not yield significant differences between the groups, but the effect sizes were large enough for the authors to suggest that significant effects may have been found in a larger sample. MRS indicated that those with OSA had abnormal metabolites in the left hippocampus and right frontal cortex [85].

Additional factors, such as hypercarbia, architectural disturbances, including REM latency prolongation or reduction in REM sleep percentage as well as alternations in other stages of sleep may also play important roles.

It is important to emphasize that not all children with OSA exhibit cognitive deficits or behavioral problems. It has been speculated that both genetic and environmental factors may play roles in making some children more susceptible to the neurocognitive complications of OSA. Several genetic factors have been identified so far, including polymorphism within the NOX gene or its functional subunits [106]. The differences in systemic inflammatory responses, including plasma C-reactive protein (CRP) and interleukin levels may also be responsible for increased susceptibility to OSA related cognitive deficits [107]. Genetic variants of a gene critically involved in the formation of free radicals have been shown to account for discrepancies in cognitive outcomes in pediatric OSA [108]. Additional factors, such as insulin-like growth factor (IGF)-1 and apolipoprotein E allelic variants, have also been identified to be detrimental to neurocognitive function [108,109]. Some researchers have hypothesized that changes in regional cerebral blood flow during obstructive episodes leads to neurocognitive impairments [110].

6. Conclusions

There is now a plethora of evidence that children with SDB show deficits in neurocognitive performance, behavioral impairments, and decreased school performance; however, it is still not clear which factors (e.g., sleep fragmentation, degree of respiratory disturbance, hypoventilation, or oxygenation) play the most importance roles in neurocognitive morbidity. The exact mechanisms by which OSA causes neural deficits remain unresolved.

Although sleep studies provide an objective evaluation of SDB severity, they are not predictive of OSA-associated morbidities. In addition, some children fulfilling current polysomnographic criteria for OSA do not manifest disease related morbidities. Other factors, such as individual susceptibility, co-morbid conditions, and environmental factors, appear to be important as well [14,111]. Some children with primary snoring display neurocognitive or cardiovascular sequelae and/or signs of systemic inflammation, despite normal sleep study findings [46,112].

Some SDB neurocognitive consequences are reversible while others may be irreversible if left untreated [22].

Despite some controversies, there is enough available data to support screening children with hyperactive behavior, inattentiveness, disruptive behavior, or learning disabilities for SDB and other sleep disorders. Screening for sleep disorders should be part of any well-child visit. Better education of pediatricians, general practitioners, mental health professionals, educators, and parents may help to identify and treat children at risk. An appropriate SDB diagnosis in children with ADHD symptoms may help prevent unnecessary stimulant use. Identification of the most severe SDB cases and subsequent early interventions are imperative to improve psychobehavioral short-term and long-term outcomes. Future research will help us better understand the pathophysiology of SDB and its effect on cognition and behavior in order to identify the most vulnerable children.

Conflicts of Interest: The authors declare no conflict of interest.

References

1. Carroll, J.L.; McLoughlin, G.M. Diagnostic criteria for obstructive sleep apnea in children. *Pediatr. Pulmonol.* **1992**, *14*, 71–74. [CrossRef] [PubMed]
2. Marcus, C.L.; Chapman, D.; Ward, S.D.; McColley, S.A.; Herrerias, C.T.; Stillwell, P.C.; Howenstine, M.; Light, M.J.; Schaeffer, D.A.; Wagener, J.S.; et al. Pediatric Pulmonology Subcommittee on Obstructive Sleep Apnea Syndrome. *Pediatrics* **2002**, *109*, 704–712.
3. Lumeng, J.C.; Chervin, R.D. Epidemiology of pediatric obstructive sleep apnea. *Proc. Am. Thorac. Soc.* **2008**, *5*, 242–252. [CrossRef] [PubMed]
4. Sateia, M.J. International classification of sleep disorders—Third Edition Highlights and Modification. *Chest J.* **2014**, *146*, 1387–1394. [CrossRef] [PubMed]
5. Loughlin, G.M.; Brouillette, R.T.; Brooke, L.J.; Carroll, J.L.; Chipps, B.E.; England, S.J.; Ferber, P.; Ferraro, N.F.; Gaultier, C.; Givan, D.C.; et al. Standards and indications for cardiopulmonary sleep studies in children. *Am. J. Respir. Crit. Care Med.* **1996**, *153*, 866–878.
6. Kheirandish-Gozal, L.; Gozal, D. (Eds.) *Sleep Disordered Breathing in Children A Comprehensive Clinical Guide to Evaluation and Treatment*; Springer Science & Business Media: New York, NY, USA, 2012.
7. Owens, J.A. Sleep in children: Cross-cultural perspectives. *Sleep Biol. Rhythm.* **2004**, *2*, 165–173. [CrossRef]
8. Bixler, E.O.; Vgontzas, A.N.; Lin, H.M.; Liao, D.; Calhoun, S.; Vela-Bueno, A.; Fedok, F.; Vlasic, V.; Graff, G. Sleep disordered breathing in children in a general population sample: Prevalence and risk factors. *Sleep* **2009**, *32*, 731–736. [CrossRef] [PubMed]
9. Marcus, C.L.; Brooks, L.J.; Ward, S.D.; Draper, K.A.; Gozal, D.; Halbower, A.C.; Jones, J.; Lehmann, C.; Schechter, M.S.; Sheldon, S.; et al. Diagnosis and management of childhood obstructive sleep apnea syndrome. *Pediatrics* **2012**, *130*, e714–e755. [CrossRef] [PubMed]
10. Rosen, C.L.; Larkin, E.K.; Kirchner, H.L.; Emancipator, J.L.; Bivins, S.F.; Surovec, S.A.; Martin, R.J.; Redline, S. Prevalence and risk factors for sleep-disordered breathing in 8- to 11-year-old children: Association with race and prematurity. *J. Pediatr.* **2003**, *142*, 383–389. [CrossRef] [PubMed]
11. Teculescu, D.B.; Caillier, I.; Perrin, P.; Rebstock, E.; Rauch, A. Snoring in French preschool children. *Pediatr. Pulmonol.* **1992**, *13*, 239–244. [CrossRef] [PubMed]
12. Brunetti, L.; Rana, S.; Lospalluti, M.L.; Pietrafesa, A.; Francavilla, R.; Fanelli, M.; Armenio, L. Prevalence of obstructive sleep apnea syndrome in a cohort of 1,207 children of Southern Italy. *Chest* **2001**, *120*, 1930–1935. [CrossRef] [PubMed]
13. American Academy of Sleep Medicine. *International Classification of Sleep Disorders: Diagnostic and Coding Manual*, 2nd ed.; American Academy of Sleep Medicine: Westchester, IL, USA, 2005.

14. Tan, H.L.; Gozal, D.; Kheirandish-Gozal, L. Obstructive sleep apnea in children: A critical update. *Nat. Sci. Sleep* **2013**, *5*, 109–123. [PubMed]

15. Yoon, S.Y.R.; Jain, U.; Shapiro, C. Sleep in attention-deficit/hyperactivity disorder in children and adults: Past, present, and future. *Sleep Med. Rev.* **2012**, *16*, 371–388. [CrossRef] [PubMed]

16. Berry, R.B.; Budhiraja, R.; Gottlieb, D.J.; Gozal, D.; Iber, C.; Kapur, V.K.; Marcus, C.L.; Mehra, R.; Parthasarathy, S.; Quan, S.F.; et al. Rules for scoring respiratory event in Sleep: Update of the 2007 AASM Manual. *J. Clin. Sleep Med.* **2012**, *13*, 597–619.

17. Castronovo, V.; Zucconi, M.; Nosetti, L.; Marazzini, C.; Hensley, M.; Veglia, F.; Nespoli, L.; Ferini-Strambi, L. Prevalence of habitual snoring and sleep-disordered breathing in preschool-aged children in an Italian community. *J. Pediatr.* **2003**, *142*, 377–382. [CrossRef] [PubMed]

18. Owen, G.O.; Canter, R.J.; Robinson, A. Snoring, apnoea and ENT symptoms in the paediatric community. *Clin. Otolaryngol.* **1996**, *21*, 130–134. [CrossRef] [PubMed]

19. Gozal, E.; Row, B.W.; Schurr, A.; Gozal, D. Developmental difference in cortical and hippocampal vulnerability to intermittent hypoxia in the rat. *Neurosci. Lett.* **2001**, *305*, 197–201. [CrossRef]

20. Row, B.W.; Kheirandish, L.; Neville, J.J.; Gozal, D. Impaired spatial learning and hyperactivity in developing rats exposed to intermittent hypoxia. *Pediatr. Res.* **2002**, *52*, 449–453. [CrossRef] [PubMed]

21. Gozal, D. Sleep-disordered breathing and school performance in children. *Pediatrics* **1998**, *102*, 616–620. [CrossRef] [PubMed]

22. Gozal, D.; Pope, D.W., Jr. Snoring during early childhood and academic performance at ages thirteen to fourteen years. *Pediatrics* **2001**, *107*, 1394–1399. [CrossRef] [PubMed]

23. Marcus, C.L.; Moore, R.H.; Rosen, C.L.; Giordani, B.; Garetz, S.L.; Taylor, H.G.; Mitchell, R.B.; Amin, R.; Katz, E.S.; Arens, R.; et al. Childhood Adenotonsillectomy Trial (CHAT). *N. Engl. J. Med.* **2013**, *368*, 2366–2376. [CrossRef] [PubMed]

24. Chervin, R.D.; Ruzicka, D.L.; Hoban, T.F.; Fetterolf, J.L.; Garetz, S.L.; Guire, K.E.; Dillon, J.E.; Felt, B.T.; Hodges, E.K.; Giordani, B.J. Esophageal pressures, polysomnography, and neurobehavioral outcomes of adenotonsillectomy in children. *Chest J.* **2012**, *142*, 101–110. [CrossRef] [PubMed]

25. Giordani, B.; Hodges, E.K.; Guire, K.E.; Ruzicka, D.L.; Dillon, J.E.; Weatherly, R.A.; Garetz, S.L.; Chervin, R.D. Changes in neuropsychological and behavioral functioning in children with and without obstructive sleep apnea following Tonsillectomy. *J. Int. Neuropsychol. Soc.* **2012**, *18*, 212–222. [CrossRef] [PubMed]

26. Landau, Y.E.; Bar-Yishay, O.; Greenberg-Dotan, S.; Goldbart, A.D.; Tarasiuk, A.; Tal, A. Impaired behavioral and neurocognitive function in preschool children with obstructive sleep apnea. *Pediatr. Pulmonol.* **2012**, *47*, 180–188. [CrossRef] [PubMed]

27. Bourke, R.; Anderson, V.; Yang, J.S.; Jackman, A.R.; Killedar, A.; Nixon, G.M.; Davey, M.J.; Walker, A.M.; Trinder, J.; Horne, R.S. Cognitive and academic functions are impaired in children with all severities of sleep-disordered breathing. *Sleep Med.* **2011**, *12*, 489–496. [CrossRef] [PubMed]

28. Garetz, S.L. Behavior, cognition, and quality of life after adenotonsillectomy for pediatric sleep-disordered breathing: Summary of the literature. *Otolaryngol. Head Neck Surg.* **2008**, *138* (Suppl. 1), S19–S26. [CrossRef] [PubMed]

29. Wei, J.L.; Bond, J.; Mayo, M.S.; Smith, H.J.; Reese, M.; Weatherly, R.A. Improved behavior and sleep after adenotonsillectomy in children with sleep-disordered breathing: Long-term follow-up. *Arch. Otolaryngol. Head Neck Surg.* **2009**, *135*, 642–646. [CrossRef] [PubMed]

30. Wei, J.L.; Mayo, M.S.; Smith, H.J.; Reese, M.; Weatherly, R.A. Improved behaviour and sleep after adenotonsillectomy in children with sleep-disordered breathing. *Arch. Otolaryngol. Head Neck Surg.* **2007**, *133*, 974–979. [CrossRef] [PubMed]

31. Golan, N.; Shahar, E.; Ravid, S.; Pillar, G. Sleep disorders and daytime sleepiness in children with attention-deficit/hyperactive disorder. *Sleep* **2004**, *15*, 261–266. [CrossRef]

32. Gozal, D. Obstructive Sleep Apnea in Children: Implications for the Developing Central Nervous System. In *Seminars in Pediatric Neurology*; WB Saunders: Philadelphia, PA, USA, 2008; Volume 15, pp. 100–106.

33. Carroll, J.L.; McColley, S.A.; Marcus, C.L.; Curtis, S.; Loughlin, G.M. Inability of clinical history to distinguish primary snoring from obstructive sleep apnea syndrome in children. *Chest* **1995**, *108*, 610–618. [CrossRef] [PubMed]

34. Carskadon, M.A.; Dement, W.C. Sleep tendency: An objective measure of sleep loss. *Sleep Res.* **1977**, *6*, 940.

35. Chervin, R.D.; Weatherly, R.A.; Ruzicka, D.L.; Burns, J.W.; Giordani, B.J.; Dillon, J.E.; Marcus, C.L.; Garetz, S.L.; Hoban, T.F.; Guire, K.E. Subjective sleepiness and polysomnographic correlates in children scheduled for adenotonsillectomy vs other surgical care. *Sleep* **2006**, *29*, 495–503. [PubMed]

36. Gozal, D.; Wang, M.; Pope, D.W., Jr. Objective sleepiness measures in pediatric obstructive sleep apnea. *Pediatrics* **2001**, *108*, 693–697. [CrossRef] [PubMed]

37. Melendres, M.C.; Lutz, J.M.; Rubin, E.D.; Marcus, C.L. Daytime sleepiness and hyperactivity in children with suspected sleep-disordered breathing. *Pediatrics* **2004**, *114*, 768–775. [CrossRef] [PubMed]

38. Born, J.; Rasch, B.; Gais, S. Sleep to Remember. *Neuroscientist* **2006**, *12*, 410–424. [CrossRef] [PubMed]

39. Daneman, M.; Carpenter, P.A. Individual differences in working memory and reading. *J. Verbal Learn. Verbal Behav.* **1980**, *19*, 450–466. [CrossRef]

40. Daneman, M.; Merikle, P.M. Working memory and language comprehension: A meta-analysis. *Psychon. Bull. Rev.* **1996**, *3*, 422–433. [CrossRef] [PubMed]

41. Conway, A.R.A.; Kane, M.J.; Bunting, M.F.; Hambrick, D.Z.; Wilhelm, O.; Engle, R.W. Working memory span tasks: A methodological review and user's guide. *Psychon. Bull. Rev.* **2005**, *12*, 769–786. [CrossRef] [PubMed]

42. Beebe, D.W.; Groesz, L.; Wells, C.; Nichols, A.; McGee, K. The neuropsychological effects of obstructive sleep apnea: A meta-analysis of norm-referenced and case-controlled data. *Sleep* **2003**, *26*, 298–307. [CrossRef] [PubMed]

43. Kaemingk, K.L.; Pasvogel, A.E.; Goodwin, J.L.; Mulvaney, S.A.; Martinez, F.; Enright, P.L.; Rosen, G.M.; Morgan, W.J.; Fregosi, R.F.; Quan, S.F. Learning in children and sleep disordered breathing: Findings of the Tucson Children's Assessment of Sleep Apnea (TuCASA) prospective cohort study. *J. Int. Neuropsychol. Soc.* **2003**, *9*, 1016–1026. [CrossRef] [PubMed]

44. Goodwin, J.L.; Kaemingk, K.L.; Fregosi, R.F.; Rosen, G.M.; Morgan, W.J.; Sherrill, D.L.; Quan, S.F. Clinical outcomes associated with sleep-disordered breathing in Caucasian and Hispanic children—The Tucson Children's Assessment of Sleep Apnea study (TuCASA). *Sleep* **2003**, *26*, 587–591. [CrossRef] [PubMed]

45. Gottlieb, D.J.; Chase, C.; Vezina, R.M.; Heeren, T.C.; Corwin, M.J.; Auerbach, S.H.; Weese-Mayer, D.E.; Lesko, S.M. Sleep-disordered breathing symptoms are associated with poorer cognitive function in 5-year-old children. *J. Pediatr.* **2004**, *145*, 458–464. [CrossRef] [PubMed]

46. O'Brien, L.M.; Mervis, C.B.; Holbrook, C.R.; Bruner, J.L.; Klaus, C.J.; Rutherford, J.; Raffield, T.J.; Gozal, D. Neurobehavioral implications of habitual snoring in children. *Pediatrics* **2004**, *114*, 44–49. [CrossRef] [PubMed]

47. O'Brien, L.M.; Mervis, C.B.; Holbrook, C.R.; Bruner, J.L.; Smith, N.H.; McNally, N.; Catherine McClimment, M.; Gozal, D. Neurobehavioral correlates of sleep-disordered breathing in children. *J. Sleep Res.* **2004**, *13*, 165–172. [CrossRef] [PubMed]

48. Lau, E.Y.; Choi, E.W. Working memory impairment and its associated sleep-related respiratory parameters in children with obstructive sleep apnea. *Sleep Med.* **2015**, *16*, 1109–1115. [CrossRef] [PubMed]

49. Blunden, S.; Lushington, K.; Kennedy, D.; Martin, J.; Dawson, D. Behavior and neurocognitive performance in children aged 5–10 years who snore compared to controls. *J. Clin. Exp. Neuropsychol.* **2000**, *22*, 554–568. [CrossRef]

50. Rhodes, S.K.; Shimoda, K.C.; Wald, L.R.; O'Neil, P.M.; Oexmann, M.J.; Collop, N.A.; Willi, S.M. Neurocognitive deficits in morbidly obese children with obstructive sleep apnea. *J. Pediatr.* **1995**, *127*, 741–744. [CrossRef]

51. Owens-Stively, J.; McGuinn, M.; Berkelhammer, L.; Marcotte, A.; Nobile, C.; Spirito, A. Neuropsychological and behavioral correlates of obstructive sleep apnea in children. *Sleep Res.* **1997**, *26* (Suppl. 1), 452.

52. Archbold, K.H.; Pituch, K.J.; Panahi, P.; Chervin, R.D. Symptoms of sleep disturbances among children at two general pediatric clinics. *J. Pediatr.* **2002**, *140*, 97–102. [CrossRef] [PubMed]

53. Ali, N.J.; Pitson, D.; Stradling, J.R. Sleep disordered breathing: Effects of adenotonsillectomy on behaviour and psychological functioning. *Eur. J. Pediatr.* **1996**, *155*, 56–62. [CrossRef] [PubMed]

54. Goldstein, N.A.; Fatima, M.; Campbell, T.F.; Rosenfeld, R.M. Child behavior and quality of life before and after tonsillectomy and adenoidectomy. *Arch. Otolaryngol. Head Neck Surg.* **2002**, *128*, 770–775. [CrossRef] [PubMed]

55. Owens, J.; Opipari, L.; Nobile, C.; Spirito, A. Sleep and daytime behavior in children with obstructive sleep apnea and behavioral sleep disorders. *Pediatrics* **1998**, *102*, 1178–1184. [CrossRef] [PubMed]

56. Stradling, J.R.; Thomas, G.; Warley, A.R.; Williams, P.; Freeland, A. Effect of adenotonsillectomy on nocturnal hypoxaemia, sleep disturbance, and symptoms in snoring children. *Lancet* **1990**, *335*, 249–253. [CrossRef]
57. Brouillette, R.T.; Fernbach, S.K.; Hunt, C.E. Obstructive sleep-apnea in infants and children. *J. Pediatr.* **1982**, *100*, 31–40. [CrossRef]
58. Lewin, D.S.; Rosen, R.C.; England, S.J.; Dahl, R.E. Preliminary evidence of behavioral and cognitive sequelae of obstructive sleep apnea in children. *Sleep Med.* **2002**, *3*, 5–13. [CrossRef]
59. Gottlieb, D.J.; Vezina, R.M.; Chase, C.; Lesko, S.M.; Heeren, T.C.; Weese-Mayer, D.E.; Auebarch, S.H.; Corwin, M.J. Symptoms of sleep-disordered breathing in 5-year-old children are associated with sleepiness and problem behaviors. *Pediatrics* **2003**, *1112*, 870–877. [CrossRef]
60. Mulvaney, S.A.; Goodwin, J.L.; Morgan, W.J.; Rosen, G.R.; Quan, S.F.; Kaemingk, K.L. Behavior problems associated with sleep disordered breathing in school-aged children—The Tuscon children's assessment of sleep apnea study. *J. Pediatr. Psychol.* **2006**, *31*, 322–330. [CrossRef] [PubMed]
61. O'Brien, L.M.; Lucas, N.H.; Felt, B.T.; Hoban, T.F.; Ruzicka, D.L.; Jordan, R.; Guire, K.; Chervin, R.D. Aggressive behavior, bullying, snoring, and sleepiness in schoolchildren. *Sleep Med.* **2011**, *12*, 652–658. [CrossRef] [PubMed]
62. Hvolby, A. Associations of sleep disturbance with ADHD: Implications for treatment. *ADHD Atten. Defic. Hyperact. Disord.* **2015**, *7*, 1–18. [CrossRef] [PubMed]
63. Chervin, R.D.; Archbold, K.H.; Dillon, J.E.; Panahi, P.; Pituch, K.J.; Dahl, R.E.; Guilleminault, C. Inattention, hyperactivity, and symptoms of sleep-disordered breathing. *Pediatrics* **2002**, *109*, 449–456. [CrossRef] [PubMed]
64. Chervin, R.D.; Archbold, K.H. Hyperactivity and polysomnographic findings in children evaluation for sleep disordered breathing. *Sleep* **2001**, *24*, 313–320. [CrossRef] [PubMed]
65. Goldstein, N.A.; Post, J.C.; Rosenfeld, R.M.; Campbell, T.F. Impact of tonsillectomy and adenoidectomy on child behavior. *Arch. Otolaryngol. Head Neck Surg.* **2000**, *126*, 494–498. [CrossRef] [PubMed]
66. Chervin, R.D.; Ruzicka, D.L.; Giordani, B.J.; Weatherly, R.A.; Dillon, J.E.; Hodges, E.K.; Marcus, C.L.; Guire, K.E. Sleep-disordered breathing, behavior and cognition in children before and after adenotonsillectomy. *Pediatrics* **2006**, *117*, 769–778. [CrossRef] [PubMed]
67. Beebe, D.W.; Gozal, D. Obstructive sleep apnea and the prefrontal cortex: Towards a comprehensive model linking nocturnal upper airway obstruction to daytime cognitive and behavioral deficits. *J. Sleep Res.* **2002**, *11*, 1–16. [CrossRef] [PubMed]
68. Beebe, D.W. Neurobehavioral morbidity associated with disordered breathing during sleep in children: A comprehensive review. *Sleep* **2006**, *29*, 1115–1134. [CrossRef] [PubMed]
69. Picchetti, D.L.; Walters, A.S. Moderate to severe periodic limb movement disorder in childhood and adolescence. *Sleep* **1999**, *22*, 297–300. [CrossRef]
70. Chervin, R.D.; Archbold, K.H.; Dillon, J.E.; Pituch, K.J.; Panahi, P.; Dahl, R.E.; Guilleminault, C. Associations between symptoms of inattention, hyperactivity, restless legs, and periodic leg movements. *Sleep* **2002**, *25*, 213–218. [PubMed]
71. Gaultney, J.F.; Terrell, D.F.; Gingras, J.L. Parent-reported periodic limb movement, sleep disordered breathing, bedtime resistance behaviors, and ADHD. *Behav. Sleep Med.* **2005**, *3*, 32–43. [CrossRef] [PubMed]
72. Gruber, R.; Sadeh, A.V.I.; Raviv, A. Instability of sleep patterns in children with ADHD. *J. Am. Acad. Child Adolesc. Psychiatr.* **2000**, *39*, 495–501. [CrossRef] [PubMed]
73. Hvolby, A. Actigraphic and parental reports of sleep difficulties in children with attention-deficit/hyperactivity disorder. *J. Abnorm. Child Psychol.* **2008**, *162*, 323–329. [CrossRef] [PubMed]
74. Sedky, K.; Bennett, D.S.; Carvalho, K.S. Attention deficit hyperactivity disorder and sleep disordered breathing in pediatric populations: A meta-analysis. *Sleep Med. Rev.* **2014**, *18*, 349–356. [CrossRef] [PubMed]
75. Carotenuto, M.; Esposito, M.; Parisi, L.; Gallai, B.; Marotta, R.; Pascotto, A.; Roccella, M. Depressive symptoms and childhood sleep apnea syndrome. *Neuropsychiatr. Dis. Treat.* **2012**, *8*, 369–373. [CrossRef] [PubMed]
76. Rezaeitalab, F.; Moharrari, F.; Saberi, S.; Asadpour, H.; Rezaeetalab, F. The correlation of anxiety and depression with obstructive sleep apnea syndreom. *J. Res. Med. Sci.* **2014**, *19*, 205–210. [PubMed]
77. Bardwell, W.A.; Berry, C.C.; Ancoli-Israel, S.; Dimsdale, J.E. Psychological correlates of sleep apnea. *J. Psychosom. Res.* **1999**, *47*, 583–596. [CrossRef]

78. Crabtree, V.M.; Varni, J.W.; Gozal, D. Health-related quality of life and depressive symptoms in children with suspected sleep-disordered breathing. *Sleep* **2004**, *27*, 1131–1138. [CrossRef] [PubMed]
79. Yilmaz, E.; Sedky, K.; Bennett, D.S. The relationship between depressive symptoms and obstructive sleep apnea in pediatric populations: A meta-analysis. *J. Clin. Sleep Med.* **2013**, *9*, 1213–1219. [CrossRef] [PubMed]
80. American Academy of Otolaryngology—Head and Neck Surgery. *Position Statement: Tonstillectomy and OSAs*; adopted 5/3/17, revised 3/2/2014; American Academy of Otolaryngology—Head and Neck Surgery: Alexandria, VA, USA, 2014.
81. Tauman, R.; Gulliver, T.E.; Krishna, J.; Montgomery-Downs, H.E.; O'Brien, L.M.; Ivanenko, A.; Gozal, D. Persistence of obstructive sleep apnea syndrome in children after adenotonsillectomy. *J. Pediatr.* **2006**, *149*, 803–808. [CrossRef] [PubMed]
82. Mitchell, R.B. Adenotonsillectomy for obstructive sleep apnea in children: Outcome evaluated by pre- and postoperative polysomnography. *Laryngoscope* **2007**, *117*, 1844–1854. [CrossRef] [PubMed]
83. Montgomery-Downs, H.E.; Crabtree, V.M.; Gozal, D. Cognition, sleep and respiration in at-risk children treated for obstructive sleep apnoea. *Eur. Respir. J.* **2005**, *25*, 336–342. [CrossRef] [PubMed]
84. Kohler, M.J.; Lushington, K.; van den Heuvel, C.J.; Martin, J.; Pamula, Y.; Kennedy, D. Adenotonsillectomy and neurocognitive deficits in children with sleep disordered breathing. *PLoS ONE* **2009**, *4*, e7343. [CrossRef] [PubMed]
85. Halbower, A.C.; Degaonkar, M.; Barker, P.B.; Earley, C.J.; Marcus, C.L.; Smith, P.L.; Prahme, M.C.; Mahone, E.M. Childhood obstructive sleep apnea associates with neuropsychological deficits and neuronal brain injury. *PLoS Med.* **2006**, *3*, e301. [CrossRef] [PubMed]
86. Cortese, S.; Faraone, S.V.; Konofal, E.; Lecendreux, M. Sleep in children with attention-deficit/hyperactivity disorder: Meta-analysis of subjective and objective studies. *J. Am. Acad. Child Adolesc. Psychiatr.* **2009**, *48*, 894–908. [CrossRef]
87. Korkman, N.; Kirk, U.; Kemp, S. *NEPSY: A Developmental Neuropsychological Assessment Manual*; The Psychological Corp: New York, NY, USA, 1998.
88. Taylor, H.G.; Bowen, S.R.; Beebe, D.W.; Hodges, E.; Amin, R.; Arens, R.; Chervin, R.D.; Garetz, S.L.; Katz, E.S.; Moore, R.H.; et al. Cognitive effects of adenotonsillectomy for obstructive sleep apnea. *Pediatrics* **2016**, *138*, e20154458. [CrossRef] [PubMed]
89. Burton, M.J.; Goldstein, N.A.; Rosenfeld, R.M. Cochrane Corner: Extracts from The Cochrane Library: Tonsillectomy or Adenotonsillectomy versus Non-Surgical Management for Obstructive Sleep-Disordered Breathing in Children. *Otolaryngol. Head Neck Surg.* **2016**, *154*, 581–585. [CrossRef] [PubMed]
90. Marcus, C.L.; Rosen, G.; Ward, S.L.D.; Halbower, A.C.; Sterni, L.; Lutz, J.; Stading, P.J.; Bolduc, D.; Gordon, N. Adherence to and effectiveness of positive airway pressure therapy in children with obstructive sleep apnea. *Pediatrics* **2006**, *117*, e442–e451. [CrossRef] [PubMed]
91. Beebe, D.W.; Byars, K.C. Adolescents with obstructive sleep apnea adhere poorly to positive airway pressure (PAP), but PAP users show improved attention and school performance. *PLoS ONE* **2011**, *6*, e16924. [CrossRef] [PubMed]
92. O'Donnell, A.R.; Bjornson, C.L.; Bohn, S.G.; Kirk, V.G. Compliance rates in children using noninvasive continuous positive airway pressure. *Sleep* **2006**, *29*, 651–658. [PubMed]
93. Marcus, C.L.; Radcliffe, J.; Konstantinopoulou, S.; Beck, S.E.; Cornaglia, M.A.; Traylor, J.; DiFeo, N.; Karamessinis, L.R.; Gallagher, P.R.; Meltzer, L.J. Effects of Positive Airway Pressure Therapy on Neurobehavioral Outcomes in Children with Obstructive Sleep Apnea. *Am. J. Respir. Crit. Care Med.* **2012**, *185*, 998–1003. [CrossRef] [PubMed]
94. Bass, J.L.; Corwin, M.; Gozal, D.; Moore, C.; Nishida, H.; Parker, S.; Schonwald, A.; Wilker, R.E.; Stehle, S.; Kinane, T.B. The effect of chronic or intermittent hypoxia on cognition in childhood: A review of the evidence. *Pediatrics* **2004**, *114*, 805–816. [CrossRef] [PubMed]
95. O'Brien, L.M.; Gozal, D. Neurocognitive dysfunction and sleep in children: From human to rodent. *Pediatr. Clin. N. Am.* **2004**, *51*, 187–202. [CrossRef]
96. Gozal, D.; Serpero, L.D.; Sans Capdevila, O.; Kheirandish-Gozal, L. Systemic inflammation in non-obese children with obstructive sleep apnea. *Sleep Med.* **2008**, *9*, 254–259. [CrossRef] [PubMed]
97. Tauman, R.; O'Brien, L.M.; Gozal, D. Hypoxemia and obesity modulate plasma C-reactive protein and interleukin-6 levels in sleep-disordered breathing. *Sleep Breath.* **2007**, *11*, 77–84. [CrossRef] [PubMed]

98. Gozal, D.; Serpero, L.D.; Kheirandish-Gozal, L.; Capdevila, O.S.; Khalyfa, A.; Tauman, R. Sleep measures and morning plasma TNF-alpha levels in children with sleep-disordered breathing. *Sleep* **2010**, *33*, 319–325. [CrossRef] [PubMed]

99. Tam, C.S.; Wong, M.; McBain, R.; Bailey, S.; Waters, K.A. Inflammatory measures in children with obstructive sleep apnoea. *J. Paediatr. Child Health* **2006**, *42*, 277–282. [CrossRef] [PubMed]

100. Hogan, A.M.; Hill, C.M.; Harrison, D.; Kirkham, F.J. Cerebral blood flow velocity and cognition in children before and after adenotonsillectomy. *Pediatrics* **2008**, *122*, 75–82. [CrossRef] [PubMed]

101. Gozal, D.; Kheirandish-Gozal, L.; Bhattacharjee, R.; Spruyt, K. Neurocognitive and endothelial dysfunction in children with obstructive sleep apnea. *Pediatrics* **2010**, *126*, e1161–e1167. [CrossRef] [PubMed]

102. Levin, H.S.; Culhane, K.A.; Hartmann, J.; Evankovich, K.; Mattson, A.J.; Harward, H.; Ringholz, G.; Ewing-Cobbs, L.; Fletcher, J.M. Developmental changes in performance on tests of purported frontal lobe functioning. *Dev. Neuropsychol.* **1991**, *7*, 377–395. [CrossRef]

103. Welch, M.C.; Pennington, B.F.; Groisser, D.B. A normative-developmental study of executive function. A window on prefrontal function in children. *Dev. Neuropsychol.* **1991**, *7*, 131–149.

104. Denckla, M.B. Research on executive function in a neurodevelopmental context: Application of clinical measures. *Dev. Neuropsychol.* **1996**, *12*, 5–15. [CrossRef]

105. Jones, K.; Harrison, Y. Frontal lobe function, sleep loss and fragmented sleep. *Sleep Med. Rev.* **2001**, *5*, 463–475. [CrossRef] [PubMed]

106. Gozal, D.; Khalyfa, A.; Capdevila, O.S.; Kheirandish-Gozal, L.; Khalyfa, A.A.; Kim, J. Cognitive function in prepubertal children with obstructive sleep apnea: A modifying role for NADPH Oxidase p22 subunit gene polymorphism? *Antioxid. Redox Signal.* **2011**, *16*, 171–177. [CrossRef] [PubMed]

107. Gozal, D.; Crabtree, V.M.; Sans Capdevila, O.; Witcher, L.A.; Kheirandish-Gozal, L. C-reactive protein, obstructive sleep apnea, and cognitive dysfunction in school-aged children. *Am. J. Respir. Crit. Care Med.* **2007**, *176*, 188–193. [CrossRef] [PubMed]

108. Gozal, D.; Sans Capdevila, O.; McLaughlin Crabtree, V.; Serpero, L.D.; Witcher, L.A.; Kheirandish-Gozal, L. Plasma IGF-1 levels and cognitive dysfunction in children with obstructive sleep apnea. *Sleep Med.* **2009**, *10*, 167–173. [CrossRef] [PubMed]

109. Gozal, D.; Capdevila, O.S.; Kheirandish-Gozal, L.; Crabtree, V.M. APOE epsilon 4 allele, cognitive dysfunction, and obstructive sleep apnea in children. *Neurology* **2007**, *69*, 243–249. [CrossRef] [PubMed]

110. Khadra, M.A.; McConnell, K.; VanDyke, R.; Somers, V.; Fenchel, M.; Quadri, S.; Jefferies, J.; Cohen, A.P.; Rutter, M.; Amin, R. Determinants of regional cerebral oxygenation in children with sleep-disordered breathing. *Am. J. Respir. Crit. Care Med.* **2008**, *178*, 870–875. [CrossRef] [PubMed]

111. Kheirandish-Gozal, L.; Gozal, D. The multiple challenges of obstructive sleep apnea in children: Diagnosis. *Curr. Opin. Pediatr.* **2008**, *20*, 650–653. [CrossRef] [PubMed]

112. Khalyfa, A.; Gharib, S.A.; Kim, J.; Capdevila, O.S.; Kheirandish-Gozal, L.; Bhattacharjee, R.; Hegazi, M.; Gozal, D. Peripheral blood leukocyte gene expression patterns and metabolic parameters in habitually snoring and non-snoring children with normal polysomnographic findings. *Sleep* **2011**, *34*, 153–160. [CrossRef] [PubMed]

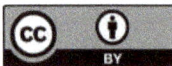

medical sciences

MDPI

Review

The Association between Sleep and Theory of Mind in School Aged Children with ADHD

Rackeb Tesfaye and Reut Gruber *

Department of Psychiatry, McGill University and Attention, Behavior and Sleep Lab, Douglas Mental Health University Institute, Montreal, QC H4H 1R3, Canada; rackeb.tesfaye@mail.mcgill.ca
* Correspondence: reut.gruber@douglas.mcgill.ca; Tel.: +1-514-761-6131 (ext. 3476)

Academic Editors: Ujjwal Ramtekkar and Anna Ivanenko
Received: 3 July 2017; Accepted: 16 August 2017; Published: 21 August 2017

Abstract: Theory of Mind (ToM) is defined as the ability to infer a range of internal mental states of others, including beliefs, intentions, desires, and emotions. These abilities are associated with children's ability to socialize effectively with peers. ToM impairments are associated with peer rejection and psychiatric disorders such as Attention-Deficit/Hyperactivity Disorder (ADHD). Previous studies have found poor sleep negatively impacts executive functioning (EF) and emotional information processing, which are essential for the effective use of ToM. Youth with ADHD have EF deficits and sleep problems. However, the relationship between sleep, executive functioning, and ToM in children with ADHD has not been studied. In this review, we propose that the poor social and interpersonal skills characterizing individuals with ADHD could be explained by the impact of poor sleep on the emotional and cognitive mechanisms underlying ToM.

Keywords: Theory of Mind; sleep; attention deficit hyperactivity disorder; executive functions; emotional information processing cognition; social functioning

---

1. Introduction

Theory of Mind (ToM) is defined as the ability to infer a range of internal mental states including beliefs, intentions, desire, and emotions [1,2]. It is central to the development of social cognition in children, referring to the psychological processes needed for an individual to integrate and be a part of a social group. Children's capacity to successfully use ToM has been shown to be a positive predictor of their ability to socialize effectively [3–5]. ToM impairments are associated with poor social interactions [6,7] and various psychiatric [8–10] and neuro-developmental disorders [11]. Very little is known about the factors or mechanisms that influence the development of successful ToM in school aged children. Previous studies have found poor or insufficient sleep negatively impacts executive functioning and emotional functioning. Both of these impairments are associated with deficits in ToM. However, the relationship between sleep and ToM has not been studied. Youth with Attention-Deficit/Hyperactivity Disorder (ADHD) experience lower sleep quality and duration compared to their typically developing peers [12,13]. We propose that poor and insufficient sleep found in 50%–80% of children with ADHD contributes to the documented social impairments found in youth with ADHD. Examining the relationship between sleep and social impairments in youth with ADHD is of particular importance. First, ADHD is one of the most common neuro-developmental disorders found in childhood, with approximately 5% of school aged children diagnosed [14] and higher estimated rates found in various United States community samples [15]. Second, youth with ADHD have documented social impairments, including greater peer rejection [16,17], impaired expression of empathy [18], and poorer social competence skills [19], compared to their typically developing peers. These social impairments in youth are associated with negative future outcomes, like increased school dropout and psychopathology [20,21]. Furthermore, pharmacological interventions, such as stimulant medication, are shown to not be effective in reducing social information processing impairments in youth with ADHD [22] and have been reported to exacerbate deficits in successfully processing information from social scenarios when compared to ADHD youth in a placebo group [23]. Therefore, examining other potential factors, such as sleep, that may be associated with improving social impairments in youth with ADHD is imperative.

2. Theory of Mind

An implicit form of ToM refers to a spontaneous detection of other's mental states that is not deliberate or consciously inferred [24,25]. Implicit ToM presents early in childhood, with children correctly anticipating actions based on others' mental states [24,25]. This can be seen in infants as young as 7 months, whose eye gazes correctly anticipate the goal-directed behaviors of others based on their personal beliefs [26]. Explicit ToM emerges around the age of 4 with the mastery of first order false belief tasks, signifying their awareness that individuals can hold beliefs that contrast with reality and their own beliefs [27–29]. ToM has been recognized as a pivotal milestone in social development for children across cultures [30–32]. Children develop more complex higher order ToM abilities as they age [33]. This includes successfully completing second order false-belief tasks, demonstrating an understanding of another person's thoughts about a third person(s) [34]. For instance, a child demonstrating second-order false belief will predict that his/her friend will behave differently in a situation if their friend does not have the same new information as someone else (e.g., if the teacher changes the class location and the friend has not been informed, they will go to their regular class room, but the rest of the class who has been informed will go to the new room).

Recognizing that two people can have different understandings of the same situation, and that someone's underlying understanding might be different from what is apparent in reality [28], is implicated in several everyday tasks. These tasks include detecting deception and others' emotions, and understanding the use of non-literal language (e.g., metaphors and sarcasm) [35], all of which are critical to social skills. Social skills are broadly defined as the ability to interact with others appropriately and effectively [36,37]. Such ToM skills, like detecting if someone is lying to you or understanding if someone is upset and why, are crucial to knowing how to appropriately engage in social situations.

ToM ability is a predictor of social skills [3], as well as pro-social behavior [5,6,38] and emotional regulation [39,40]; whereas impairments in ToM are associated with higher rates of peer rejection [6,7], aggressive behavior [41,42], and diverse psychiatric disorders, including depression and anxiety [8–10], and neuro-developmental disorders, like autism [11].

ToM has cognitive and affective components [43–45]. Cognitive ToM refers to inferences about others' beliefs and intentions, while affective ToM refers to inferences about others' emotions and feelings. The distinction between the affective and cognitive components of ToM has been supported by studies showing performance can vary among ToM tasks, and impairments of one ToM component may not correspond to impairments of the other (see references [46–51] for examples).

Neuroimaging studies support the existence of a 'core neural network' for ToM, which includes the medial prefrontal cortex and the bilateral posterior temporo-parietal junction. This network has been proposed because these neural areas are activated during all ToM tasks, irrespective of modality or stimuli, as they require thinking about the mental states of other persons [52]. Within this network, distinctions between affective and cognitive ToM have been made (for a comprehensive review, see refs [45,53]). Affective ToM engages the ventral medial prefrontal cortex, the inferior lateral frontal cortex, the ventral striatum, the ventral temporal pole, the ventral anterior cingulate cortex, the orbitofrontal cortex, and the amygdala [45,53]. Cognitive ToM recruits the dorsal medial prefrontal cortex, the dorsal lateral prefrontal cortex, the dorsal striatum, the dorsal temporal lobe, and the dorsal anterior cingulate cortex [45,53].

Tasks used to measure affective and cognitive ToM vary in types of stimuli and modality. They include situational narrative tasks and picture identification formats. The Reading the Mind in the

Eyes Task [54,55] assesses affective ToM. It requires the identification of a word that best describes how a person is thinking or feeling based on photographs presented to them of the eye regions of human faces. It is dependent on emotional facial processing. The neural pathways involved in affective facial recognition and emotional information processing that include the amygdala and fusiform gyriare are implicated in the performance of this task [56,57]. Affective ToM tasks also require the ability to detect and regulate one's own emotions. Emotional regulation refers to the intrinsic and extrinsic processes responsible for monitoring, evaluating, and modifying one's own emotional reactions [58]. This ability enables a person to make inferences based on the feelings and emotions of others, while having an awareness of their own differing emotional state and regulating it appropriately in a situation.

The Faux Pas Recognition Task [59] measures both cognitive and affective ToM abilities. It presents a story to a participant who is asked to determine if a character has said something socially inappropriate, a "faux pas" that would insult or hurt someone's feelings (affective component), and asked if the "faux pas" was intended to hurt the listener's feelings, and to determine the character's intention to cause harm (the cognitive component).

Although neural mechanisms underlying ToM have been characterized, behavioral and psychological factors that may influence or interact with these networks are still poorly understood. The most prevalent explanatory psychological mechanism put forth to account for ToM performance is executive functioning.

Executive Functioning and Theory of Mind

Executive functioning (EF) is an umbrella term that describes the cognitive processes that enable one to engage in deliberate, goal-directed thought and action [60,61]. The components of EF include: working memory, inhibitory control, and cognitive flexibility [60–63]. Working memory is the capacity to retain information in the short-term to guide future actions [60,61]. Inhibitory control is the ability to override prepotent responses, which involves being able to control one's attention, behaviors, and/or emotions [61]. Cognitive flexibility (also known as 'cognitive shifting', 'task shifting', or 'set-shifting') refers to the ability to shift between tasks and adapt to new information [60]. Moderate to strong associations have been found between EF subcomponents and ToM in childhood [64]. The two constructs—EF and ToM—are reported to be dependent on the prefrontal cortex [65], and they both develop in a similar fashion from early to middle childhood [66–68]. EF and its subcomponents have been related to subcomponents of ToM (see Figure 1 for details) [67]. Inhibitory control is needed to inhibit salient knowledge of one's current reality and one's own emotions, beliefs, or intentions, in order to successfully respond to others' mental states that are needed for both cognitive and affective ToM [69]. Cognitive flexibility is needed in order to shift between perspectives and mental states of others and oneself. Lastly, the capacity to actively retain multiple perspectives and information as one processes information requires working memory capacity. Collectively, EF abilities, including inhibitory control, cognitive flexibility, and working memory are simultaneously needed to successfully detect the mental states of others' ToM.

Although, the majority of research connecting EF and ToM has been conducted in pre-school children, there is evidence to suggest that this link extends into school age [70]. For instance, cognitive flexibility in school-age children predicts performance on social understanding tasks requiring affective and cognitive ToM abilities [71]. Cognitive flexibility, along with working memory, has also been shown to longitudinally predict affective and cognitive ToM ability on social scenario tasks in school aged children [70]. While very strong associations exist between inhibitory control and ToM in pre-school years [32,69,72], very little is known about this relationship as children develop.

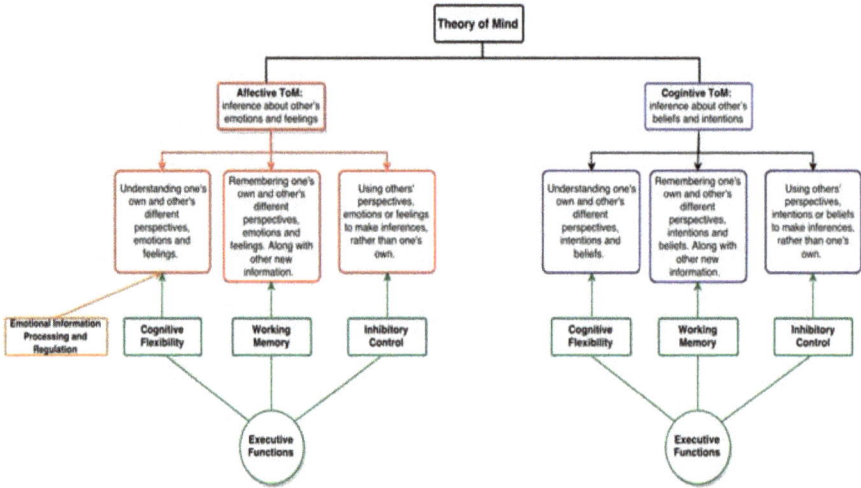

Figure 1. Flowchart demonstrating links between Theory of Mind (ToM) and executive functions (EF). Theory of mind is split into cognitive ToM, the ability to understand and make inferences about others' beliefs and intentions; and affective ToM, the ability to understand and make inference about others' emotions and feelings. Presented are the links found in literature [64,67,70] between affective and cognitive ToM in youth, with three EF subtypes: (1) cognitive flexibility; (2) working memory; and (3) inhibitory control. In addition to associations with EF, affective ToM is also associated with emotional information processing and regulation, needed to understand various feelings and emotions of others and oneself.

3. Sleep

3.1. Sleep and Executive Functioning

According to the two-process model, sleep timing and duration is regulated by two distinct yet interacting biological processes, (1) the sleep-wake homeostasis (process S) and (2) the circadian rhythm (process C) [73]. A homeostatic sleep drive (i.e., the biological need for sleep) accumulates the longer a person is awake, causing pressure to fall asleep. The circadian rhythm controls the timing of sleep. It is an oscillatory rhythm that fluctuates with an approximate daily cycle of 24 h. The circadian rhythm is driven by an internal pacemaker, the biological clock, located in the superchiasmatic nucleus. External environmental stimuli known as zeitgerbers, which include light-dark cycles and temperature, influence circadian rhythms. Expert consensus recommends school children aged 6–12 years sleeping a duration of 9 to 11 h a night consistently to promote optimal health outcomes [74–76].

Insufficient and inadequate sleep are associated with poor executive functioning [77–84]. Insufficient sleep refers to getting less sleep than needed [85]. Inadequate sleep refers to poor-quality sleep, which includes low sleep efficiency, defined as the percentage of time in bed spent sleeping [86]. Neuroimaging studies reveal that sleep deprivation negatively disrupts the prefrontal cortex, a neural system central to EF [65,87]. Individuals with insomnia who experience poor sleep, characterized by frequent night awakenings, low sleep efficiency, troubles falling asleep at bedtime, and early morning awakenings [88,89], are shown to have altered connectivity in the frontostriatal networks [90]. Impaired frontostriatal connections are associated with EF deficits [91].

Shortened sleep duration and low sleep efficiency are associated with impaired inhibitory control abilities in youths and adults [92–97]. Behavioral tasks measuring the ability to suppress prepotent responses, known as inhibitory control, are negatively impacted by one to two nights of moderate sleep deprivation in adults [92,93]. After sleep deprivation an adult's performance on the Go/No-Go

Task, a computerized task whereby inhibitory control is measured by a participant's ability to withhold responses to a known target, significantly deteriorates [92,93]. Similarly, six nights of moderate sleep deprivation, measured using actigraphy in typically developing school aged children and children diagnosed with ADHD, is shown to significantly impair their performance on the Continuous Performance Task (CPT) [94]. The CPT measures impulsivity and inhibitory control [98] by testing a participant's ability to suppress their responses to a known target (i.e., the letter X), just like the Go/No-Go Task. One week of moderate sleep deprivation also alters brain activity measured by event-related potentials in school aged children compared to non-sleep deprived school aged children preforming the same inhibitory control task [96].

In addition to sleep deprivation, extending sleep duration by less than an hour has been found to improve inhibitory control abilities in children [99]. One study randomized school aged children into a sleep extension or sleep deprivation group [99]. They reported children in the sleep extension group, who slept an average of 35 min longer than their sleep-deprived peers, performed significantly better on the CPT.

Typically developing children with low sleep efficiency, measured with actigraphy, are also shown to perform poorly on the CPT, compared to peers with higher sleep efficiency [95]. Taken together, these results provide a strong case for the impact sleep has on inhibitory control ability.

The capacity to retain working memory is also affected by insufficient and poor-quality sleep in youth [99–103]. After going to bed one hour later than usual for four nights, school aged children's working memory ability deteriorated compared to when they went to bed an hour earlier than their regular sleep schedule [103]. Two nights of actigraphy and one night of polysomnography (a gold standard biophysiological sleep measure, monitoring electroencephalography signals in the brain and other physiological movement during sleep) data of school aged children also revealed lower sleep duration was associated with poorer working memory ability compared to peers with higher sleep duration, as reported by their teachers on the revised Conners Teacher Rating Scale [100]. Sadeh et al. [99] found that extending school aged children's sleep duration, monitored by actigraphy, significantly improved their performance of the Digital Span task. Low sleep efficiency in children, measured for 72 h using actigraphy, is also shown to be associated with poor auditory and visual working memory performance on the n-back task [102]. Overall, evidence to date demonstrates short sleep duration and low sleep efficiency significantly impairs working memory ability.

Cognitive flexibility in youth is shown to be affected by sleep duration [104]; however, limited research exists and its relation to sleep efficiency is unknown. In adolescents, two weeks of extending sleep duration 5 min a night, measured using actigraphy, was found to have positive performance effects on the Divided Attention task [104]. The task requires participants to actively shift their attention between an initial stimulus while simultaneously processing others in order to correctly detect different target sequences corresponding to cognitive flexibility. This demonstrates a link between longer sleep duration and better cognitive flexibility performance in youth.

In all, a great deal of evidence directly links sleep duration and efficiency with all three EF subcomponents: working memory, inhibitory control, and cognitive flexibility (see Figure 2 for an overview).

3.2. Sleep and Emotional Information Processing

Sleep has been shown to be associated with emotional information processing and regulation, key processes needed for the proper function of affective ToM.

Sleep deprivation is associated with altered brain activation when viewing negative salient emotional stimuli [57]. Those who are sleep-deprived experience a greater magnitude of amygdala activation when seeing aversive stimuli. This demonstrates that shortened sleep duration intensifies emotional reactivity, which challenges the ability to successfully regulate ones' own emotions. Also, compared to non-sleep deprived individuals, sleep-deprived participants who viewed emotional stimuli on pictures showed reduced functional connectivity between the amygdala and medial prefrontal cortex, an area found to be involved in the top-down modulation of emotional processing and responses [57].

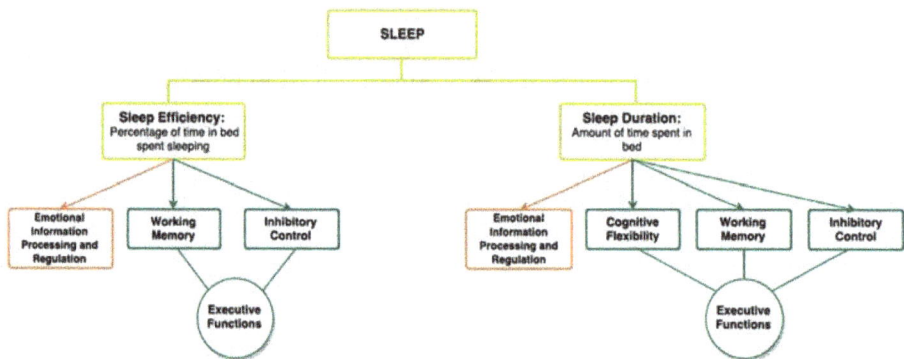

Figure 2. Conceptual framework demonstrating links between ToM and EF. The present chart demonstrates the links found in the literature between two sleep variables, the sleep efficiency (percentage of time in bed spent sleeping) and the sleep duration (amount of time spent in bed sleeping), and EF subtypes. Sleep duration is associated with cognitive flexibility [104], working memory [99,100,103], and inhibitory control [92–94,99]. Sleep efficiency is associated with working memory [102] and inhibitory control [97]. Both sleep duration and efficiency have been shown to be associated with emotional information processing and regulation [57,105,108,109].

Additionally, sleep deprivation elevates the activation of the ventral anterior cingulate cortex [105]. Increased activation of the ventral anterior cingulate cortex is linked to detecting and regulating emotions in school aged children [106].

Shorter sleep duration and poor-sleep quality has been associated with reduced emotional information processing abilities in both adults and youth [103,107,108]. This includes an impaired ability to match emotions to faces [109], a ToM deficit. A 2011 study [109] found that elevated night awakenings and decreased sleep efficiency predicted poor performance in identifying simple facial emotions (e.g., happy and sad) in school aged children.

Furthermore, neuroimaging studies have found longer sleep duration and sleep credit (sleeping more than the minimal duration needed to avoid impairment) are related to greater grey matter volume of the medial frontal and orbitofrontal cortex regions, and are also associated with higher emotional intelligence [110,111]. Emotional intelligence includes the ability to respond flexibly to changing emotional information and understanding others' emotions [110,111].

All of these emotional processing and regulating abilities disrupted by poor-sleep duration and efficiency are directly needed for successful affective ToM.

Overall, shorter sleep duration and lower sleep efficiency are associated with an impaired ability to regulate one's own emotions and process emotional information, which are central to successfully understanding other people's emotional mental states.

4. Sleep and ToM: Are They Associated?

A large body of evidence has shown that poor sleep is associated with impaired EF and with poor emotional information processing abilities. Both of these impairments correspond to ToM deficits. Neural networks disrupted by poor sleep also correspond to brain areas involved in the affective and cognitive ToM network.

Given EF is strongly entrenched in the development of ToM, and poor sleep impairs EF ability, we propose that poor sleep may be associated with poor cognitive ToM. Based on evidence demonstrating that poor sleep worsens the ability to process emotional information (such as emotions on faces), we propose that poor sleep will be associated with poor affective ToM.

Future research should examine the relationship between sleep and ToM to determine if any casual associations can be identified. This information can then eventually be applied to forming the basis of developing innovative approaches to support children with dysfunctional ToM and improve their future social cognitive development.

5. Attention Deficit/Hyperactivity Disorder

5.1. ADHD, EF, and Social Functioning

Attention-Deficit/Hyperactivity Disorder is a prevalent developmental disorder that affects children and adults. It is defined by atypical levels of inattention, impulsivity, and hyperactivity, and occurs in 5% of school aged children [14]. Children diagnosed with ADHD are characterized as having impaired EF [112,113]. They exhibit significant impairment in all subcomponents of EF, including cognitive flexibility and working memory [114]; however, the most robust deficits are seen in the inhibitory control [114]. Brain regions corresponding to EF performance, like the prefrontal cortex, are shown to activate atypically in youth diagnosed with ADHD [115–117].

Literature on ADHD has mostly focused on its impact on cognition and academic performance [118–120], reading [121], or organizational skills needed for academic success [122,123], but has sparsely focused on social cognition. This is despite well-documented reports of youth with ADHD having severe social impairments [124,125]. Children diagnosed with ADHD are more often rejected by their peers and have fewer friends compared to typically developing children [16,126]. In fact, within a few hours or even minutes of a social interaction with unfamiliar peers, youth with ADHD are often disliked and make negative impressions [17,127,128]. Additionally, children with ADHD have been found to express impaired empathy [18], are socially intrusive [125], have fewer reciprocal dyadic friendships [129], and are rated as less socially competent compared to typically developing peers by parents and teachers [19] relative to non-ADHD youth. Although youth with ADHD struggle with interpersonal and social competence skills, they inaccurately perceive their own abilities, overestimating their social competence when self-evaluating [130]. Such interpersonal and social skill impairments, like peer rejection, are troubling, as they are associated with negative future outcomes including dropping out of school, substance abuse, delinquency, and higher rates of psychopathology [20,21].

5.2. ADHD and ToM

Studies have found ToM deficits are present in youth diagnosed with ADHD [131,132]. Research findings indicate youth with ADHD exhibit emotional regulation deficits [133] and impaired affective information processing [134,135] needed for successful ToM. In comparison to typically developing peers, youth with ADHD show reduced amygdala activation when processing fearful expressions [135] and perform poorly on social decision problems requiring the processing of others' facial emotions to appropriately solve a social problem [136]. Additionally, youth with ADHD have difficulties detecting positive and negative cues in social stories, including interpreting other people's intentions [137]. One study [131] found children with ADHD performed worse than typically developing children on the Reading the Mind in the Eyes Task and the Faux Pas Recognition Task, testing affective and cognitive ToM. Poor inhibitory control and attention deficits predicted performance on the Faux Pas Recognition and Reading the Mind in the Eyes tasks, respectively, in youth with ADHD.

5.3. ADHD and Sleep

Sleep problems are common in children with ADHD [12], with parents reporting 2- to 3-times higher prevalence of sleep disturbances compared to normal controls [13]. Sleep disorders that have been reported to be more prevalent in children with ADHD compared to their typically developing peers include Periodic Leg Movement Disorder and Restless Leg Syndrome (PLMS), and sleep disordered breathing [138–140]. Poor sleep negatively impacts EFs, which are already disrupted in children with ADHD. Hence, these sleep issues can contribute to exacerbating existing cognitive, emotional, and social deficits in youth with ADHD [141].

The novel link proposed between sleep and ToM in section 4 can provide insight into the associations between sleep issues and social deficits observed in youth with ADHD. Current literature has associated ADHD and ToM with deficits in EF. Inadequate and insufficient sleep negatively affect EF, and sleep issues are found to be prevalent in youth diagnosed with ADHD. As youth with ADHD exhibit deficits with interpersonal skills and social cognitive functioning, including impaired ToM, sleep may be a key factor contributing to these deficits by impairing EF and emotional information processing. Future research is warranted to examine the interplay between sleep, ToM, and socio-emotional cognition in children with and without ADHD. If casual associations are uncovered, this information can then eventually be applied to forming the basis of developing innovative approaches in the treatment of social dysfunction in youth.

6. Conclusions

This paper has presented substantial evidence that poor and inadequate sleep may be associated with ToM impairments in youth with and without ADHD. Sleep deprivation causes impairments in EF and emotional information processing, both of which are associated with poor ToM ability. EF deficits are a core impairment in youth with ADHD, who also experience greater sleep issues compared to their typically developing peers. Since youth with ADHD are known to experience social dysfunction, which includes ToM deficits, sleep may be a contributing factor by impairing EF. Therefore, examining the role of sleep in relation to the social deficits that characterize youth with ADHD may provide helpful insights into understanding and treating the social impairments identified.

Author Contributions: Rackeb Tesfaye proposed the conceptual framework and wrote the manuscript. Reut Gruber refined and edited the manuscript.

Conflicts of Interest: The authors declare no conflict of interest.

References

1. Premack, D.; Woodruff, G. Does the chimpanzee have a theory of mind? *Behav. Brain Sci.* **1978**, *1*, 515–526. [CrossRef]
2. Wellman, H.M. *The child's Theory of Mind*; The MIT Press: Cambridge, MA, USA, 1990.
3. Peterson, C.; Slaughter, V.; Moore, C.; Wellman, H.M. Peer social skills and theory of mind in children with autism, deafness, or typical development. *Dev. Psychol.* **2016**, *52*, 46–57. [CrossRef] [PubMed]
4. Watson, A.C.; Nixon, C.L.; Wilson, A.; Capage, L. Social interaction skills and theory of mind in young children. *Dev. Psychol.* **1999**, *35*, 386–391. [CrossRef] [PubMed]
5. Imuta, K.; Henry, J.D.; Slaughter, V.; Selcuk, B.; Ruffman, T. Theory of mind and prosocial behavior in childhood: A meta-analytic review. *Dev. Psychol.* **2016**, *52*, 1192–1205. [CrossRef] [PubMed]
6. Banerjee, R.; Watling, D.; Caputi, M. Peer relations and the understanding of faux pas: Longitudinal evidence for bidirectional associations. *Child Dev.* **2011**, *82*, 1887–1905. [CrossRef] [PubMed]
7. Slaughter, V.; Imuta, K.; Peterson, C.C.; Henry, J.D. Meta-analysis of theory of mind and peer popularity in the preschool and early school years. *Child Dev.* **2015**, *86*, 1159–1174. [CrossRef] [PubMed]
8. Bora, E.; Berk, M. Theory of mind in major depressive disorder: A meta-analysis. *J. Affect. Disord.* **2016**, *191*, 49–55. [CrossRef] [PubMed]
9. Lee, L.; Harkness, K.L.; Sabbagh, M.A.; Jacobson, J.A. Mental state decoding abilities in clinical depression. *J. Affect. Disord.* **2005**, *86*, 247–258. [CrossRef] [PubMed]
10. Hezel, D.M.; McNally, R.J. Theory of mind impairments in social anxiety disorder. *Behav. Ther.* **2014**, *45*, 530–540. [CrossRef] [PubMed]

11. Baron-Cohen, S. Theory of mind and autism: A review. *Int. Rev. Res. Ment. Retard.* **2000**, *23*, 169–184. [CrossRef]

12. Corkum, P.; Tannock, R.; Moldofsky, H.; Hogg-Johnson, S.; Humphries, T. Actigraphy and parental ratings of sleep in children with attention-deficit/hyperactivity disorder. *Sleep* **2001**, *24*, 303–312. [CrossRef] [PubMed]

13. Owens, J.A. The ADHD and sleep conundrum: A review. *J. Dev. Behav. Pediatr.* **2005**, *26*, 312–322. [CrossRef] [PubMed]

14. American Psychiatric Association. *Diagnostic and Statistical Manual of Mental Disorders, (DSM-5®)*; American Psychiatric Pub: Washington, DC, USA, 2013.

15. Visser, S.N.; Danielson, M.L.; Bitsko, R.H.; Holbrook, J.R.; Kogan, M.D.; Ghandour, R.M.; Blumberg, S.J. Trends in the parent-report of health care provider-diagnosed and medicated attention-deficit/hyperactivity disorder: United States, 2003–2011. *J. Am. Acad. Child Adolesc. Psychiatry* **2014**, *53*, 34–46. [CrossRef] [PubMed]

16. Hoza, B.; Mrug, S.; Gerdes, A.C.; Hinshaw, S.P.; Bukowski, W.M.; Gold, J.A.; Arnold, L.E. What aspects of peer relationships are impaired in children with attention-deficit/hyperactivity disorder? *J. Consult. Clin. Psychol.* **2005**, *73*, 411. [CrossRef] [PubMed]

17. Mikami, A.Y. The importance of friendship for youth with attention-deficit/hyperactivity disorder. *Clin. Child Fam. Psychol. Rev.* **2010**, *13*, 181–198. [CrossRef] [PubMed]

18. Braaten, E.B.; Rosén, L.A. Self-regulation of affect in attention deficit-hyperactivity disorder (ADHD) and non-ADHD boys: Differences in empathic responding. *J. Consult. Clin. Psychol.* **2000**, *68*, 313. [CrossRef] [PubMed]

19. Ronk, M.J.; Hund, A.M.; Landau, S. Assessment of social competence of boys with attention-deficit/hyperactivity disorder: Problematic peer entry, host responses, and evaluations. *J. Abnorm. Child Psychol.* **2011**, *39*, 829–840. [CrossRef] [PubMed]

20. Greene, R.W.; Biederman, J.; Faraone, S.V.; Sienna, M.; Garcia-Jetton, J. Adolescent outcome of boys with attention-deficit/hyperactivity disorder and social disability: Results from a 4-year longitudinal follow-up study. *J. Consult. Clin. Psychol.* **1997**, *65*, 758. [CrossRef] [PubMed]

21. Klein, R.G.; Mannuzza, S. Long-term outcome of hyperactive children: A review. *J. Am. Acad. Child Adolesc. Psychiatry* **1991**, *30*, 383–387. [CrossRef] [PubMed]

22. Derefinko, K.J.; Bailey, U.L.; Milich, R.; Lorch, E.P.; Riley, E. The effects of stimulant medication on the online story narrations of children with ADHD. *School Ment. Health* **2009**, *1*, 171–182. [CrossRef]

23. King, S.; Waschbusch, D.A.; Pelham, W.E., Jr.; Frankland, B.W.; Andrade, B.F.; Jacques, S.; Corkum, P.V. Social information processing in elementary-school aged children with ADHD: Medication effects and comparisons with typical children. *J. Abnorm. Child Psychol.* **2009**, *37*, 579–589. [CrossRef] [PubMed]

24. Sodian, B.; Schuwerk, T.; Kristen, S. Implicit and spontaneous theory of mind reasoning in autism spectrum disorders. In *Autism Spectrum Disorder-Recent Advances*; InTech: Rijeka, Croatia, 2015. [CrossRef]

25. Schuwerk, T.; Vuori, M.; Sodian, B. Implicit and explicit theory of mind reasoning in autism spectrum disorders: the impact of experience. *Autism* **2015**, *19*, 459–468. [CrossRef] [PubMed]

26. Kovács, Á.M.; Téglás, E.; Endress, A.D. The social sense: Susceptibility to others' beliefs in human infants and adults. *Science* **2010**, *330*, 1830–1834. [CrossRef] [PubMed]

27. Wimmer, H.; Perner, J. Beliefs about beliefs: Representation and constraining function of wrong beliefs in young children's understanding of deception. *Cognition* **1983**, *13*, 103–128. [CrossRef]

28. Perner, J. *Understanding the Representational Mind*; The MIT Press: Cambridge, MA, US, 1991; p. 348.

29. Wellman, H.M.; Cross, D.; Watson, J. Meta-analysis of theory-of-mind development: The truth about false belief. *Child Dev.* **2001**, *72*, 655–684. [CrossRef] [PubMed]

30. Frith, C.D.; Frith, U. Interacting minds—A biological basis. *Science (New York, N.Y.)* **1999**, *286*, 1692–1695. [CrossRef]

31. Hughes, C.; Devine, R.T.; Ensor, R.; Masuo, K.; Ai, M.; Lecce, S. Lost in translation? Comparing british, japanese, and italian children's theory-of-mind performance. *Child Dev. Res.* **2014**, 1–10. [CrossRef]

32. Sabbagh, M.A.; Xu, F.; Carlson, S.M.; Moses, L.J.; Lee, K. The development of executive functioning and theory of mind. A comparison of Chinese and U.S. Preschoolers. *Psychol. Sci.* **2006**, *17*, 74–81. [CrossRef] [PubMed]

33. Miller, S.A. Children's understanding of second-order mental states. *Psychol. Bull.* **2009**, *135*, 749–773. [CrossRef] [PubMed]

34. Perner, J.; Wimmer, H. "John thinks that mary thinks that . . . " attribution of second-order beliefs by 5- to 10-year-old children. *J. Exp. Child Psychol.* **1985**, *39*, 437–471. [CrossRef]

35. Happe, F. Theory of mind and the self. *Ann. N. Y. Acad. Sci.* **2003**, *1001*, 134–144. [CrossRef] [PubMed]

36. Segrin, C. Social skills deficits associated with depression. *Clin. Psychol. Rev.* **2000**, *20*, 379–403. [CrossRef]

37. Spitzberg, B.H.; Cupach, W.R. Issues in interpersonal competence research. In *Handbook of Interpersonal Competence Research*; Springer: New York, NY, USA, 1989; pp. 52–75.

38. Caputi, M.; Lecce, S.; Pagnin, A.; Banerjee, R. Longitudinal effects of theory of mind on later peer relations: The role of prosocial behavior. *Dev. Psychol.* **2012**, *48*, 257–270. [CrossRef] [PubMed]

39. Baurain, C.; Nader-Grosbois, N. *Compétences Sociales et émotionnelles: Enfant Typique et Déficient Intellectuel*; Presses Académiques Francophones: Saarbrücken, Germany, 2013.

40. Riggs, N.R.; Greenberg, M.T.; Kusche, C.A.; Pentz, M.A. The mediational role of neurocognition in the behavioral outcomes of a social-emotional prevention program in elementary school students: Effects of the paths curriculum. *Prev. Sci. Off. J. Soc. Prev. Res.* **2006**, *7*, 91–102. [CrossRef] [PubMed]

41. Harvey, R.J.; Fletcher, J.; French, D.J. Social reasoning: A source of influence on aggression. *Clin. Psychol. Rev.* **2001**, *21*, 447–469. [CrossRef]

42. Renouf, A.; Brendgen, M.; Parent, S.; Vitaro, F.; David Zelazo, P.; Boivin, M.; Dionne, G.; Tremblay, R.E.; Pérusse, D.; Séguin, J.R. Relations between theory of mind and indirect and physical aggression in kindergarten: Evidence of the moderating role of prosocial behaviors. *Soc. Dev.* **2010**, *19*, 535–555. [CrossRef]

43. Kalbe, E.; Schlegel, M.; Sack, A.T.; Nowak, D.A.; Dafotakis, M.; Bangard, C.; Brand, M.; Shamay-Tsoory, S.; Onur, O.A.; Kessler, J. Dissociating cognitive from affective theory of mind: A tms study. *Cortex* **2010**, *46*, 769–780. [CrossRef] [PubMed]

44. Shamay-Tsoory, S.G.; Shur, S.; Barcai-Goodman, L.; Medlovich, S.; Harari, H.; Levkovitz, Y. Dissociation of cognitive from affective components of theory of mind in schizophrenia. *Psychiatry Res.* **2007**, *149*, 11–23. [CrossRef] [PubMed]

45. Abu-Akel, A.; Shamay-Tsoory, S. Neuroanatomical and neurochemical bases of theory of mind. *Neuropsychologia* **2011**, *49*, 2971–2984. [CrossRef] [PubMed]

46. Bottiroli, S.; Cavallini, E.; Ceccato, I.; Vecchi, T.; Lecce, S. Theory of mind in aging: Comparing cognitive and affective components in the faux pas test. *Arch. Gerontol. Geriatr.* **2016**, *62*, 152–162. [CrossRef] [PubMed]

47. Roca, M.; Parr, A.; Thompson, R.; Woolgar, A.; Torralva, T.; Antoun, N.; Manes, F.; Duncan, J. Executive function and fluid intelligence after frontal lobe lesions. *Brain J. Neurol.* **2010**, *133*, 234–247. [CrossRef] [PubMed]

48. Sebastian, C.L.; Fontaine, N.M.; Bird, G.; Blakemore, S.J.; Brito, S.A.; McCrory, E.J.; Viding, E. Neural processing associated with cognitive and affective theory of mind in adolescents and adults. *Soc. Cognit. Affect. Neurosci.* **2012**, *7*, 53–63. [CrossRef] [PubMed]

49. Shamay-Tsoory, S.G.; Aharon-Peretz, J. Dissociable prefrontal networks for cognitive and affective theory of mind: A lesion study. *Neuropsychologia* **2007**, *45*, 3054–3067. [CrossRef] [PubMed]

50. Shamay-Tsoory, S.G.; Tibi-Elhanany, Y.; Aharon-Peretz, J. The ventromedial prefrontal cortex is involved in understanding affective but not cognitive theory of mind stories. *Soc. Neurosci.* **2006**, *1*, 149–166. [CrossRef] [PubMed]

51. Van Overwalle, F.; Baetens, K. Understanding others' actions and goals by mirror and mentalizing systems: A meta-analysis. *NeuroImage* **2009**, *48*, 564–584. [CrossRef] [PubMed]

52. Frith, C.D.; Frith, U. The neural basis of mentalizing. *Neuron* **2006**, *50*, 531–534. [CrossRef] [PubMed]

53. Schurz, M.; Radua, J.; Aichhorn, M.; Richlan, F.; Perner, J. Fractionating theory of mind: A meta-analysis of functional brain imaging studies. *Neurosci. Biobehav. Rev.* **2014**, *42*, 9–34. [CrossRef] [PubMed]

54. Baron-Cohen, S.; Jolliffe, T.; Mortimore, C.; Robertson, M. Another advanced test of theory of mind: Evidence from very high functioning adults with autism or asperger syndrome. *J. Child Psychol. Psychiatry* **1997**, *38*, 813–822. [CrossRef]

55. Baron-Cohen, S.; Wheelwright, S.; Hill, J.; Raste, Y.; Plumb, I. The "reading the mind in the eyes" test revised version: A study with normal adults, and adults with asperger syndrome or high-functioning autism. *J. Child Psychol. Psychiatry* **2001**, *42*, 241–251. [CrossRef]

56. Adolphs, R.; Sears, L.; Piven, J. Abnormal processing of social information from faces in autism. *J. Cognit. Neurosci.* **2001**, *13*, 232–240. [CrossRef]

57. Yoo, S.S.; Gujar, N.; Hu, P.; Jolesz, F.A.; Walker, M.P. The human emotional brain without sleep—A prefrontal amygdala disconnect. *Curr. Biol.* **2007**, *17*, R877–R878. [CrossRef] [PubMed]

58. Thompson, R.A. Emotion regulation: A theme in search of definition. *Monogr. Soc. Res. Child Dev.* **1994**, *59*, 25–52. [CrossRef] [PubMed]

59. Stone, V.E.; Baron-Cohen, S.; Knight, R.T. Frontal lobe contributions to theory of mind. *J. Cognit. Neurosci.* **1998**, *10*, 640–656. [CrossRef]

60. Carlson, S.M.; Zelazo, P.D.; Faja, S. Executive function. In *The Oxford Handbook of Developmental Psychology*; Zelazo, P.D., Ed.; Oxford University Press: New York, NY, USA, 2013; Volume 1, pp. 706–743.

61. Diamond, A. Executive functions. *Annu. Rev. Psychol.* **2013**, *64*, 135–168. [CrossRef] [PubMed]

62. Friedman, N.P.; Miyake, A. The relations among inhibition and interference control functions: A latent-variable analysis. *J. Exp. Psychol. Gen.* **2004**, *133*, 101–135. [CrossRef] [PubMed]

63. Miyake, A.; Friedman, N.P.; Emerson, M.J.; Witzki, A.H.; Howerter, A.; Wager, T.D. The unity and diversity of executive functions and their contributions to complex "frontal lobe" tasks: A latent variable analysis. *Cognit. Psychol.* **2000**, *41*, 49–100. [CrossRef] [PubMed]

64. Devine, R.T.; Hughes, C. Relations between false belief understanding and executive function in early childhood: A meta-analysis. *Child Dev.* **2014**, *85*, 1777–1794. [CrossRef] [PubMed]

65. Fuster, J.M. *The Prefrontal Cortex*, 4th ed.; Academic Press: Boston, MA, USA, 2008.

66. Davidson, M.C.; Amso, D.; Anderson, L.C.; Diamond, A. Development of cognitive control and executive functions from 4 to 13 years: Evidence from manipulations of memory, inhibition, and task switching. *Neuropsychologia* **2006**, *44*, 2037–2078. [CrossRef] [PubMed]

67. Apperly, I.A.; Warren, F.; Andrews, B.J.; Grant, J.; Todd, S. Developmental continuity in theory of mind: Speed and accuracy of belief-desire reasoning in children and adults. *Child Dev.* **2011**, *82*, 1691–1703. [CrossRef] [PubMed]

68. Devine, R.T.; Hughes, C. Silent films and strange stories: Theory of mind, gender, and social experiences in middle childhood. *Child Dev.* **2013**, *84*, 989–1003. [CrossRef] [PubMed]

69. Carlson, S.M.; Moses, L.J. Individual differences in inhibitory control and children's theory of mind. *Child Dev.* **2001**, *72*, 1032–1053. [CrossRef] [PubMed]

70. Austin, G.; Groppe, K.; Elsner, B. The reciprocal relationship between executive function and theory of mind in middle childhood: A 1-year longitudinal perspective. *Front. Psychol.* **2014**, *5*, 655. [CrossRef] [PubMed]

71. Bock, A.M.; Gallaway, K.C.; Hund, A.M. Specifying links between executive functioning and theory of mind during middle childhood: Cognitive flexibility predicts social understanding. *J. Cognit. Dev.* **2015**, *16*, 509–521. [CrossRef]

72. Perner, J.; Lang, B. Theory of mind and executive function: Is there a developmental relationship? In *Understanding Other Minds: Perspectives from Developmental Cognitive Neuroscience*, 2nd ed.; Oxford University Press: New York, NY, USA, 2000; pp. 150–181.

73. Borbely, A.A. A two process model of sleep regulation. *Hum. Neurobiol.* **1982**, *1*, 195–204. [CrossRef] [PubMed]

74. Hirshkowitz, M.; Whiton, K.; Albert, S.M.; Alessi, C.; Bruni, O.; DonCarlos, L.; Neubauer, D.N. National Sleep Foundation's sleep time duration recommendations: Methodology and results summary. *Sleep Health* **2015**, *1*, 40–43. [CrossRef]

75. Paruthi, S.; Brooks, L.J.; D'Ambrosio, C.; Hall, W.A.; Kotagal, S.; Lloyd, R.M.; Rosen, C.L. Recommended amount of sleep for pediatric populations: A consensus statement of the American Academy of Sleep Medicine. *J. Clin. Sleep Med. JCSM Off. Publ. Am. Acad. Sleep Med.* **2016**, *12*, 785. [CrossRef] [PubMed]

76. Tremblay, M.S.; Carson, V.; Chaput, J.P.; Connor Gorber, S.; Dinh, T.; Duggan, M.; Janssen, I. Canadian 24-Hour Movement Guidelines for Children and Youth: An Integration of Physical Activity, Sedentary Behaviour, and Sleep 1. *Appl. Physiol. Nutr. Metab.* **2016**, *41*, S311–S327. [CrossRef] [PubMed]

77. Beebe, D.W.; Wells, C.T.; Jeffries, J.; Chini, B.; Kalra, M.; Amin, R. Neuropsychological effects of pediatric obstructive sleep apnea. *J. Int. Neuropsychol. Soc. JINS* **2004**, *10*, 962–975. [CrossRef] [PubMed]

78. Bourke, R.; Anderson, V.; Yang, J.S.; Jackman, A.R.; Killedar, A.; Nixon, G.M.; Davey, M.J.; Walker, A.M.; Trinder, J.; Horne, R.S. Cognitive and academic functions are impaired in children with all severities of sleep-disordered breathing. *Sleep Med.* **2011**, *12*, 489–496. [CrossRef] [PubMed]

79. Dahl, R.E. The impact of inadequate sleep on children's daytime cognitive function. *Semin. Pediatr. Neurol.* **1996**, *3*, 44–50. [CrossRef]

80. Friedman, N.P.; Corley, R.P.; Hewitt, J.K.; Wright, K.P., Jr. Individual differences in childhood sleep problems predict later cognitive executive control. *Sleep* **2009**, *32*, 323–333. [CrossRef] [PubMed]

81. Gregory, A.M.; Caspi, A.; Moffitt, T.E.; Poulton, R. Sleep problems in childhood predict neuropsychological functioning in adolescence. *Pediatrics* **2009**, *123*, 1171–1176. [CrossRef] [PubMed]

82. Nelson, T.D.; Nelson, J.M.; Kidwell, K.M.; James, T.D.; Espy, K.A. Preschool sleep problems and differential associations with specific aspects of executive control in early elementary school. *Dev. Neuropsychol.* **2015**, *40*, 167–180. [CrossRef] [PubMed]

83. Nilsson, J.P.; Soderstrom, M.; Karlsson, A.U.; Lekander, M.; Akerstedt, T.; Lindroth, N.E.; Axelsson, J. Less effective executive functioning after one night's sleep deprivation. *J. Sleep Res.* **2005**, *14*, 1–6. [CrossRef] [PubMed]

84. Taveras, E.M.; Rifas-Shiman, S.L.; Bub, K.L.; Gillman, M.W.; Oken, E. Prospective study of insufficient sleep and neurobehavioral functioning among school-age children. *Acad. Pediatr.* **2017**, *17*, 625–632. [CrossRef] [PubMed]

85. Owens, J. Insufficient sleep in adolescents and young adults: An update on causes and consequences. *Pediatrics* **2014**, *134*, e921–e932. [CrossRef] [PubMed]

86. Ohayon, M.; Wickwire, E.M.; Hirshkowitz, M.; Albert, S.M.; Avidan, A.; Daly, F.J.; Dauvilliers, Y.; Ferri, R.; Fung, C.; Gozal, D.; et al. National sleep foundation's sleep quality recommendations: First report. *Sleep Health* **2017**, *3*, 6–19. [CrossRef] [PubMed]

87. Durmer, J.S.; Dinges, D.F. Neurocognitive consequences of sleep deprivation. *Semin. Neurol.* **2005**, *25*, 117–129. [CrossRef] [PubMed]

88. Edinger, J.D.; Bonnet, M.H.; Bootzin, R.R.; Doghramji, K.; Dorsey, C.M.; Espie, C.A.; Stepanski, E.J. Derivation of research diagnostic criteria for insomnia: Report of an American Academy of Sleep Medicine Work Group. *Sleep* **2004**, *27*, 1567–1596. [CrossRef] [PubMed]

89. Morin, C.M.; Benca, R. Chronic insomnia. *Lancet* **2012**, *379*, 1129–1141. [CrossRef]

90. Lu, F.M.; Liu, C.H.; Lu, S.L.; Tang, L.R.; Tie, C.L.; Zhang, J.; Yuan, Z. Disrupted topology of frontostriatal circuits is linked to the severity of insomnia. *Front. Neurosci.* **2017**, *11*, 214. [CrossRef] [PubMed]

91. Riley, J.D.; Moore, S.; Cramer, S.C.; Lin, J.J. Caudate atrophy and impaired frontostriatal connections are linked to executive dysfunction in temporal lobe epilepsy. *Epilepsy Behav.* **2011**, *21*, 80–87. [CrossRef] [PubMed]

92. Chuah, Y.M.; Venkatraman, V.; Dinges, D.F.; Chee, M.W. The neural basis of interindividual variability in inhibitory efficiency after sleep deprivation. *J. Neuroscience Off. J. Soc. Neurosci.* **2006**, *26*, 7156–7162. [CrossRef] [PubMed]

93. Drummond, S.P.; Paulus, M.P.; Tapert, S.F. Effects of two nights sleep deprivation and two nights recovery sleep on response inhibition. *J. Sleep Res.* **2006**, *15*, 261–265. [CrossRef] [PubMed]

94. Gruber, R.; Wiebe, S.; Montecalvo, L.; Brunetti, B.; Amsel, R.; Carrier, J. Impact of sleep restriction on neurobehavioral functioning of children with attention deficit hyperactivity disorder. *Sleep* **2011**, *34*, 315–323. [CrossRef] [PubMed]

95. Maski, K.P.; Kothare, S.V. Sleep deprivation and neurobehavioral functioning in children. *Int. J. Psychophysiol.* **2013**, *89*, 259–264. [CrossRef] [PubMed]

96. Molfese, D.L.; Ivanenko, A.; Key, A.F.; Roman, A.; Molfese, V.J.; O'Brien, L.M.; Gozal, D.; Kota, S.; Hudac, C.M. A one-hour sleep restriction impacts brain processing in young children across tasks: Evidence from event-related potentials. *Dev. Neuropsychol.* **2013**, *38*, 317–336. [CrossRef] [PubMed]

97. Sadeh, A.; Gruber, R.; Raviv, A. Sleep, neurobehavioral functioning, and behavior problems in school-age children. *Child Dev.* **2002**, *73*, 405–417. [CrossRef] [PubMed]

98. Halperin, J.M.; Sharma, V.; Greenblatt, E.; Schwartz, S.T. Assessment of the continuous performance test: Reliability and validity in a nonreferred sample. *Psychol. Assess. A J. Consult. Clin. Psychol.* **1991**, *3*, 603–608. [CrossRef]

99. Sadeh, A.; Gruber, R.; Raviv, A. The effects of sleep restriction and extension on school-age children: What a difference an hour makes. *Child Dev.* **2003**, *74*, 444–455. [CrossRef] [PubMed]

100. Gruber, R.; Michaelsen, S.; Bergmame, L.; Frenette, S.; Bruni, O.; Fontil, L.; Carrier, J. Short sleep duration is associated with teacher-reported inattention and cognitive problems in healthy school-aged children. *Nat. Sci. Sleep* **2012**, *4*, 33–40. [CrossRef] [PubMed]

101. Kopasz, M.; Loessl, B.; Hornyak, M.; Riemann, D.; Nissen, C.; Piosczyk, H.; Voderholzer, U. Sleep and memory in healthy children and adolescents—A critical review. *Sleep Med. Rev.* **2010**, *14*, 167–177. [CrossRef] [PubMed]

102. Steenari, M.R.; Vuontela, V.; Paavonen, E.J.; Carlson, S.; Fjallberg, M.; Aronen, E. Working memory and sleep in 6- to 13-year-old schoolchildren. *J. Am. Acad. Child Adolesc. Psychiatry* **2003**, *42*, 85–92. [CrossRef] [PubMed]

103. Vriend, J.L.; Davidson, F.D.; Corkum, P.V.; Rusak, B.; Chambers, C.T.; McLaughlin, E.N. Manipulating sleep duration alters emotional functioning and cognitive performance in children. *J. Pediatr. Psychol.* **2013**, *38*, 1058–1069. [CrossRef] [PubMed]

104. Dewald-Kaufmann, J.F.; Oort, F.J.; Meijer, A.M. The effects of sleep extension on sleep and cognitive performance in adolescents with chronic sleep reduction: An experimental study. *Sleep Med.* **2013**, *14*, 510–517. [CrossRef] [PubMed]

105. Wu, J.C.; Buchsbaum, M.; Bunney, W.E., Jr. Clinical neurochemical implications of sleep deprivation's effects on the anterior cingulate of depressed responders. *Neuropsychopharmacology* **2001**, *25*, S74–S78. [CrossRef]

106. Perlman, S.B.; Pelphrey, K.A. Developing connections for affective regulation: Age-related changes in emotional brain connectivity. *J. Exp. Child Psychol.* **2011**, *108*, 607–620. [CrossRef] [PubMed]

107. Berger, R.H.; Miller, A.L.; Seifer, R.; Cares, S.R.; LeBourgeois, M.K. Acute sleep restriction effects on emotion responses in 30- to 36-month-old children. *J. Sleep Res.* **2012**, *21*, 235–246. [CrossRef] [PubMed]

108. Deliens, G.; Gilson, M.; Peigneux, P. Sleep and the processing of emotions. *Exp. Brain Res.* **2014**, *232*, 1403–1414. [CrossRef] [PubMed]

109. Soffer-Dudek, N.; Shahar, G. Daily stress interacts with trait dissociation to predict sleep-related experiences in young adults. *J. Abnorm. Psychol.* **2011**, *120*, 719–729. [CrossRef] [PubMed]

110. Killgore, W.D. Self-reported sleep correlates with prefrontal-amygdala functional connectivity and emotional functioning. *Sleep* **2013**, *36*, 1597–1608. [CrossRef] [PubMed]

111. Weber, M.; Webb, C.A.; Deldonno, S.R.; Kipman, M.; Schwab, Z.J.; Weiner, M.R.; Killgore, W.D. Habitual 'sleep credit' is associated with greater grey matter volume of the medial prefrontal cortex, higher emotional intelligence and better mental health. *J. Sleep Res.* **2013**, *22*, 527–534. [CrossRef] [PubMed]

112. Doyle, A.E. Executive functions in attention-deficit/hyperactivity disorder. *J. Clin. Psychiatry* **2005**, *67*, 21–26.

113. Barkley, R.A. Behavioral inhibition, sustained attention, and executive functions: Constructing a unifying theory of ADHD. *Psychol. Bull.* **1997**, *121*, 65. [CrossRef] [PubMed]

114. Willcutt, E.G.; Doyle, A.E.; Nigg, J.T.; Faraone, S.V.; Pennington, B.F. Validity of the executive function theory of attention-deficit/hyperactivity disorder: A meta-analytic review. *Biol. Psychiatry* **2005**, *57*, 1336–1346. [CrossRef] [PubMed]

115. Schoemaker, K.; Bunte, T.; Wiebe, S.A.; Espy, K.A.; Deković, M.; Matthys, W. Executive function deficits in preschool children with ADHD and DBD. *J. Child Psychol. Psychiatry* **2012**, *53*, 111–119. [CrossRef] [PubMed]

116. Durston, S.; Mulder, M.; Casey, B.J.; Ziermans, T.; van Engeland, H. Activation in ventral prefrontal cortex is sensitive to genetic vulnerability for attention-deficit hyperactivity disorder. *Biol. Psychiatry* **2006**, *60*, 1062–1070. [CrossRef] [PubMed]

117. Shaw, P.; Rabin, C. New insights into attention-deficit/hyperactivity disorder using structural neuroimaging. *Curr. Psychiatry Rep.* **2009**, *11*, 393–398. [CrossRef] [PubMed]

118. Schulz, K.P.; Newcorn, J.H.; Fan, J.I.N.; Tang, C.Y.; Halperin, J.M. Brain activation gradients in ventrolateral prefrontal cortex related to persistence of ADHD in adolescent boys. *J. Am. Acad. Child Adolesc. Psychiatry* **2005**, *44*, 47–54. [CrossRef] [PubMed]

119. Loe, I.M.; Feldman, H.M. Academic and educational outcomes of children with ADHD. *J. Pediatr. Psychol.* **2007**, *32*, 643–654. [CrossRef] [PubMed]

120. Biederman, J.; Monuteaux, M.C.; Doyle, A.E.; Seidman, L.J.; Wilens, T.E.; Ferrero, F.; Faraone, S.V. Impact of executive function deficits and attention-deficit/hyperactivity disorder (ADHD) on academic outcomes in children. *J. Consult. Clin. Psychol.* **2004**, *72*, 757. [CrossRef] [PubMed]

121. Savitz, J.B.; Jansen, P. The Stroop Color-Word Interference Test as an indicator of ADHD in poor readers. *J. Genet. Psychol.* **2003**, *164*, 319–333. [CrossRef] [PubMed]

122. Langberg, J.M.; Epstein, J.N.; Urbanowicz, C.; Simon, J.; Graham, A. Efficacy of an organization skills intervention to improve the academic functioning of students with ADHD. *School Psychol. Q.* **2008**, *23*, 407–417. [CrossRef]

123. Gureasko-Moore, S.; Dupaul, G.J.; White, G.P. The effects of self-management in general education classrooms on the organizational skills of adolescents with ADHD. *Behav. Modif.* **2008**, *30*, 159–183. [CrossRef] [PubMed]

124. DuPaul, G.J.; McGoey, K.E.; Eckert, T.L.; VanBrakle, J. Preschool children with attention-deficit/hyperactivity disorder: impairments in behavioral, social, and school functioning. *J. Am. Acad. Child Adolesc. Psychiatry* **2001**, *40*, 508–515. [CrossRef] [PubMed]

125. Frankel, F.; Feinberg, D. Social problems associated with ADHD vs. ODD in children referred for friendship problems. *Child Psychiatry Hum. Dev.* **2002**, *33*, 125–146. [CrossRef] [PubMed]

126. Grygiel, P.; Humenny, G.; Rębisz, S.; Bajcar, E.; Świtaj, P. Peer Rejection and Perceived Quality of Relations With Schoolmates Among Children With ADHD. *J. Atten. Disord.* **2014**. [CrossRef] [PubMed]

127. Erhardt, D.; Hinshaw, S.P. Initial sociometric impressions of attention-deficit hyperactivity disorder and comparison boys: Predictions from social behaviors and from nonbehavioral variables. *J. Consult. Clin. Psychol.* **1994**, *62*, 833. [CrossRef] [PubMed]

128. Pelham, W.E.; Bender, M.E. Peer relationships in hyperactive children: Description and treatment. *Adv. Learn. Behav. Disabil.* **1982**, *1*, 365–436.

129. Gresham, F.M.; MacMillan, D.L.; Bocian, K.M.; Ward, S.L.; Forness, S.R. Comorbidity of hyperactivity-impulsivity-inattention and conduct problems: Risk factors in social, affective, and academic domains. *J. Abnorm. Child Psychol.* **1998**, *26*, 393–406. [CrossRef] [PubMed]

130. Hoza, B.; Gerdes, A.C.; Hinshaw, S.P.; Arnold, L.E.; Pelham, W.E., Jr.; Molina, B.S.; Odbert, C. Self-perceptions of competence in children with ADHD and comparison children. *J. Consult. Clin. Psychol.* **2004**, *72*, 382. [CrossRef] [PubMed]

131. Mary, A.; Slama, H.; Mousty, P.; Massat, I.; Capiau, T.; Drabs, V.; Peigneux, P. Executive and attentional contributions to Theory of Mind deficit in attention deficit/hyperactivity disorder (ADHD). *Child Neuropsychol.* **2016**, *22*, 345–365. [CrossRef] [PubMed]

132. Papadopoulos, T.C.; Panayiotou, G.; Spanoudis, G.; Natsopoulos, D. Evidence of poor planning in children with attention deficits. *J. Abnorm. Child Psychol.* **2005**, *33*, 611–623. [CrossRef] [PubMed]

133. Wheeler Maedgen, J.; Carlson, C.L. Social functioning and emotional regulation in the attention deficit hyperactivity disorder subtypes. *J. Clin. Child Psychol.* **2000**, *29*, 30–42. [CrossRef] [PubMed]

134. Williams, L.M.; Hermens, D.F.; Palmer, D.; Kohn, M.; Clarke, S.; Keage, H.; Gordon, E. Misinterpreting emotional expressions in attention-deficit/hyperactivity disorder: Evidence for a neural marker and stimulant effects. *Biol. Psychiatry* **2008**, *63*, 917–926. [CrossRef] [PubMed]

135. Marsh, A.A.; Blair, R.J.R. Deficits in facial affect recognition among antisocial populations: A meta-analysis. *Neurosci. Biobehav. Rev.* **2008**, *32*, 454–465. [CrossRef] [PubMed]

136. Humphreys, K.L.; Galán, C.A.; Tottenham, N.; Lee, S.S. Impaired social decision-making mediates the association between ADHD and social problems. *J. Abnorm. Child Psychol.* **2016**, *44*, 1023–1032. [CrossRef] [PubMed]

137. Andrade, B.F.; Waschbusch, D.A.; Doucet, A.; King, S.; MacKinnon, M.; McGrath, P.J.; Corkum, P. Social information processing of positive and negative hypothetical events in children with ADHD and conduct problems and controls. *J. Atten. Disord.* **2012**, *16*, 491–504. [CrossRef] [PubMed]

138. Chervin, R.D.; Archbold, K.H.; Dillon, J.E.; Pituch, K.J.; Panahi, P.; Dahl, R.E.; Guilleminault, C. Associations between symptoms of inattention, hyperactivity, restless legs, and periodic leg movements. *Sleep* **2002**, *25*, 213–218. [CrossRef] [PubMed]

139. Picchietti, D.L.; England, S.J.; Walters, A.S.; Willis, K.; Verrico, T. Periodic limb movement disorder and restless legs syndrome in children with attention-deficit hyperactivity disorder. *J. Child Neurol.* **1998**, *13*, 588–594. [CrossRef] [PubMed]

140. Golan, N.; Shahar, E.; Ravid, S.; Pillar, G. Sleep disorders and daytime sleepiness in children with attention-deficit/hyperactive disorder. *Sleep* **2004**, *27*, 261–266. [CrossRef] [PubMed]

141. Konofal, E.; Lecendreux, M.; Cortese, S. Sleep and ADHD. *Sleep Med.* **2010**, *11*, 652–658. [CrossRef] [PubMed]

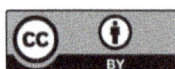

MDPI

St. Alban-Anlage 66

4052 Basel

Switzerland

Tel. +41 61 683 77 34

Fax +41 61 302 89 18

www.mdpi.com

Medical Sciences Editorial Office

E-mail: medsci@mdpi.com

www.mdpi.com/journal/medsci

www.ingramcontent.com/pod-product-compliance
Lightning Source LLC
Chambersburg PA
CBHW051904210326
41597CB00033B/6024